Recent Advances in Nervous System Toxicology

NATO ASI Series

Advanced Science Institutes Series

A series presenting the results of activities sponsored by the NATO Science Committee, which aims at the dissemination of advanced scientific and technological knowledge, with a view to strengthening links between scientific communities.

The series is published by an international board of publishers in conjunction with the NATO Scientific Affairs Division

A	**Life Sciences**	Plenum Publishing Corporation
B	**Physics**	New York and London
C	**Mathematical and Physical Sciences**	D. Reidel Publishing Company Dordrecht, Boston, and Lancaster
D	**Behavioral and Social Sciences**	Martinus Nijhoff Publishers
E	**Engineering and Materials Sciences**	The Hague, Boston, and Lancaster
F	**Computer and Systems Sciences**	Springer-Verlag
G	**Ecological Sciences**	Berlin, Heidelberg, New York, and Tokyo

Recent Volumes in this Series

Volume 95—Drugs Affecting Leukotrienes and Other Eicosanoid Pathways
edited by B. Samuelsson, F. Berti, G. C. Folco, and G. P. Velo

Volume 96—Epidemiology and Quantitation of Environmental Risk in Humans from Radiation and Other Agents
edited by A. Castellani

Volume 97—Interactions between Electromagnetic Fields and Cells
edited by A. Chiabrera, C. Nicolini, and H. P. Schwan

Volume 98—Structure and Function of the Genetic Apparatus
edited by Claudio Nicolini and Paul O. P. Ts'o

Volume 99—Cellular and Molecular Control of Direct Cell Interactions
edited by H.-J. Marthy

Volume 100—Recent Advances in Nervous System Toxicology
edited by Corrado L. Galli, Luigi Manzo, and Peter S. Spencer

Volume 101—Chromosomal Proteins and Gene Expression
edited by Gerald R. Reeck, Graham H. Goodwin, and Pedro Puigdomènech

Series A: Life Sciences

Recent Advances in Nervous System Toxicology

Edited by

Corrado L. Galli

Institute of Pharmacology and Pharmacognosy
Milan, Italy

Luigi Manzo

Institute of Pharmacology
Pavia, Italy

and

Peter S. Spencer

Albert Einstein College of Medicine of Yeshiva University
Bronx, New York

Plenum Press
New York and London
Published in cooperation with NATO Scientific Affairs Divison

Proceedings of a NATO Advanced Study Institute on
Toxicology of the Nervous System,
held September 10–20, 1984,
in Belgirate, Italy

Library of Congress Cataloging in Publication Data

NATO Advanced Study Institute on Toxicology of the Nervous System (1984: Belgirate, Italy)
Recent advances in nervous system toxicology.

(NATO ASI series. Series A, Life sciences; v. 100)
"Proceedings of a NATO Advanced Study Institute on Toxicology of the Nervous System, held September 10–20, 1984, in Belgirate, Italy"—Verso of t.p.
"Published in cooperation with NATO Scientific Affairs Division."
Bibliography: p.
Includes index.
1. Nervous system—Diseases—Congresses. 2. Neurotoxic agents—Congresses. 3. Toxicology—Congresses. I. Galli, C. L. (Corrado L.) II. Manzo, L. III. Spencer, Peter S. IV. Title. V. Series.
RC347.N37 1984 616.8 85-25805
ISBN 0-306-42209-3

A Division of Plenum Publishing Corporation
233 Spring Street, New York, N.Y. 10013

Printed in the United States of America

PREFACE

This volume addresses some facets of the adverse actions of chemical agents on the central and peripheral nervous systems in developing and mature states. Some of the effects of these chemicals are short-lasting and rapidly reversible; others, especially those that cause structural damage to the nervous system, may result in permanent damage to the organism.

The nervous system has several levels of vulnerability to toxic substances. Some substances perturb ion channels or synaptic mechanisms required for the orderly transfer of electrochemical information within the nervous system. Others disrupt sites required for the maintenance of cellular integrity, and these variably result in degenerative responses of neurons and myelinating cells. Further sites of vulnerability include the delicate neural vasculature and neurohumeral mechanisms responsible for physiological homeostasis.

The science of neurotoxicology inevitably is a multidisciplinary endeavor, with contributions from biochemistry, physiology, morphology and behavior, to name a few. The challenge is to apply appropriate techniques to investigate neurotoxic phenomena. The first logical step in this analysis is to determine from the point of view of the nervous system the nature of the exposure. Is the chemical a single or multiple entity; is it metabolized; how does it gain access to neural tissue? Once these factors are understood, changes induced by the exposure can be described at various levels from the biochemical to the behavioral. Here one must strive to correlate the findings from one level of analysis to another, otherwise time is wasted in describing phenomena that are unrelated to the problem at hand. Is this biochemical alteration connected with the observed pathological change? Does this experimentally observed behavioral alteration relate to clinical neurological findings in similarly exposed humans? Do these tissue-culture changes really represent alterations that occur in the whole organism? Care in addressing these types of questions will ensure that neurotoxicology is kept on track in its principal mission of predicting, preventing, and ameliorating toxic disorders that plague mankind.

CONTENTS

NEUROTOXIC EFFECTS OF PROLONGED EXPOSURE TO TOXIC AGENTS

The Nervous System as a Target for Toxic Agents
S Norton 3

Towards the Molecular Basis of Toxic Neuropathies
J B Cavanagh 23

Biochemical Contributions to Neurotoxicology
S C Bondy 43

Metabolic Activation of Neurotoxicants
E Perucca, L Manzo 67

Membrane Effects of Neurotoxic Chemicals
J van den Bercken 87

Mode of Action of Pyrethroid Insecticides
J van den Bercken, H P M Vijverberg 91

Excitotoxins and Animal "Models" of Human Disease
E G McGeer, P L McGeer 107

Retinotoxic Agents and Its Pathogenesis
W Meier-Ruge 133

NEUROTOXIC AGENTS IN THE HUMAN ENVIRONMENT

Analysis of Neurotoxic Disease: The Acrylamide Experience
P S Spencer, H H Schaumburg 163

Neurotoxic Effects of Metals and Their Interactions
J B Cavanagh 177

Organophosphorus Compounds
L G Costa 203

The Delayed Polyneuropathy Caused by Some Organophosphorus Esters
M Lotti 247

Central Nervous System Effects of Lead: a Study Model in Neurotoxicology
S Govoni, F Battaini, R A Rius, C Fernicola, L Coniglio, M Trabucchi 259

EXPERIMENTAL MODELS AND ASSESSMENT OF NEUROTOXIC MECHANISMS

Criteria and Strategies for Neurobehavioral Assessment
S Norton 279

The Role of Neurochemistry in Behavioural Teratology and Toxicology
V Cuomo, G Racagni 297

Receptor Binding Techniques in Neurotoxicology
L G Costa, M Marinovich, C L Galli 307

The Use of Neurotransmitter Indices and the Deoxyglucose Technique to Assess Neurotoxic Effects
E G McGeer 351

Recent Electrophysiological Techniques in Experimental Neurotoxicology
P L Chambers 365

Index 377

NEUROTOXIC EFFECTS of PROLONGED EXPOSURE

to TOXIC AGENTS

THE NERVOUS SYSTEM AS A TARGET FOR TOXIC AGENTS

Stata Norton

Pharmacology, Toxicology and Therapeutics
University of Kansas College of Health Sciences
Kansas City, Kansas

INTRODUCTION

Damage to cells from toxic agents is of most serious consequence in those tissues where restoration of function through cell division or regeneration of cell processes is difficult or impossible. This situation is most characteristic of the nervous system. Mature neurons undergo cell division either rarely or not at all and restoration of complex cell processes interacting with other cell processes may be impossible even if the neuron does not die. In addition the large size and specialized biochemistry of some of the neurons makes them uniquely susceptible to specific toxic agents, especially those interfering with availability of oxygen.

The focus of this discussion will be on the effect of toxic agents which cause irreversible damage to the nervous system, although functional recovery following exposure to these agents may occur through partial regrowth of axons and dendritic processes. Other neuronal pathways may take over the function. Damage to, or death of, some neurons may not result in detectable loss of function if remaining neurons can adapt to carrying out the function. Usually complete recovery of function can occur at one exposure level, while larger doses result in permanent functional damage. Acute, reversible effects of toxic agents, resembling the brief response to therapeutic actions of most drugs will not be the major consideration here.

Because of the potential breadth of the topic of this presentation, only a survey will be attempted. Subsequent presentations by others will cover, in depth and sophistication, areas just touched upon briefly at this point.

PERIPHERAL NERVOUS SYSTEM

The peripheral nervous system is a target for various toxic chemicals. Neuropathies usually are a result of repeated exposure, although neuropathy may result from single large doses of some of these chemicals.

Acute, pharmacological effects are characteristic of chemicals interacting reversibly at the neuromuscular junction. Neuropathy is more likely to result from effects on components of axons, myelin or nerve cell bodies in sensory ganglia or the spinal cord.

Morphology

The typical peripheral nerve contains nerve fibers of various sizes, from the very large myelinated sensory fibers and large myelinated motor fibers to small, unmyelinated sensory and motor fibers. The designation of fiber size is more determined by thickness of myelin than by difference in cross-sectional size of the axon in different nerve fibers. Nevertheless some of the largest nerve fibers are associated with the largest cell bodies, such as the alpha motor neurons in the ventral horn of the spinal cord. Some cell bodies associated with large fibers are small, such as the granule cells of the dorsal root sensory ganglia. One characteristic of large fibers is that they carry impulses for long distances and this function is tied to the presence of thick myelin sheaths.

Irreversible damage to the myelin sheath eventually results in loss of the axon and vice versa. There is a post-damage period during which slow regrowth of damaged axons may occur if the myelin sheath has not degenerated or if the pathway to the peripheral target can be followed by the regenerating axon.

The axons contain large quantities of neurofilaments, demonstrable with electron microscopy, and showing characteristic alterations with some toxic agents.

Biochemistry

As noted above, the neuromuscular junction and associated neurotransmitter, acetylcholine, are not the primary targets of most agents causing irreversible neuropathies. However, biochemical interest has focused recently on an enzyme in the axonal membrane which interacts with various esterases. This enzyme is labeled neurotoxic esterase (Johnson, 1982). Its function in the normal animal is not known.

The high energy requirement of the neuron and its dependence on oxidative metabolism is also a unique biochemical state. The axon is involved in active transport of essential nutrients as well as cell organelles both from the cell body down the axon and retrograde transport to the cell body. This complex process is often interfered with by toxic agents.

Table 1. Peripheral Neuropathies

1. Neurofilamentous accumulations
   a. acrylamide
   b. 2,5-hexanedione
   c. carbon disulfide
2. Inhibition of tubulin polymerization
   a. colchicine
   b. vincristine
   c. methyl mercury
3. Inhibition of neurotoxic esterase
   a. TOCP
   b. leptophos
4. Hypoxia
   a. cyanide
   b. carbon monoxide
5. Thiamine-reversible neuropathy
   a. alcohol
   b. carbon disulfide
6. Heavy metals
   a. mercury
   b. lead
   c. arsenic
   d. thallium

Toxic Agents

There is no simple way with which to classify the various agents which cause peripheral neuropathies. Table 1 classifies the toxic chemicals discussed here into several categories which, except for the category of "metals", are based on possible mechanisms responsible for the neuropathic effects.

Neuropathies resulting from exposure to toxic chemicals are usually both sensory and motor in nature. Large fibers are commonly more often damaged than small fibers and long-axoned neurons more than short-axoned cells. Thus the long hind legs are more vulnerable than the forelimbs.

Three neurotoxic agents which cause nodal or internodal swelling and block of axonal transport are acrylamide, 2,5-hexanedione and a group of organophosphates (See Fig. 1). The latter group causes a delayed neuropathy. Exposure, even to a high dose of these organophosphates results in signs of nerve damage and muscle weakness only after more than a week has elapsed following exposure. There is no correlation between neuropathy from these compounds and block of cholinesterase but there is a good correlation with block of neurotoxic esterase. No specific causation has been established. Examples of chemicals in this group are triorthocresylphosphate, leptophos and mipafox. As with many toxic agents, there are marked species differences in sensitivity. Age within a susceptible species is also a factor.

Several neuropathic chemicals share an effect which may be related to the mechanism of the neuropathy. Acrylamide, 2,5-hexanedione, carbon disulfide and iminodipropionitrile all cause neurofilamentous accumulations in the axons, proximal to nodes of Ranvier (Mendell and Sahenk, 1980). The neurofilament is a 10 nm protein filament organized in the perikaryon and transported down the axon (Hoffman and Lasek, 1975). It is a stable protein which is probably degraded by calcium-activated proteases (Cavanagh, 1982). Retrograde as well as anterograde axonal transport is slowed in neuropathies (Miller et al., 1983). It has been proposed that the mechanism of neurofilamentous neuropathy involves the cross-linking of the neurofilament protein by the neuropathic chemical and formation of neurofilamentous aggregates which impair axonal transport (Graham et al., 1982; Anthony et al., 1983). An alternate hypothesis is that the significant effect is a failure of maintenance of the axonal membrane and the slowing of axonal transport is secondary to failure of utilization of transported substances (Cavanagh, 1982). Proposals for a unitary hypothesis of mechanism of action are clouded by the fact that they do not explain differences in the site of action and the selective cell toxicity of compounds sharing a common toxic manifestation.

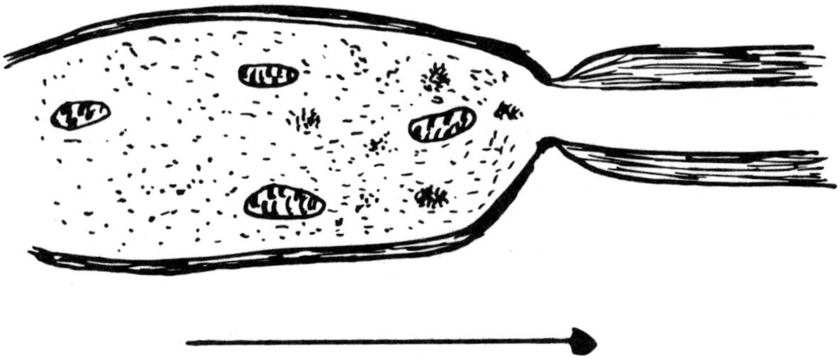

Fig. 1. Example of selective toxicity: representation of axonopathy with perinodal swelling and accumulation of organelles affecting anterograde and retrograde transport.

Repeated episodes of anoxia may damage the axon or myelin and result in neuropathies. This has been reported from repeated ingestion of improperly prepared cassava root which may contain toxic amounts of a cyanogen. A single severe exposure to carbon monoxide (and hence anoxia from accumulation of carboxyhemoglobin) may cause a severe or fatal neuropathy, associated with generalized damage to myelin (Lumsden, 1970). A possible mechanism for impairment of cells by hypoxia has been proposed (Savolainen, 1982). The harmful consequences of hypoxia, caused by impairment of oxygen utilization by the cell, may be the generation of superoxide anions resulting in lipid peroxidation (Fridovich, 1978). Lipid peroxidation may be catalyzed by hemolysis products and be self-perpetuating (Miller et al., 1980).

Chronic exposure to alcohol or carbon disulfide can cause neuropathies which are reversible, at least in part, by administration of thiamine. Neuropathy in dietary deficiency of thiamine is also well known but the causal mechanism is unknown (Walsh and McLeod, 1970).

Some metals can be included among the agents known to cause neuropathy through action on the peripheral nervous system. Thallium in toxic doses causes a generalized neuropathy. The physiological and biochemical resemblance of thallium to potassium is the basis for treatment of thallium poisoning with Prussian blue

(Heydlauf, 1969) but the mechanism of the neuropathy has not been causally linked to interference with potassium. One characteristic finding in human and experimental thallium intoxication is mitochondrial swelling and vacuolation (Herman and Bensch, 1967) and other types of mitochondrial damage (Spencer et al., 1973; Bank, 1980) Roizin (1977) has noted that the mitochondrion shows changes in shape, number of cristae and inclusions in various chronic neuropathological conditions but no classification of these changes has been proposed (See Fig. 2).

Methyl mercury causes damage to the visual system and also peripheral sensory neuropathy through damage to the small sensory cell bodies in the dorsal root ganglia of the spinal cord (Jacobs et al., 1975). A mechanism of methyl mercury toxicity has been proposed which relates to the action of organic sulfhydryl blocking agents, such as organomercury compounds. The polymerization of the protein, tubulin, in the formation of microtubules is dependent on available sulfhydryl groups. Miura and co-workers (1984) have compared methyl mercury to colchicine in inhibiting tubulin polymerization and suggest that this action of methyl mercury plays an important role in its neurotoxicity. An alternative mechanism is that methyl mercury may be cytotoxic through lipid peroxidation, however, evidence has recently been presented showing that lipid peroxidation and cytotoxicity of inorganic Hg^{2+} can be dissociated (Stacey and Kappus, 1982).

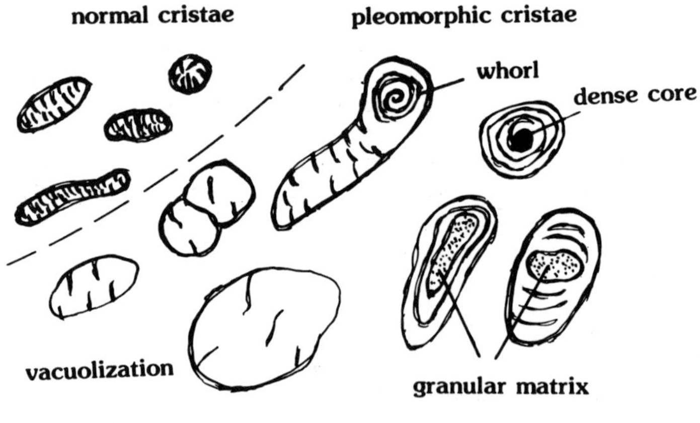

Fig. 2. Example of selective toxicity: representation of mitochondrial changes associated with several types of neurotoxicity.

Arsenic in the trivalent form combines, like mercury, with sulfhydryl groups. Chronic exposure to arsenic or acute intoxication results in a sensory neuropathy as the earliest change. Affected individuals describe numbness, burning and tingling in the hands, feet and lower legs followed by distal muscle weakness with foot drop (Heyman et al., 1956; Dinman, 1960). There is a sensory-distal axonopathy progressing to motor-proximal damage. Degeneration of myelin is secondary (Feldman et al., 1979).

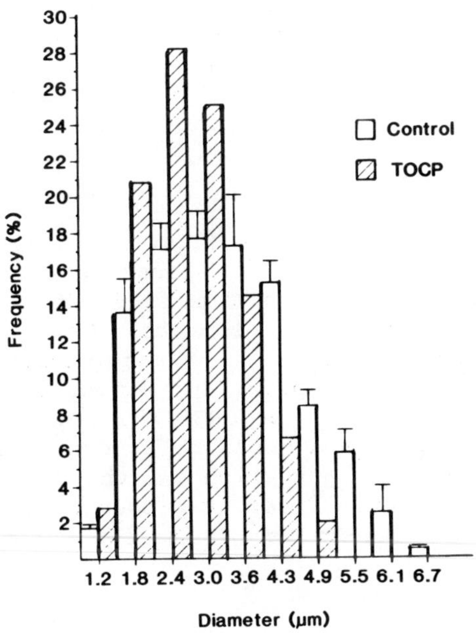

Fig. 3. Example of selective toxicity: loss of large diameter nerve fibers following treatment of chicks with triorthocresyl phosphate (TOCP).

One characteristic of all these neuropathies is that they go through a period of exacerbation within a few days or weeks after exposure, followed by partial or complete recovery if the individual survives the initial period. Recovery may progress slowly over one to two years after exposure. The slow rate of growth of long axons may account for the long period over which gradual recovery occurs. If damage is not too extensive, the axonal swelling associated with neurofilamentous aggregations may also be resolved (Cavanagh, 1982). In the early stages of damage the preferential damage to large axons can be detected in measurements of fiber diameters (Fig. 3).

In considering the effects of all of these agents, the focus on neurotoxicity of some chemicals should not diminish recognition of the other effects on the body. For example, ketone has been studied intensively for its axonal effects, but also causes a syndrome which includes depression of white blood cells and testicular germinal cell atrophy (O'Donaghue et al., 1984). Chronic carbon disulfide poisoning results in atherosclerotic changes in addition to the neurotoxic action. Arsenic acutely damages capillaries in the brain and elsewhere and petechial hemorrhages may be responsible for considerable neuronal damage, regardless of other mechanisms which may exist.

CENTRAL NERVOUS SYSTEM

The central nervous system (CNS) in the adult animal can restore or maintain function in response to damage, in a limited way, as noted before. Cell division is limited to the supporting cells or glia and the vascular elements. Cell swelling, a common response to anoxia, presents unique problems to the central nervous system because of space limitations in the skull. However, the marked ability of the CNS to recover functionally from irreversible structural damage can be accounted for by redundancy of neurons involved in a function or the recruitment of other neurons for the function. Recovery processes may be particularly marked in the immature nervous system but undoubtedly exists in the adult.

Morphology

Retention of function in the presence of structural damage is not equally likely in all part of the nervous system. The sensory and motor pathways leading to and from the brain are particularly vulnerable in lacking alternate pathways. They can be considered "hard-wired" so that sufficient irreversible damage results in complete loss of function. In contrast, irreversible damage to large portions of forebrain structures, particularly unilateral damage, may result in no recognized functional alteration.

In addition to the specific sensory and motor pathways, toxic agents may selectively damage cells in the cerebral cortex, hippocampus, hypothalamus, basal ganglia and cerebellum. Large neurons, for example, cortical layer V pyramidal cells and cerebellar Purkinje cells, are sensitive to agents which do not selectively affect small granule cells in the cortex or cerebellum, while other agents preferentially damage these small neurons.

Oligodendrocytes and astrocytes are targets for some toxic chemicals which thereby interfere with neuronal function. Agents which cause edema and splitting of the spiral wrapping of myelin, produced by the oligodendrocyte, cause secondary damage to the myelinated axon. Astrocytes play a significant role in protection of the neuron from some chemicals by their contribution to the structure of the blood-brain barrier.

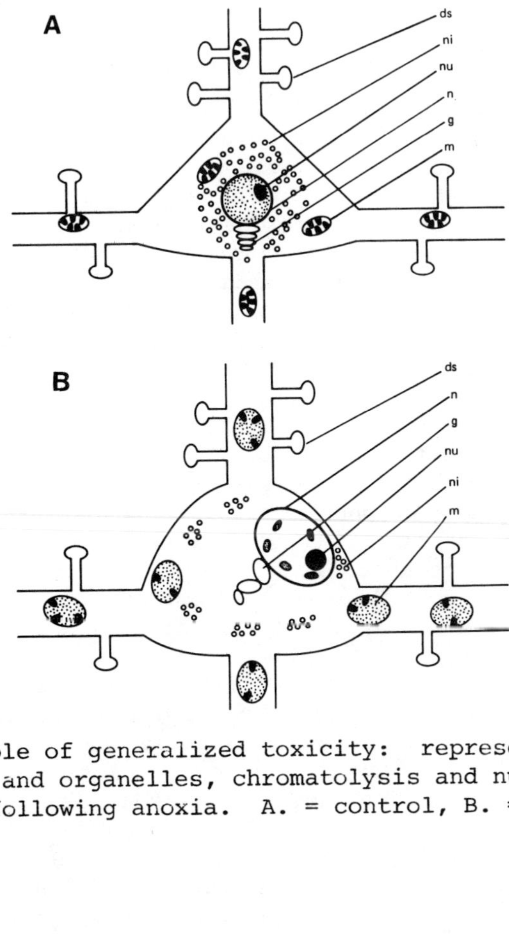

Fig. 4. Example of generalized toxicity: representation of cell body and organelles, chromatolysis and nuclear eccentricity following anoxia. A. = control, B. = anoxia.

Subcellular organelles may show changes in response to toxic agents as they do in the peripheral nervous system, including the neurofibrils and microtubules. Synaptic contacts, distributed on axons, dendrites and soma, may be altered. Unique synaptic structures, the dendritic spines, may show alterations in number or distribution (Fig. 4). It is likely that synapses are the most mutable of neuronal structures; it has been estimated that the half-life of a dendritic spine may be as short as 4 days (Cragg, 1974).

Biochemistry

The distribution of various neurotransmitters and putative transmitters in the brain is the subject of continuing research. Major pathways involving acetylcholine, norepinephrine and dopamine are well known. Various amino acids and polypeptides are widely distributed and presumably many of them serve as transmitters or modulators of neuronal function. Some toxic agents may damage neurons through acting as agonists or irreversible blockers of transmitters.

The dependence of the neuron on a constant supply of glucose not only makes this a special target for agents which interfere with energy production from glucose, but has allowed specialized techniques to be developed to study cell metabolism *in situ*. The ^{14}C-2-deoxyglucose (2-DG) technique developed by Sokoloff (1981) depicts the brain as a map of clusters of cells with high energy requirements. Under differing conditions, cells utilizing glucose at high rates pick up excess quantities of 2-DG, visible on autoradiography. Alterations in metabolism may be detected in the presence of toxic substances.

Two specialized structures combine to produce the blood-brain barrier. One is the tight junction or desmosome joining adjacent capillary endothelial cells and the other is the "foot-process" of the astrocyte which surrounds most of the capillary endothelium in the brain. The effect of these structures is to prevent many polar or ionized substances from penetrating to the neuron, since the cell membranes of the endothelial cell and astrocyte, like other membranes, are relatively impermeable to highly charged chemicals.

Loss of available oxygen, as noted before, presents particular problems to the adult nervous system since many neuron types have high oxygen requirements and, once damaged, function may not be restored by neuronal regeneration or mitosis. Toxic agents may produce hypoxia in a variety of direct and indirect ways. Hypoxia may result from failure of oxygen-carrying capacity of blood (e.g. from the formation of carboxyhemoglobin), ischemia or failure of the blood vessels to carry oxygen to tissues (e.g. from capillary damage or hypotension) or cytotoxic anoxia from failure of the cells to utilize oxygen (e.g. from inhibition of cytochrome oxidase by cyanide). Morphological changes characteristic of hypoxia (cell and organelle swelling, chromatolysis and nuclear eccentricity) result in association with accumulation of anaerobic oxidative products (e.g. lactic acid) and decreased pH (Fig. 4). Rate of decrease in pH is somewhat related to the adequacy of the blood supply in removing end products of anaerobic metabolism. Irreversible damage and cell death may result if the process is carried to the point of lysosomal fragmentation and release of hydrolases activated at low pH. The cascade effect of superoxide formation in some hypoxic conditions has already been mentioned.

Some cells have high concentrations of enzymes associated with special functions which may result in selective toxicity from agents which interfere with or otherwise alter enzyme activity. Examples are the high concentrations of glutamine synthetase in astrocytes in the caudate nucleus and cerebellum; transketolase in the mammillary body; and succinic dehydrogenase in the hippocampus.

Toxic Agents

The responses of the CNS to toxic agents is divided arbitrarily into two categories: generalized responses and selective toxicity (Table 2). The distinction is based on the site of action. Chemicals which damage the vasculature, myelin or cell membranes generally cause encephalopathies which represent a generalized response. Interaction of toxic agents with specialized structures with limited distribution in the CNS or specific components results in selective toxicity to those cell groups.

Table 2. Central Neuropathies

I. Generalized toxicity (encephalopathies)

- a. Leukencephalopathies
  - triethyltin
  - carbon monoxide
- b. Vascular encephalopathies
  - lead
  - arsenic
  - methyl bromide

II. Selective toxicity

- a. chemical Parkinsonism
- b. sensory damage
- c. motor damage
- d. cognitive/affective damage

Leukencephalopathies are characterized by damage to oligodendrocytes. Splitting and swelling of myelin spirals around axons increases intracranial pressure and subsequently causes generalized damage. Triethyltin is known to cause this type of encephalopathy (Watanabe, 1980). A possible mechanism for the effect on the oligodendrocyte has been related to an inhibitory action on taurine transfer by glia (Martin et al., 1983). A similar leukencephalopathy has been described as a sequela of serious carbon monoxide exposure (Lumsden, 1970; Miyagishi et al., 1969). Arsenic poisoning and exposure to methyl bromide gas can each cause encephalopathy. These agents damage the capillary and cause multiple hemorrhages in the brain. Encephalopathy develops as a result of the generalized damage to the capillary and subsequent anoxia. A comparable vascular condition probably initiates the development of lead-induced encephalopathy.

Selective damage to the basal ganglia can result from exposure to various unrelated chemicals. Basal ganglia damage is expressed as motor rigidities and tremor. There may be an emotional disturbance as well. The prevalence of chemical Parkinsonism, as this chemically-induced syndrome has been called, is somewhat surprising. The system includes the dopamine pathway involving the caudate nucleus, globus pallidus and substantia nigra. Chronic exposure to manganese, carbon disulfide or MPTP (1-methyl-4-phenyl-1,2,5,6-tetrahydropyridine) (Heikkila et al., 1984) may result in Parkinsonian dysfunction. It has been proposed that the toxicity of manganese on the corpora striata may be related to the observed increase in lysosomes in these areas in manganese intoxication and the possibility of cell damage from lysosomal rupture (Suzuki et al., 1983).

Among the other selective chemical toxicities, central sensory damage is notable from exposure to methyl mercury. Vision, hearing and other sensory disturbances have been proposed to result from loss of granule cells in the sensory cortex and sensory cells in the dorsal root ganglia. The reason for the sensitivity of small neurons to mercury has not been established. It has been suggested that the binding of mercury to cytoplasmic elements is more damaging to small cells with fewer non-specific binding sites on protein-containing elements (Jacobs et al., 1975).

Central motor systems may be affected by cortical or cerebellar damage, in addition to the motor component of basal ganglia damage seen in chemical Parkinsonism. The large pyramidal cells in the motor cortex and Purkinje cells in the cerebellum are damaged by agents which cause central nervous system anoxia.

Emotional disturbances are common sequalae of encephalopathies but may also develop more insidiously in certain toxic conditions. In cases of chronic mercury poisoning the emotional disturbance has often taken a form of paranoia and labile responses given the label, "erethism" (Gerstner and Huff, 1977).

DEVELOPING NERVOUS SYSTEM

The developing nervous system differs from the adult in response to toxic agents in several important ways. At some points in development the young animal may be more able to recover from damage. The over-production of neurons during embryology is well known. For example, in the chick embryo only about 1 out of 4 or 5 ventral horn neurons survives past incubation day 10 to innervate the developing skeletal muscle of the body (Okado and Oppenheim, 1984). It may be that death of some of these cells prior to day 10 from a toxic agent would still result in normal innervation by survival of the requisite number of neurons. On the other hand, the developing fetal nervous system may be at greater risk than the maternal nervous system from conditions which cause hypoxia. The most common cause of neurologic damage in the human at birth may well be periventricular hemorrhage prior to birth (Volpe, 1978; Lou, 1984; Scott, 1984) and it has been said that the fetus "lives on Mount Everest in utero" in regard to oxygen tension in the normal condition. Hence any decrease in maternal placental oxygen may have serious fetal consequences, particularly brain hemorrhages. Another major difference is the formation of neurons from the germinal matrix around the ventricles. The period of neuronal cell formation lasts from early embryology to the early postnatal period and during this entire period agents which inhibit mitosis may alter brain formation. This aspect is particularly important since the formation of brain structures follows an orderly sequence, building upon earlier structures in a rostrad direction. The formation of the layers of the cerebral cortex offers a good example of this since the layers form in an outward sequence with layer VI the first formed and with subsequent layers formed by migrations of neuroblasts successively through the earlier layers. Finally, the adult blood-brain barrier is lacking in the fetus and develops gradually in the early postnatal period. Most glial cell division occurs postnatally while most neuronal cell division is prenatal. The above considerations apply to the stages of development of atricial mammals like the rat and man. In both of these species the brain is still very immature at birth and considerable development takes place postnatally.

Toxic agents which affect the immature CNS can be divided into four categories: mitotic inhibitors, agents causing vascular damage, agents damaging through neuroendocrine effects and agents causing selective cell death.

Mitotic inhibitors, such as chemotherapeutic agents, or any agents which damage DNA and subsequently cause cell death, produce varying effects on the developing organism. Damage early in embryology results in failure to implant or loss of the embryo. During the period of major organogenesis, CNS damage from these agents is accompanied by gross abnormalities of many organs. During the third trimester when organogenesis is well advanced, the CNS is a selective target for these agents because cell division is proceeding rapidly and the requirement for an orderly sequence of development of brain structures during the late period of fetal development makes the brain particularly vulnerable. Instead of the classic teratogenesis of major organs during the second trimester, the brain shows changes in layered structures in response to block of cell division. For example, X-radiation at doses which cause death of dividing cells can cause formation of cortical islands below the corpus callosum instead of above (Norton, 1979).

Agents which damage fetal brain capillaries and cause hemorrhage through anoxia include carbon monoxide. Maternal exposure to agents which cause hypoxia may result in no recognizable harm to the mother. Areas such as the basal ganglia may be at particular risk because of the combination of high oxygen requirement and poor vascularity. Permanent structural damage may result (Daughtrey and Norton, 1982).

The late fetal and early postnatal nervous system is dependent on the neuroendocrine system for normal development. The role of the thyroid gland in the differentiation of neurons to the mature state is well known. In the absence of the hormone, neuronal and functional development is severely retarded. There is a long list of agents which can interfere with thyroxine synthesis or can otherwise reduce circulating levels and these agents have a potential for affecting the offspring of mothers exposed during late gestation. Early postnatal exposure also represents a greater threat to the young than to the mature organism. Examples of agents with goitrogenic potential are some halogenated hydrocarbons (e.g. DDT, DDE, PBB, and PCB), oxalate ion, lead (Comer and Norton, 1984) and the herbicide, aminotriazole (Murphy, 1980). Other ways in which neuroendocrine effects may occur are through damage to the developing hypothalamus or pituitary. It has been shown that the hypothalamic neurons are damaged by excitatory amino acids, such as kainic acid (Olney, 1974), although possible neuroendocrine consequences have not been reported. In other studies, however, long term changes in the pituitary following fetal exposure to ionizing radiation have been found (Donoso and Norton, 1984). This is an area of concern for possible subtle consequences to the developing organism.

CONCLUSIONS

The functional consequences of damage to the adult or immature nervous system are of great importance. It is necessary to consider the implications of different levels of nervous system damage.

1. Parallels exist between the functional consequences of marked nervous system damage in animals and humans. These have been divided into five general categories relating to marked functional changes.

a. Peripheral neuropathy
b. Encephalopathy
c. Parkinsonism
d. Sensorimotor damage
e. Emotional disturbance

Each of these functional categories can be related to morphological damage.

2. In addition to marked functional effects, more subtle changes may occur. These are more difficult to detect and quantify in animal experiments but quantification is essential. Dose-response relationships characterize nervous system effects of toxic agents as they do other organs or systems, and consideration should be given to the consequences of a range of doses.

3. Some types of nervous system damage may not be reflected in any recognized functional change. The potential importance of undetectable (or undetected) functional damage is worth considering. This type of damage may deplete reserve capacity and therefore make the nervous system more vulnerable to additional insult. Normal loss with aging may be accelerated and result in functional changes at a future period when the relationship to earlier damage is unrecognized. Morphological damage may be found in the absence of functional changes.

In addition to the importance of the study of neurotoxicology as directly applied to human health, there is interest in the use of toxic agents to learn more about the relationship of structure to function of the nervous system. In this connection it is interesting that most toxic agents, except for those acting on sensory or motor systems, produce generalized behavioral changes (i.e. nonspecific emotional disturbances or hyperactivity). Either there is a lack of selectivity in much of brain function in regard to morphology and biochemistry or the selective tools have not yet been found among the neurotoxic agents.

REFERENCES

Anthony, D. C., Boekelheide, V., Anderson, C. W. and Graham, D. G. The effect of 3,4,-dimethyl substitution on the neurotoxicity of 2,5-hexanedione. Toxicol. Appl. Pharmacol. 71: 372-382, 1983.

Bank, W. J. Thallium. In, Experimental and Clinical Neurotoxicology. Eds. P.S. Spencer and H. H. Schaumburg. Williams and Wilkins, Baltimore, 1980, pp. 570-527.

Cavanagh, J. B. The patho-kinetics of acrylamide intoxication: a reassessment of the problem. Neuropath. Appl. Neurobiol. 8: 315-336, 1982.

Comer, C. P. and Norton, S. Behavioral consequences of perinatal hypothyroidism in postnatal and adult rats. Pharmacol. Biochem. Behav. 22: in press, 1985.

Cragg, B. G. Plasticity of synapses. Brit. Med. Bull. 30: 141-147, 1974.

Daughtrey, W. C. and Norton, S. Morphological damage to the premature fetal rat brain after acute carbon monoxide exposure. Exp. Neurol. 78: 26-37, 1982.

Dinman, B. D. Arsenic: chronic human intoxication. J. Occup. Med. 2: 137-144, 1960.

Donoso, J. A. and Norton, S. Morphological and functional damage following fetal exposure to X-irradiation. Fed. Proc. 43: 928, 1984.

Feldman, R. G., Niles, C. A., Kelly-Hayes, M., Sax, D. S., Dixon, W. J., Thompson, D. J. and Landau, E. Peripheral neuropathy in arsenic smelter workers. Neurology 29: 939-944, 1979.

Fridovich, T. The biology of oxygen radicals. Science 201: 875-880, 1978.

Gerstner, H. B. and Huff, J. E. Clinical toxicology of mercury. J. Toxicol. Env. Health 2: 491-526, 1977.

Graham, D. G., Anthony, D. C., Boekelheide, K., Maschmann, N. A., Richards, R. G., Wolfram, J. W. and Shaw, B. R. Studies of the molecular pathogenesis of hexane neuropathy. II. Evidence that the pyrrole derivatization of lysyl residues leads to protein cross-linking. Toxicol. Appl. Pharmacol. 64; 415-422, 1982.

Heikkila, R. E., Hess, A. and Duvoisin, R. C. Dopaminergic neurotoxicity of 1-methyl-4-phenyl-1,2,5,6-tetrahydropyridine in mice. Science 224: 1451-1453, 1984.

Herman, M. M. and Bensch, K. G. Light and electron microscope studies of acute and chronic thallium intoxication in rats. Toxicol. Appl. Pharmacol. 10: 199-222, 1967.

Heydlauf, H. Ferric-cyanoferrate (II): an effective antidote in thallium poisoning. Eur. J. Pharmacol. 6: 340-344, 1969.

Heyman, A., Pfeiffer, Jr., J. B., Willett, R. W. and Taylor, H. M. Peripheral neuropathy caused by arsenical intoxication. New Eng. J. Med. 254: 401-409, 1956.

Hoffman, P. N. and Lasek, R. J. The slow component of axonal transport: identification of major structural polypeptides of the axon and their generality among mammalian neurons. J. Cell Biol. 66: 351-366, 1975.

Jacobs, J. M., Carmichael, N. and Cavanagh, J. B. Ultrastructural changes in the dorsal root and trigeminal ganglia of rats poisoned with methyl mercury. Neuropathol. Appl. Neurobiol. 1: 1-19, 1975.

Johnson, M. K. The target for initiation of delayed neurotoxicity by organophosphorus esters: biochemical studies and toxicological applications. Rev. Biochem. Toxicol. 4: 141-212, 1982.

Lou, H. C., Hendriksen, L. and Bruhn, P. Focal cerebral hypoperfusion in children with dysphasia and/or attention deficit disorder. Arch. Neurol. 41 : 825-829, 1984.

Lumsden, C. B. Delayed carbon monoxide encephalopathy. In, Handbook of Clinical Neurology, Vol. 9. Eds. P. J. Vinken and G. W. Bruyn. North Holland Publ. Co., Amsterdam, 1980, pp. 628-632.

Martin, D. L., Waniewski, R. A. and Wolpaw, E. W. Inhibitory effect of triethyltin and taurine transfer by glioma cells. Toxicol. Appl. Pharmacol. 71: 155-162, 1983.

Mendell, J. R., and Sahenk, Z. Interference of neuronal processing and axoplasmic transport by toxic chemicals. In, Experimental and Clinical Neurotoxicology. Eds. P. S. Spencer and H. Schaumburg. Williams and Wilkins, Baltimore, 1980, pp. 139-160.

Miller, M. S., Miller, M. J., Burks, T. F. and Sipes, I. G. Altered retrograde axonal transport of nerve growth factor after single and repeated doses of acrylamide in the rat. Toxicol. Appl. Pharmacol. 69: 96-101, 1983.

Miller, S. M., Cottrell, J. E. and Turndorf, H. Cerebral protection by barbiturates and loop diuretics in head trauma: possible modes of action. Bull. N. Y. Acad. Med. 56: 305-313, 1980.

Miura, K., Inokawa, M. and Imura, N. Effects of methyl mercury and some metal ions on microtubule network in mouse glioma cells and in vitro tubulin polymerization. Toxicol. Appl. Pharmacol. 73: 218-231, 1984.

Miyagishi, T. Electron microscope studies on cerebral lesions of rats in experimental CO poisoning. Acta Neuropathol. 14: 118-125, 1969.

Murphy, S. D. Pesticides. In, Casarett and Doull's Toxicology. Eds. J. Doull, C. D. Klaassen and M. O. Amdur. Macmillan Co., New York, 1980, pp. 357-408.

Norton, S. Development of rat telencephalic neurons after prenatal X-irradiation. J. Environ. Sci. Health. C13: 121-134, 1979.

Norton, S. Toxic responses of the central nervous system. In, Casarett and Doull's Toxicology. Eds. J. Doull, C. D. Klaassen and M. O. Amdur. Macmillan Co., New York, 1980, pp. 179-205.

Norton, S. and Sheets, L. Neuropathy in the chick from embryonic exposure to organophosphorus compounds. NeuroToxicology 4: 137-142, 1983.

O'Donaghue, G. L., Krasavage, W. J., DiVincenzo, G. D. and Katz, G. V. Further studies on ketone neurotoxicity and interactions. Toxicol. Appl. Pharmacol. 72: 201-209, 1984.

Okado, N. and Oppenheim, R. W. Cell death of motoneurons in the chick embryo spinal cord. J. Neuroscience 4: 1639-1652, 1984.

Olney, J. W., Rhee, V. and Ho, O. L. Kainic acid: a powerful neurotoxic analogue of glutamate. Brain Res. 77: 507-512, 1974.

Roizin, L. Chemogenic lesion: a multifactor pathogenic concept. In, Neurotoxicology. Eds. L. Roizin, H. Shiraki and N. Grcević. Raven Press, New York, 1977, pp. 613-648.

Savolainen, H. Toxicological mechanisms in acute and chronic nervous system degeneration. Acta neurol. Scand. 66 (Suppl. 92): 23-35, 1982.

Scott, D. T., Ment, L. R., Ehrenkranz, R. A. and Warshaw, J. B. Evidence for late developmental deficit in very low birth weight infants surviving intraventricular hemorrhage. Child's Brain. 11: 261-269, 1984.

Sheets, L. and Norton, S. Peripheral nerve damage in chicks following treatment with triorthocresyl phosphate in vivo. Submitted for publication, 1984.

Sokoloff, L. The relationship between function and energy metabolism: its use in the localization of functional activity in the nervous system. Neurosci. Res. Prog. Bull. 19: 159-210, 1981.

Spencer, P. S., Peterson, E. R., Madrid, R. and Raine, C. S. Effects of thallium salts on neuronal mitochondria in organotypic cord-ganglia-muscle combination cultures. J. Cell Biol. 58: 79-95, 1973.

Stacey, N. H. and Kappus, H. Cellular toxicity and lipid peroxidation in response to mercury. Toxicol. Appl. Pharmacol. 63: 29-35, 1982.

Suzuki, H., Wada, O., Inoue, K., Tosaka, H. and Ono, T. Role of brain lysosomes in the development of manganese toxicity in mice. Toxicol. Appl. Pharmacol. 71: 422-429, 1983.

Volpe, J. J. Neonatal periventricular hemorrhage: past, present and future. J. Pediat. 92: 693-696, 1978.

Walsh, J. C. and McLeod, J. J. Alcoholic neuropathy. An electrophysiological and histological study. J. Neurol. Sci. 10: 457-465, 1970.

Watanabe, I. Organotins (triethyltin). In, Experimental and Clinical Neurotoxicology. Eds. P. S. Spencer and H. H. Schaumburg. Williams and Wilkins, Baltimore, 1980, pp. 545-557.

TOWARDS THE MOLECULAR BASIS OF TOXIC NEUROPATHIES

J.B. Cavanagh
Institute of Neurology, Queen Square
London WC1N 3BG , U.K.

By comparison with all other kinds of cells in the animal body, neurons have unique logistical problems. No other cell has to maintain such a large surface area nor to provide working materials over such long distances for something like 1500 times its own volume (Table 1). Under conditions of normality, the support mechanisms are adequate and enable almost perfect survival during a whole lifetime, and in addition they also allow for occasional repair and regeneration in the event of accidents. There is a large number of clinical conditions, however, where this system breaks down with the production of a symmetrical distal peripheral neuropathy. Among these conditions are genetic vitamin disorders, deficiencies, particularly of the B group vitamins, and chemical intoxications (Table 2). While we have known of the existence of most of the first two for a long time, and of the occurrence of those of the last group, understanding of the mechanisms that lead to the breakdown of longer axons has been dependent upon the understanding of the normal physiological and metabolic background to the logistical support and maintainance by the perikaryon of the cell's very large axon and neurites of the projection field.

Before, therefore, any detailed analysis of the pathological events in these intoxications can be made, it is essential that we look at a little of what is involved in the normal process of axon maintenance.

Table 1. Some Volume and Surface Relationships between Cell Body and Axon in Human Dorsal Root Ganglion Cells. (All figures are only approximations)

DORSAL ROOT GANGLION CELL :			
CELL SIZE - up to 50 micra diam.			
	-vol.	65450	$micra^3$
	-surface	31416	$micra^2$
NUCLEAR SIZE - up to 20 micra diam.			
	-vol.	4188	$micra^3$
	-surface	5020	$micra^2$
NUCLEOLAR SIZE - up to 6 micra diam.			
	-vol.	113	$micra^3$
	-surface	452	$micra^2$
PROXIMAL AXON (spinal cord-1000 mm long) -up to 5 micra diam			
	-vol.	19635000	$micra^3$
	-surface	15708000	$micra^2$
DISTAL AXON (peripheral-1000 mm long) -up to 10 micra diam.			
	-vol.	78540000	$micra^3$
	-surface	31416000	$micra^2$
TOTAL AXON (2 metres long)			
	-vol.	98175900	$micra^3$
	-surface	47124000	$micra^2$
Ratio of Cell Volume / Axon Volume	- 1/1500		
Ratio of Cell Surface / Axon Surface	- 1/1500		

Table 2. Examples of Long Axon Diseases and Possible Mechanisms

CONDITION	Cause	Effect
Genetic		
Friedreich's Disease		? energy defect
Werdnig-Hoffman Disease		?
Giant Axonal Neuropathy		?filament cross linking defect
Acute Intermittent Porphyria		? consumptive depletion of PLP
Vitamin Deficiency		
Beri-beri	B_1 defic.	energy defect
Pellagra	Nicotinic acid defic.	?NAD/NADP defect
Riboflavin	B_2 defic.	FAD defect
Pyridoxine	B_6 defic.	?GSH/Cysteine defect
Subacute Combined degeneration	B_{12} defic.	?methylation defect
Toxic Chemicals		
Arsenic (As^{+++})	Lipoate inactivation	energy defect
5'-nitroimidazoles	?electron "sink" effect	energy defect
Thallium (Tl^{+})	riboflavin inactivation	energy defect
Isoniazid,etc.	PLP inactivation	GABA defic.-fits. ?GSH/cysteine defic.
Hexacarbon, CS_2, IDPN	cross-linking defect	cyto-skeleton defect

PLP = Pyridoxal phosphate

Very little de novo synthesis of new materials occurs in the axon for there are no ribosomes in the mammalian axon nor any Golgi apparatus : these are confined to the cell body and, to a lesser extent, the dendrites. Assembly of macromolecules and their minor modification must, however be able to take place within the axon and for this, the smooth endoplasmic reticulum (SER) network that may be particularly emphasised by Droz and his colleagues (Rambourg and Droz 1980), who pointed to the existence of this network along the axon. This system is able to move large molecular weight proteins at rates approximating to 400 mm/day just as the microtubules with the aid of myosin and actin can move organelles, such as mitochondria and synaptic vesicles, at this rate. Primary synthesis of enzymes, glycoproteins, lipoproteins and cofactors necessary for the continued maintainance of metabolism in the axon must be from the perikaryon. Moreover, the transport rate of these products must be regulated by their use in axonal functions. The example of thiamine pyrophosphate, essential for the provision of energy in nervous tissue from oxidative sources, is illuminating. The complete cofactor cannot enter the nervous system from the blood stream, but must be made in the cell body. The pyrophosphate, as probably with other cofactors such as lipoate, pyridoxal phosphate, etc., made in the perikaryon are passed down the axon to the site of utilisation (Tanaka et al.,1976). More recent studies of Rindi et al.(1980) have shown that the thiamine content of nervous tissue is high, particularly in the cerebellum. In the sciatic nerve the thiamine content is low, but the turnover rate is high, equal to that in the cerebellum (Table 3). This rather surprising finding is explicable in terms of the relatively short half life of thiamine in the peripheral nerves. Whether, the same occurs also for other cofactors is not known but from what we know of other tissues this would probably be true.

The calculations from axoplasmic transport studies of Ochs (1975) and of Munoz-Martinez (1982) strongly indicate that more than 90% of the materials made in the perikaryon and passed into the axon never in fact reach the periphery. They appear to be used up along the route, presumably in axonal maintainance. If not for this purpose, it is difficult to see what activity within the axon is so energy and material consuming. Indeed, Munoz-Martinez (1981) suggests rather pertinently that a shortage of materials in the further parts of the axon may well account for the distal degeneration of axons in the "dying back" process.

Table 3. Thiamine Content and Calculated Turn-over in Liver, Brain and Nerve

Tissue	Thiamine Content (g/g w.t) Free	Phosph[d]	Total	Calculated turnover (g/g. h)
Liver	0.29	8.78	9.07	0.952
Cerebellum	0.14	4.24	4.38	0.551
Medulla	0.12	2.78	2.90	0.541
Cortex	0.12	2.50	2.62	0.159
Spinal Cord	0.11	1.96	2.07	0.389
Sciatic nerve	0.06	1.39	1.41	0.582

turn-over times 5 - 10 hours

(taken from Rindi et al. (1980), Brain Res. 181:369)

In an important sense, axons in the resting state have many similarities with red blood corpuscles, although clearly the identity between these two cells is by no means absolute (Cavanagh, 1984). Axons are still attached to their cell body, while red cells have lost their nucleus before or soon after leaving the site of their formation. Their connection with their source of essential materials has been cut (Table 4) . This analogy needs to be borne in mind, if only because there are a number of red cell diseases that are also associated with neurological disease, in which longer nerve fibres show distal degeneration. Such conditions are related to defects either in the metabolism of GSH or in the availability of α-tocopherol, and will be discussed in more detail later. Both cell types are critically concerned with transmembrane ionic exchanges. Both are in danger from free radical damage for this reason. While the analogy between the two cell types must not be taken too closely, they have enough features in common to make it very probable that the occurrence of peripheral neuropathy in genetic and other diseases of the red cell is not fortuitous.

Table 4. Some Properties Shared by Red Blood Cells and Axons

Red Blood Cells	Axons
Nucleus separated early in time	Nucleus separated by space
Protein synthesis absent -after reticulocyte stage	Protein synthesis absent -only in perikaryon
Essential function - O_2 and CO_2 transmembrane exchanges	Essential function - Na^+ and K^+ transmembrane exchanges
Energy mechanisms - running down	Energy mechanisms - need constant replacement
Survival depends on - Ca^{++} exclusion	Survival depends on - Ca^{++} exclusion
Integrity depends on - anti-oxidants	Integrity depends on - anti-oxidants

PERIPHERAL NEUROPATHY AND DISTURBED METABOLISM

A. Energy Depletion

With that brief general background to some of the peculiarities of neurons with long axons, let us now look at the various forms of disturbed metabolism that are known to be associated with peripheral neuropathy. Three distinct kinds of metabolic disorders can be made out that seem able to do this; in time there may be others that will become defined as we learn more of the details of the complexities of axonal transport and maintainance mechanisms, just as there are several different kinds of metabolic "lesion" in red cell diseaes which ultimately lead to irreversible membrane damage and a corresponding shortening of their half life. One fairly closely related group is that dependent upon energy depletion (Table 5) (Cavanagh, 1979). Clinically these conditions are remarkably similar, and indeed chronic vitamin B_1

deficiency and arsenical intoxication have long been known to be clinically indistinguishable from their neurological features alone. Thallium, too, presents the same restriction of symptomatology to the sensory and then the motor long nerves (Cavanagh et al., 1974). With the electron affinic radiosensitising and bacteriocidal drugs, the 5-nitroimidazoles and the nitrofurans, the same distal sensory and milder motor neuropathy is seen. Long spinal tracts except for the dorsal columns are not involved in this group of conditions. In some species we see also symmetrical vasculo-necrotic lesions in the brain stem with the electronic affinic substances (Griffin et al., 1979), though they have not been seen in man. These vasculonecrotic lesions have a close structural similarity to the lesions of acute B_1 deficiency (Wernicke's encephalopathy).

Table 5. Metabolic Background to Peripheral Neuropathy

A. Energy Deprivation

Cause	Leading to	Effect
Thiamine deficiency in beri-beri in alcoholism	defect in thiamine pyrophosphate	reduction in pyruvate decarbox^n.
Arsenic Poisoning (As^{+++})	covalent linkage to lipoate	reduction in pyruvate decarbox^n.
Thallium Poisoning (Tl^+)	inactivation of riboflavin, reduction in tissue FAD etc.	?reduction in pyruvate decarbox^n.
Overdosage with :		
Misonidazole, Metronidazole, Nitrofurantoin	high electron affinity, -electron "sink" effect	?reduction in ATP generation from electron transport chain.

The close clinical identity between these syndromes is paralleled by the probable lesion sites along the pyruvate decarboxylation pathway that occurs in these conditions. This pathway is the most important energy–yielding route that is used by nervous tissue. It is a tightly linked sequence of metabolic steps with B_1 deficiency blocking the first step, trivalent arsenic blocking the second by combination with lipoate, thallium probably interfering with the third step from the removal of flavin cofactors, and the electron affinic substances probably being capable of deviating electrons from passing along the electron transport chain, with consequent reduction of the yield of available ATP in the cell at all these steps. While the third and fourth steps are still admittedly speculative, the first two are now well established. It is noteworthy that experimental production of riboflavin deficiency in monkeys, not only produces a similar neuropathy, but there are also the same skin and hair changes (Pentschew and Garro,1969).

There is little doubt that the longer neurons in these conditions fail to maintain their axons either because there is not enough of the cofactor to make good the normal wastage or because of their irreversible inactivation by the toxic chemicals. The ultimate effect is the same, namely those regions furthest from the source of supply inevitably suffer most and the absence of available energy leads among other things to loss of control of calcium ions with consequences similar to the early phases of wallerian degeneration after axotomy. While many of the arguments put foward here have yet to be proved, the circumstantial evidence in support of the general concept is strong.

B. Defect in Anti-oxidant Availability

A second more controversial group of disorders, in which damage may be occurring in axons in quite another manner, stands in marked contrast to this first group, and can be perhaps related to another property that red cells have in common with axons, namely the apparent need for a sustained supply of anti-oxidant substances (Table 6) . Provision of this is vitally necessary for red cells because of the constant traffic of O_2 through their cell membrane and the consequent frequent occurrence of free radical species and the production of H_2O_2. This danger is adequately neutralised by the abundance of glutathione (GSH) and the active glutathione reductase and glutathione peroxidase normally found within the red cell. In deficiency of the former enzyme (Waller, 1968) not only is the red cell survival greatly reduced (12 - 16 days), but in these 9 patients 6 were described as "spastic" or showed evidence of mental deficiency. Regeneration of reduced glutathione is dependent upon NADPH, a product of the pentose phosphate shunt. As with most dehydrogenases, this step is sensitive to inhibition by sulphydryl agents and it is also adversely affected in sensitive persons in Primaquin Haemolytic Anaemia (Carson et al., 1956).

Table 6. Metabolic Background to Peripheral Neuropathy

B. Defect in Anti-oxidant Availability

Cause	Leading to	Effect
Neuropathy of Acute Intermittent Porphyria	Consumptive deficiency	?Cysteine & GSH deficiency
Isoniazid Neuropathy	Inactivation of PLP	?Cysteine & GSH deficiency
γ-glutamyl-cysteine synth. deficiency	Block in glutathione synthesis	?GSH deficiency
Acrylamide intoxication	Inactivation of glutathione	?GSH deficiency
Chronic Liver disease	Inadequate α-tocopherol absorption	α-tocopherol deficiency
Malabsorption syndromes	Inadequate α-tocopherol absorption	α-tocopherol deficiency
Abetalipoproteinaemia	Inadequate α-tocopherol transport	α-tocopherol tissue deficiency

What is of particular importance to the axon is that glutathione and its precursor, cysteine, are dependent for their synthesis upon the co-factor pyridoxal phosphate (Table 7) . Cystathionine synthetase and cystathioninase both require this cofactor (Kashiwamata, 1971). The former enzyme is found abundantly in grey matter, while its product, cystathionine, is plentiful only in white matter (Volpe and Lester, 1970), suggesting that it has passed into the axon, where the remainder of the pathway to glutathione will be completed. At all but one step in this pathway there are cases of congenital deficiency of these enzymes known. Cystathionine synthetase deficiency (homocysteinuria) (Gerritson and Waisman, 1964; Mudd et al., 1964) and cystathioninase deficiency (cystathioninuria) (Frimpter, 1965) are both associated with mental deficiency as well as shortened red cell half-life. The reason for the mental defect is unknown. γ-glutamyl-cysteine synthetase deficiency has been reported in two siblings who both also had peripheral neuropathy and mild ataxia as well as a shortened red cell half-life (Konrad et al., 1972; Richards et al., 1974). Glutathione synthetase deficiency has no known associated neurological lesions, but it causes severe shortening of the half-life of red cells. A similar but milder haemolytic anaemia associated with excess cystathionine in the urine occurs with pyridoxal phosphate deficiency which is reversed by giving the vitamin in large doses (Horrigan and Harris, 1964; Hope, 1957).

One hereditary and two drug—induced neuropathies are known which are associated with severe tissue depletion of pyridoxal phosphate. Acute episodes of intermittent porphyria are not uncommonly followed by signs of motor, and to a lesser degree sensory, neuropathy. Sometimes there are symptoms only of mild weakness from which the patient appears to recover fairly rapidly : occasionally the denervation may be devastatingly severe and fatal (Cavanagh and Mellick, 1965). During the acute phase of the attack, plasma levels of pyridoxal phosphate (PLP) are low and there is evidence of a marked inability to metabolise tryptophan and its metabolites, as judged by high urinary levels of xanthurenic acid and kynurenic acid after a tryptophan load. These biochemical features disappear on remission from the acute episode and are probably due to a consumptive deficiency of PLP in the tissues consequent upon gross overactivity of the enzyme δ-aminolaevulinic acid synthetase (Cavanagh & Ridley, 1967). This is a PLP-requiring conjugation step which initiates and is rate limiting to the porphyrin synthesis pathway. The result is the production of a typical "dying back" type of neuropathy affecting peripheral nerves, but not spinal tracts, except the dorsal columns. It is both clinically and pathologically quite unlike that found with the energy-dependent group described above, but it is closely similar to the neuropathy that can be produced in animals by large doses of isoniazid (isonicotinic acid hydrazide : INH). This drug has a powerful capacity to interact with PLP and to prevent its formation in the tissues. The human form of the intoxication is exceedingly mild by comparison with the experimental form and thus direct clinical comparisons cannot be made between the human forms of these two conditions.

Table 7. Metabolic Route of Glutathione Synthesis
(Red cell life is severely shortened by each deficiency)

	Homocysteine + serine		
I ↓		Cystathionine synthetase,PLP	in perikaryon
	Cystathionine		↓
II ↓		Cystathioninase,PLP	in axon
	Cysteine + glutamate		↓
III ↓		γ-glutamyl-cysteine synthetase, Mn^{2+}	
	γ-glutamyl-cysteine + glycine		
IV ↓		Glutathione synthetase, Mn^{2+}	
	Glutathione		

I- site of metabolic block in homocysteinuria (Gerritson & Waisman, 1964; Mudd et al., 1964) .
II- site of metabolic block in cystathioninuria (Frimpter, 1965)
III- site of metabolic block in γ-glutamyl-cysteine synthetase deficiency (Konrad et al., 1972; Richards et al., 1974)
IV- site of metabolic block in glutathione synthetase deficiency (Mohler et al., 1970).
in I & II mental deficiency is found
in III peripheral neuropathy & ataxia is found

Although there is no direct evidence one way or another, it is difficult to believe the pathway of GSH synthesis is not affected by these two conditions seeing that its formation is so dependent upon PLP. As with the energy-dependent group of conditions the distal parts of longer fibres seem to be more susceptible to ultimate damage, presumably for the same logistical reasons of distance.

Whether intoxication by acrylamide falls into the same category is a matter for discussion. Although in the chronic form of this intoxication neurofilamentous accumulations appear in many axons, filament accumulation is not an essential feature (Cavanagh & Gysbers, 1980), and there are many other reasons for not grouping this with the primary filamentous aberrations that are discussed later (Cavanagh, 1982a). Acrylamide combines avidly with GSH, but in liver and in brain as a whole there is a rapid return to GSH levels over 24 hours after each dose given (Hashimoto & Aldridge, 1970). I would like to raise the question as to whether the regeneration of GSH in the distal regions of the longer axons is adequate in the circumstances of chronic intoxication. In this condition, almost all nerve endings in both PNS and CNS show accumulations of filaments as well as other organelles, but only the longest undergo distal degeneration and sensory fibres earlier and more massively than motor fibres (Cavanagh, 1982b). There are many other defects in the functions of axons that are not found with the other intoxications, particularly inhibition of regeneration of damaged axons (Morgan Hughes et al., 1974; Griffin et al., 1977), and inhibition of terminal sprouting of motor fibres in response to partial denervation and local botulinum intoxication (Kemplay & Cavanagh, 1984). It is of interest in this connection that -SH protective agents such as dithiothreitol and GSH itself have some effect in mitigating and restoring this inhibited function. As with the red cell membrane, perhaps the flexibility and adaptability of the axon membrane also needs the protective effects of -SH groups.

The second collection of conditions in this group are those related to defects in the absorption and transport of α-tocopherol. While, so far as we know, this process has not yet been implicated in neurotoxicity, it has important implications not only for our understanding of the underlying cellular mechanisms but also in the field of possible prevention and treatment. The occurrence of these conditions also strengthens our analogy between red cell and axon membrane function, for disturbancies in red cell membrane form and flexibility occur which while not increasing the haemolysis of these cells does impair their filterability through the spleen and thus their survival (Cooper et al., 1977). These red cell changes are rapidly reversible on giving α-tocopherol (Kaydon et al., 1965). The real practical relevance of this group of conditions is that while children with these disorders will predictably develop ataxia and peripheral neuropathy due to long, large diameter axons undergoing distal degeneration in both peripheral nerves and in the spinocerebellar tracts (Miller et al., 1980; Rosenblum et al., 1981), the administration of large doses of vitamin E gives definite protection from these neurological sequelae (Muller et al., 1983). This relatively unexplored area of axon membrane function could well lead us into field of substantial interest for the understanding of underlying mechanisms of both natural and toxic peripheral neuropathies.

C. <u>Defects in the Cytoskeleton</u> (Table 8)

By the cytoskeleton in this context is meant the 10 nm intermediate (neuro-)filaments and the microtubules that run the lenght of the cell. Both these elements are synthesised in the cell body and pass slowly down (1-3 mm/day) the axons to be degraded at the periphery (Lasek, 1981). The real functions of the former are not known, but the latter form "express-ways" for the rapid transport of mitochondria, vesicles etc.

NEUROFILAMENT DEFECTS BY HEXACARBON AND CARBON DISULPHIDE

With this last group of toxic neuropathies we can begin to see the molecular basis of the toxic effects with some clarity for the first time. Doctor Spencer, from his early and extensive descriptions of the experimental production of hexacarbon intoxication (Spenser et al., (1980) has dealt with this intoxication in more detail. Here I want only to stress two points that seem to me to be central to the production of the pathological changes. Firstly, this intoxication is not just a peripheral neuropathy, and the same also goes for the effects of carbon disulphide (CS_2), a closely similar intoxication. In the other two groups of conditions discussed earlier we saw that only the peripheral nerves showed pathological changes. In hexacarbon and CS_2 poisoning axons throughout the nervous system, both PNS and CNS are found affected, and the larger the axons the greater are the filamentous accumulations found (Cavanagh and Bennetts, 1981; De Groot and Cavanagh, 1984).

Table 8. Metabolic Backgroud to Peripheral Neuropathy

C. Defects in Cytoskeleton Function

Cause	Leading to	Effect
Genetic Giant Axonal Neuropathy	Defect in filament cross-linking	Obstruction to axoplasmic transport
Toxic Hexacarbon° Carbon disulphide IDPN Intoxication	Defect in filament cross-linking	Obstruction to axoplasmic transport
Vincristine° Neuropathy	Depolymerisation of microtubules	Failure of axoplasmic transport

° - impairment of nerve regeneration after crush occurs.

The second point I wish to emphasise is also related to the reason for the selective damage to large-diameter and long fibres. Neuropathologists are always seeking to explain clinical symptoms and signs in terms of structural parameters. In hexacarbon intoxication, the binding of the 2,5 hexane dione, the proximate toxic chemical (Graham, 1980), not only changes the interactions between the neurofilaments and the microtubules so that the latter tend to be segregated into clumps at the centre or around the periphery of the axon, but also disturbs the flow characteristics of the neurofilaments (Jones and Cavanagh, 1982). In their slow normal downward movement filaments can slip readily through the constrictions at each node of Ranvier. After the cross-linking event induced by hexacarbons, and presumably also by CS_2, they appear to find it increasingly difficult to do this, particularly in larger diameter axons where the constrictions are noticeably greater than they are in the smaller axons. In the latter, the filamentous masses appear to be able to pass down to the preterminal regions where they are broken down in the normal manner (Jones and Cavanagh, 1983). With larger diameter axons the axonal constrictions imposed by the spiral winding of the Schwann cell or oligodendrocyte become increasingly difficult for the filament masses to negotiate. There is also evidence of slowing of rapidly transported materials along the axons as well as of slowing of the velocity of conduction of the nerve impulse due to the distortions of the nodal and paranodal structures. Distal dysfunction and degeneration of larger diameter axons in both PNS and CNS spinal tract are, thus, secondary consequences of the failure of the logistical support of axonal maintainance by the physical processes of axonal obstruction and distortion.

MICROTUBULE DEFECTS BY VINCRISTINE

The second toxic chemical to produce its effects by disruption of the cytoskeleton is vincristine, a drug much used in the treatment of leukaemias and lymphomas. In Man, distal neuropathy is not infrequent and is in fact the main limitation to the therapy with this drug (Casey et al., 1973). The clinical signs are those of a sensory distal neuropathy with motor weakness also affecting the more severe cases.

Experimental studies have shown other species to be less sensitive to the neurotoxicity, but electron microscopy has demonstrated loss of microtubules and accumulations of filaments in neurons affected by vincristine (Shelanski and Wisniewski, 1969). The production of neuropathy has not been particularly successful in other species though in the guinea pig some denervation and a myopathy can be produced (Bradley, 1970). In the cat loss of microtubules is associated with slowing of axonal transport (Green et al., 1977). The presence of the blood-barrier, which inhibits the entry of the drug to the CNS most certainly plays an important role in determining whether damage from this chemical occurs or not (Tomiwa et al., 1984).

Vincristine, like colchicine, binds readily to microtubules and causes the depolymerisation of the macromolecule. The main route for the rapid transport of organelles is thereby jeopardised should the drug gain access to nervous tissue. Preservation of this component of the cytoskeleton is clearly imperative for the proper function of axons. The details as to how this process takes place has still to be fully elucidated, particularly why the entrance of the drug seems to take place so relatively readily during treatment of lymphomas.

The cytoskeleton is important, too, for regeneration and regrowth of PNS axons following trauma, and toxic chemicals active against this cellular component can be markedly inhibitory to the regeneration process, even at doses below those producing overt neurotoxicity. Thus, Simonati, Rizzuto and Cavanagh (1983) found that a dose of 2,5 hexane dione that did not produce overt neurotoxic changes had a marked inhibitory effect on axons after nerve crush in the rat. Vincristine also seems to have the same effect and strikingly impairs the whole process of nerve regeneration (Shiraishi et al., 1984). Clearly further study of the effects of toxic chemical on the regeneration process could not only be valuable for determining whether a neurotoxic chemical is adversely affecting the cytoskeletal components, but the effect of this on exposed workers ia another factor to be taken into account when assessing neurotoxic effects. It may turn out in certain circumstances to be more sensitive than standard tests for neurotoxicity.

In conclusion, neurotoxic chemicals are becoming more valuable every year for leading us to a fuller understanding of the pathogenic mechanism underlying neurological disease. It is only on the basis of a combined approach from metabolic and from morphological aspects that a full understanding of the mechanisms underlying the development of the damage to these very unique cell types. Unless their special properties are fully appreciated, it will always be difficult to comprehend how toxic chemical come to cause the damage that they do.

References

Bradley, W.G., 1970, The neuropathy of vincristine in the guinea pig : an electrophysiological and pathological study, J.Neurol.Sci.,10:133

Carson, P.E., Flanagan,C.L., Ickes,C.E., and Alving,A.S., 1956, Enzymatic deficiency in primaquin sensitive erythrocytes, Science, 124:484

Casey,E.B., Jellife,A.M., LeQuesne,P.M. and Millett, Y.L., 1973, Vincristine neuropathy - clinical and electrophysiological observations, Brain, 96:69

Cavanagh,J.B., 1979, The "Dying Back" Process : a common denominator in many naturally occurring and toxic neuropathies Arch.Pathol., 103:659

Cavanagh,J.B., 1982a, Mechanisms of axon degeneration in three toxic "neuropathies" : organophosphorus, acrylamide and hexacarbon compared, in "Recent Advances in Neuropathology" , Vol. II, W.T. Smith and J.B. Cavanagh, eds., Churchill Livingstone, Edinburgh

Cavanagh,J.B., 1982b, The pathokinetics of acrylamide intoxication : a reassessment of the problem, Neuropathol. Appl. Neurobiol., 8:315

Cavanagh,J.B., 1984, The problems of neurons with long axons, Lancet, 1:1284

Cavanagh,J.B. and Mellick,R.S., 1965, On the nature of the peripheral nerve lesions associated with acute intermittent porphyria, J.Neurol.Neurosurg.Psychiatry, 28:320

Cavanagh,J.B. and Ridley,A.R., 1967, The nature of the neuropathy complicating acute intermittent porphyria, Lancet, 2:1023

Cavanagh,J.B., Fuller,N.H., Johnson,H.R.M., and Rudge,P., 1974, Effects of thallium salts with particular reference to the nervous system changes, Q.J.Med., 43:293

Cavanagh,J.B. and Bennetts,R.J., 1981, On the pattern of changes in the rat nervous system produced by 2,5 hexane diol: a topographical study by light microscopy, Brain, 104:297

Cavanagh,J.B. and Gysbers,M.F., 1980, "Dying back" above a nerve ligature produced by acrylamide, Acta Neuropathol. (Berl), 51:169

Cooper,R.A. Durocher,J.R. and Leslie,M.H., 1977, Decreased fluidity of red cell membrane lipids in abetalipoproteinemia, J.Clin.Invest., 60:115

De Groot,D.M.G. and Cavanagh,J.B., 1984, Some observations on the topography of filament accumulation in CS_2 intoxication in the rat, In preparation

Droz,B., Rambourg,A. and Koenig,H.L., 1975, The smooth endoplasmic reticulum : structure and role in the renewal of axonal membrane and synaptic vesicles, Brain Res., 93:1

Frimpter,G.W., 1965, Cystathioninuria : nature of defect, Science, 149:1095

Gerritson,T. and Waisman,H.A., 1964, Homocysteinuria : absence of cystathionine in the brain, Science, 145:588

Graham,D.G., 1980, Hexane neuropathy : a proposal for the pathogenesis of a hazard of occupational exposure and inhalant abuse, Chem.Biol.Interact., 32:339

Green,L.S., Donoso,A., Heller-Bettinger,I.E. and Samson,F. E., 1977, Axonal transport disturbances in vincristine induced peripheral neuropathy, Ann.Neurol., 1:255

Griffin,J.W., Price,D.S.L., and Drachman,D.B., 1977, Impaired axonal regeneration in acrylamide intoxication, J.Neurobiol. 8:355

Griffin,J.W., Price,D.L., Kuethe,D.O., and Goldberg,A.M., 1979, Neurotoxicity of Misonidazole in rats.I.Neuropathology Neurotoxicology, 1:299

Hashimoto, K. and Aldridge,W.N., 1970, Biochemical studies on acrylamide, a neurotoxic agent, Biochem.Pharmacol.,19:2591

Hope,D.B., 1957, Cystathionuria in vitamin B_6 deficient rats, Biochem.J., 66:486

Horrigan,D.L. and Harris,J.W., 1964, Pyridoxine responsive anaemia-prototype and variations on a theme, Vitam.Horm. , 22:721

Jones,H.B. and Cavanagh,J.B., 1982, Recovery from 2,5 Hexandiol intoxication of the retinotectal tract of the rat : an ultra structural study, Acta Neuropathol.(Berl), 58:286

Jones,H.B. and Cavanagh,J.B., 1983, Distortions of the nodes of Ranvier from axonal distension by filamentous masses in hexacarbon intoxication, J.Neurocytol., 12:439

Kashiwamata,S., 1971, Cystathionine synthetase is pyridoxal phosphate dependant, Brain Res., 30:185

Kaydon,H.J., Silber,R. and Kossman,C.E., 1965, The role of vitamin E deficiency in the abnormal autohaemolysis of acanthocytosis, Trans.Assoc.Am.Physicians, 78:334

Kempley,S. and Cavanagh,J.B., 1984, Effects of acrylamide and some other sulfhydryl reagents on spontaneous and pathologically induced terminal sprouting from motor end plates, Muscle Nerve, 7:101

Konrad,P.N., Richards,F., Valentine,N.N. and Paglia,D.E., 1972, γ-glutamyl-cysteine synthetase deficiency : a cause of hereditary haemolytic anaemia, N.Engl.J.Med., 286:557

Lasek,R.J., 1981, Dynamic ordering of the neuronal cytoskeleton in "Cytoskeleton and the Architecture of the Nervous System", R.J. Lasek and M.L. Shelanski,eds., Neurosci.Res.Bull., 19:17

Miller,R.J., Davis,C.J.F., Illingworth,D.R. and Bradley,W. G., 1980, The neuropathy of abetalipoproteinaemia, Neurology (New York), 30:1286

Mohler,D.N., Majerus,P.W., Mumich,V., Hess,C.E. and Garrick, M.D., 1970, Glutathione synthetase deficiency as a cause of hereditary haemolytic anaemia, N.Engl.J.Med., 283:1253

Morgan Hughes,J.A., Sinclair,S. and Durston,J.H., 1974, The pattern of peripheral nerve regeneration induced by crush in rats with severe acrylamide neuropathy, Brain, 97:235

Mudd,S.H., Finkelstein,J.D., Irreverre,F. and Laster,L., 1964, Homocysteinuria : an enzymatic defect, Science, 143:1443

Muller,D.P.R., Lloyd,J.K. and Wolff,O.H., 1983, Vitamin E and neurological function, Lancet, 1:225

Munoz-Martinez,E.J., 1982, Axonal retention of transported material and the lability of nerve terminals, in "Axoplasmic Transport", D.G. Weiss,ed., Springer-Verlag, Berlin

Munoz-Martinez,E.J., Nunez,R. and Sanderson,A., 1981, Axonal transport : a quantitative study of retained and transported protein fraction in the cat, J.Neurobiol., 12:15

Ochs,S., 1975, Retention and redistribution of proteins in mammalian nerve fibres by axoplasmic transport, J. Physiol., 253:459

Pentschew,A. and Garro,F., 1969, Thallium encephalopathy in monkeys, J.Neuropathol.Exp.Neurol., 28:163A

Rambourg,A. and Droz,B., 1980, Smooth endoplasmic reticulum and axonal transport, J.Neurochem., 35:16

Richards,F., Cooper,M.A., Pearce,L.A.S., Cowan,R.J. and Spur, L.L.,1974, Familial spinocerebellar degeneration, haemolytic anaemia and glutathione deficiency, Arch.Intern.Med., 134:534

Rindi,G., Patrini,C., Comincioli,V. and Reggiani,C., 1980, Thiamine content and turnover rates of some rat nervous regions using labelled thiamine as a tracer, Brain Res., 181/369

Rosenblum,J.L., Keating,J.P., Prensky,A.L. and Nelson,J.S., 1981, A progressive neurological syndrome in children with chronic liver disease, N.Engl.J.Med., 304:503

Shelanski,M.L. and Wisniewski,H., 1969, Neurofibrillary degeneration induced by vincristine neuropathy, Arch.Neurol. (Chicago), 20:199

Shiraishi,S., LeQuesne,P.M. and Cavanagh,J.B., 1984, Work in progress

Spencer,P.S., Schaumburg,H.H., Sabri,M.I. and Veronesi,B., 1980, The enlarging view of hexacarbon neurotoxicity, CRC Crit.Rev.Toxicol., 7:279

Simonati,A., Rizzuto,N. and Cavanagh,J.B., 1983, The effects of 2,5 hexanedione on axonal regeneration after nerve crush in the rat, Acta Neuropathol.(Berl), 59:216

Tanaka,C., Tanaka,S. and Itokawa,Y., 1976, Histochemical and biochemical approaches to axoplasmic transport of thiamine in "Thiamine", C.J. Grubler,M. Fujiwara and P.M. Dreyfus, eds, Wiley & Sons, New York

Tomiwa,K., Hazama,F. and Mikawa,H., 1983, Neurotoxicity of vincristine after osmotic opening of the blood-brain barrier, Neuropathol.Appl.Neurobiol., 9:345

K. Volpe,J.J. and Lester,L., 1970, Transsulphuration in primate brain : regional distribution of cystathionine synthetase, cystathionine and taurine in the brain of the rhesus monkey at various stages of development, J.Neurochem, 17:425

Waller,H.D., 1968, Glutathione reductase deficiency, in "Hereditary Disorders of Erythrocyte Metabolism", E. Beutler ed., Grune & Stratton, New York

BIOCHEMICAL CONTRIBUTIONS TO NEUROTOXICOLOGY

S.C. Bondy

Southern Occupational Health Center
Department of Community and Environmental Medicine
University of California, Irvine
Irvine, California 92715

Contents

A. The importance of research in neurotoxicology

B. The definition of a neurotoxic agent

i) Some generally acting harmful agents present as specific neurotoxicants

ii) Some apparently neurotoxic substances act by way of other organs

iii) Brain-body interactions make the definition of a neurotoxic agent arbitrary

C. The goals of neurotoxicological research

i) Problems of experimental design

ii) Relation of biochemical changes to altered behavior

D. Conclusion

E. References

A. <u>The importance of research in neurotoxicology</u>

When a closed system, such as a flask, containing a nutrient-rich broth, is inoculated with a few bacteria, a period of rapid cell division takes place. As nutrients are consumed and waste products accumulate, the rate of proliferation slows down and eventually ceases. Ultimately, the total bacterial population within the flask declines. The earth is also a closed system. In this case a rapid human population growth phase started with the onset of the industrial revolution around two hundred years ago. This exponential growth phase has reached the point where the depletion of natural resources and increasing production of toxic waste products is significantly altering a series of global characteristics. These include irreversible ecological damage and the prospect of significant climatic changes.

Waste products can be harmful in several differing ways. In the case of some types of damage such as mutagenesis, general screening tests can be relatively effectively carried out using both test animals and *in vitro* cell culture systems such as the Ames test, in order to detect genetic disruption. The study of neurotoxicity is complicated by the insidious nature of much damage to the nervous system. While carcinogenesis ultimately expresses itself as an all-or-none phenomenon, permanent but minor damage to nerve tissue may be difficult to demonstrate. The brain has a significant adaptive capacity, exemplified by the high degree of recovery that may follow a severely incapacitating stroke (cerebrovascular rupture). Broad changes across a large population might be difficult to detect, but subtle neural changes can have profound consequences. It has been calculated that a mean loss of only 5 points of I.Q. would result in a doubling of the number of people legally classified as mentally retarded. Industrially used chemicals such as mercury and organophosphates can cause obvious damage to the nervous system of a specific group of people, in manufacturing industries and in agriculture. Other neurotoxic agents in view of their widespread distribution pose a potential hazard to the general population. These include lead and carbon monoxide which may cause relatively minor neurological deficits in a large segment of the urban population. Both of these classes of compounds require neurotoxicological study for delineating their potential threat and perhaps for mitigating their harmfulness. Other chemicals that are appropriate for neurotoxicological study are highly selective agents such as pharmacological products and biological toxins such as snake venoms. A major feature of such selectively acting chemicals is their inherent design for a specific function. This design is man-made in the case of drugs and due to evolutionary pressures in the case of biological toxins. This is in marked contrast to the many industrial wastes that are not designed to affect a particular biological function. This lack of design tends to make for several biological sites of action which may be difficult to identify and more difficult to correlate with the symptomatic expression of toxicity.

B. The definition of a neurotoxic agent

The definition of a neurotoxic chemical appears to be a simple matter, but is rather complex and subjective in nature. Altered behavior is an endpoint of the effects of all toxic agents but not all poisons are classified as neurotoxicants. Neurotoxicity is generally understood to imply a direct effect upon the nervous system. However, many agents that appear to primarily damage the brain are also harmful to other tissues.

i) Some generally acting harmful agents present as specific neurotoxicants

The brain possesses a series of attributes which are not unique but which represent enhanced levels of processes common to all tissues. For example, while all mammalian cells require a nutrient and an oxygen supply, the adult brain has a distinctively high energy requirement. Furthermore, any interruption of glucose or oxygen to the brain for more than a few seconds is poorly tolerated and can lead to significant damage (Davies and Bronk, 1957). A consequence of this is that generally toxic substances interfering with oxygen or glucose supply or utilization can under some circumstances appear to be specifically neurotoxic. Thus the cyanide ion, if not immediately fatal, can cause specific and permanent cerebral lesions (Bass, 1968). Similarly, transient exposure of the young animal to carbon monoxide can result in long-term behavioral abnormality at adulthood (Mactutus and Fechter, 1984). All other tissues appear to recover from such a relatively minor insult in these cases.

All cells require B vitamins, but significant neurological deficit is an early and predominant characteristic of deficiency of most B vitamins. This is another example of a generally deleterious state having predominantly nervous expression.

Another feature of the nervous system that can be considered to be an exaggeration of a uniquitous process, is its high tubulin content associated with axonal microtubules. Microtubules are associated with intracellular transport systems and are only pronounced in most cells during mitosis. However, transport processes are permanently pronounced in nerve cells in view of their extremely long processes. Several neurotoxic chemicals are harmful to axoplasmic transport (McLean, 1984). Low levels of toxic agents that disrupt microtubules, such as colchicine or vinblastin, can under certain circumstances be shown to cause behavioral deficits in the absence of significant damage to non-nervous tissues (Clingbine, 1977; Davis et al., 1984; Tomiwa et al., 1983). The low rate of cell division in the mature brain makes this organ relatively insensitive to many antimitotic agents and to radiation. However the developing brain is especially sensitive to such agents. Systemic administration of a compound interfering with DNA synthesis, such as cytosine arabinoside can cause very selective deficits in brain structure. The nature of the damage is determined by the developmental stage at which the cytosine arabinoside is administered (Matsutani et al., 1983). The reason underlying this selectivity is the complex nature of cerebral circuitry. Assembly of the neuronal array found in a normal animal is a process which requires a precise chronology of events. Mutual interdependence and critical timing are required for successful assembly of appropriate connectivity.

Another characteristic of the mature brain is its high lipid content, largely due to the proteolipids associated with myelin. This tends to facilitate the concentration of lipophilic chemicals into the brain. The blood brain-barrier also tends to preferentially allow the passage of more lipophilic molecular species. When two neurotoxic alkyl tins are compared, triethyl tin is more specifically injurious to myelin while trimethyl tin appears to be more damaging to neurons (Chang et al., 1982; Blaker et al., 1981). The differing neurotoxic profile of these compounds may be due to the more lipophilic nature of triethyl tin (Aldridge, 1978). Triethyl tin penetrates brain more rapidly than trimethyl tin after systemic administration (Cook et al., 1984) and it also binds to myelin thirty times as powerfully as does trimethyl tin (Aldridge and Rose, 1969).

ii. Some apparently neurotoxic substances act by way of other organs

There are several means by which a compound that interacts

primarily with a non-nervous tissue can cause the appearance of neurotoxicity. Hepatic enzymes (such as mixed function oxidases), designed to facilitate excretion of xenobiotic materials by oxidation and conjugation in order to make chemicals more ionized, can actually effect the production of a much more toxic chemical than the original. The tetra-alkyl leads are not very toxic but their hepatic conversion to the trialkyl derivatives makes them very harmful. This conversion also increases the general non-nervous toxicity of these organic lead compounds. Triethyl lead is over 100 times more inhibitory toward oxidative phosphorylation than tetraethyl lead (Cremer and Callaway, 1961); it is also genotoxic (Neibuhr and Wulf, 1984) and nephrotoxic (Seawright et al., 1984). However, organolead poisoning is predominantly expressed as neurotoxicity. Another organometal illustrates how interaction with the liver may result in the formation of neurotoxic levels of a normally-occurring biological compound. Trimethyl tin causes hyperexcitability, seizure proneness and specific damage to the hippocampus (Walsh et al., 1982). However, this compound appears to damage liver function and causes large increases in circulating levels of ammonia (Wilson et al., 1984). It may be that many of the characteristics of trimethyl tin poisoning are due to hyperammonemia. Hepatic encephalopathy may underlie the damage to nerve tissue caused by several chemicals such as chloroform (Diemer, 1976).

<u>iii) Brain-body interactions make the definition of a neurotoxic agent arbitrary</u>

Several harmful agents appear to damage non-nervous tissues and also the brain. The neuroendocrine system potentially enables CNS damage to alter the output of the endocrine glands and thus can alter the metabolism of the many organs that are targets of blood-borne hormones. The neuroendocrine system functions bidirectionally so that injury to a peripheral organ or gland can alter the secretion of pituitary trophic hormones and hypothalamic release factors. The complex feedback loops involved in endocrine regulation can make the identification of primary loci of action of a xenobiotic agent very difficult. An example of this is the case of organochlorine pesticides, of which many appear to have powerful neurotoxic and endocrine properties (Guzelian, 1982; Tilson and Mactutus, 1982). Chlordecone treatment will cause endocrine changes prior to the appearance of tremor and other behavioral abnormalities (Hong et al., 1984). Serum ACTH and cortisone levels become severely depressed and FSH and testosterone levels also decline. Together with other data, a primary attack on the hypothalamo-hypophyseal system is suggested since if peripheral glands were the initial target, an initial depression of testosterone or corticosterone would lead to an elevation of the corresponding trophic hormones by relaxation of negative feedback (Hong, personal communication, Figure 1). Chlordecone exposure also causes a greatly increased level of ornithine decarboxylase in the adrenal gland (Figure 2). However, this seems to reflect a direct stimulation of the adrenal gland since it also occurs after treatment of hypophysectomized rats with chlordecone (Figure 2). Thus chlordecone may simultaneously act on a variety of tissues and a series of initial sites of interaction may exist. Many agents classed as neurotoxic affect endocrine levels. For example, testosterone has been shown to be depressed following exposure to chlordecone, acrylamide, lead, triethyl lead, monosodium glutamate and manganese (Hong et al., 1984; Nemeroff et al., 1981; Ali et al., 1983). Monosodium glutamate treatment causes rather specific lesions in the arcuate nucleus of the hypothalamus (Olney, 1971). In the case of manganese and lead, there is evidence of direct damage to the testis (Imam and Chandra, 1975) as well as to the brain, and chlordecone also seems to impact directly on peripheral glands containing steroid receptors (Bulger et al., 1978; Hammond et al., 1979). Depressed testosterone levels due to any causes, are also then likely to alter an animal's behavioral characteristics. Furthermore, testosterone can influence neurotransmitter receptors in several brain regions including the cortex (Petrovic et al., 1984), further complicating identification of primary sites of impact of chemicals.

The major brain-body interactions are funnelled through the hypothalamus and small changes here can give rise to a cascading effect and thus cause much larger somatic changes (Figure 3). The magnification factor in the sequence between release factors —> trophic hormones —> target tissues, may be around 1000-fold for each step. Thus any change of hypothalamic metabolism may have disproportionately large indirect consequences. The status of the immune system is in part regulated by the hypothalamus (Stein et al., 1976) and stress can modulate the immune response (Monjan and Collector, 1979) and thus influence many events including tumor growth (Sklar and Anisman, 1979). Altered production of trophic hormones can then cause a variety of behavioral changes. Many trophic hormones such as prolactin and

ACTH affect the nervous system directly in addition to their effect on somatic glands (Van Ree et al., 1978).

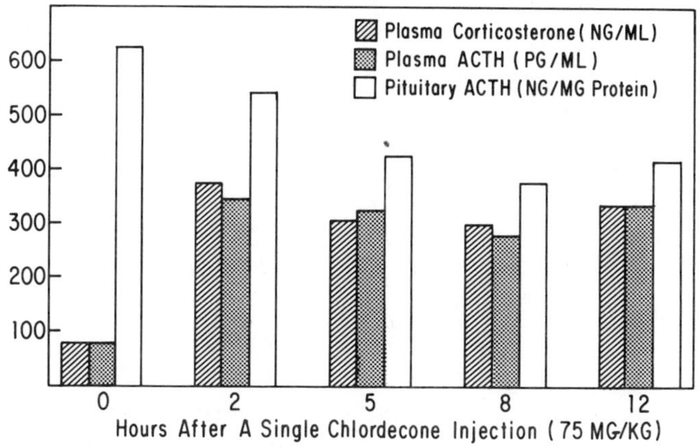

Figure 1
Circulating levels of corticosterone and ACTH and hypothalamic ACTH levels at various times after injection of chlordecone (75 mg/kg).

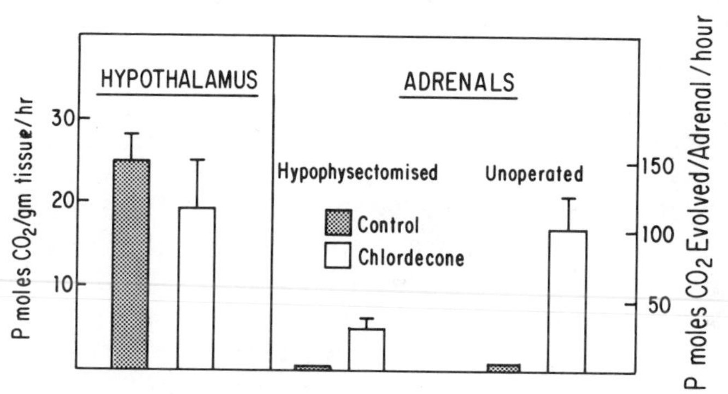

Figure 2
Ornithine decarboxylase activity in hypothalamus and adrenal glands, 4 hours after chlordecone injection (75 mg/kg).

The aspects discussed above illustrate the problems of making a clear separation of nervous from systemic toxicity. Damage to the CNS inevitably has repercussions upon the non-nervous components of an organism and thus may feed back again on the nervous system. Conversely, all toxic agents have the potential for inducing neurological abnormality. Consideration of potential interactions is essential even when an apparently selective neurotoxic agent is being studied.

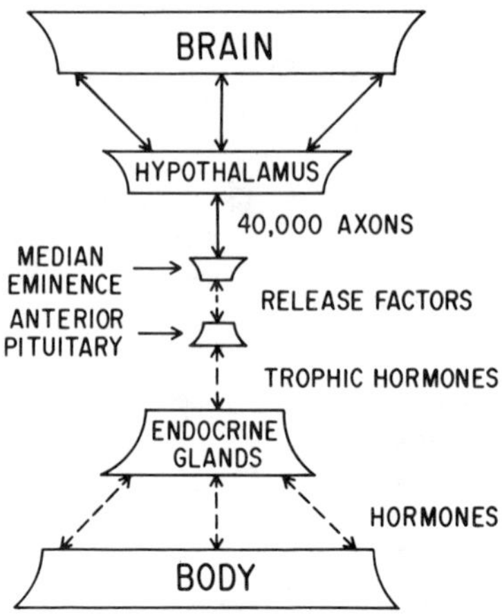

Figure 3
Magnification of molecular events by the neuro-endocrine system. Solid lines represent nerve pathways; dashed lines represent circulating hormones.

C. The goals of neurotoxicological research

The ultimate expression of damage to the nervous system is altered behavior and thus biochemical understanding of the mechanism of action of a harmful chemical ultimately implies accounting for behavioral abnormality in biochemical terms. Neurotoxicological study may often involve collaboration with behavioral scientists. Both neurochemical and behavioral responses are subject to extraneous factors. Such interdependent variables tend to be greater in number than those encountered in toxicological studies of non-nervous tissue. It is important to consider carefully a research strategy prior to the start of experimentation, as a design flaw if discovered in a study in progress, can be very costly.

i) Problems of experimental design

a) Prior experience of the animal

Coordination of biochemical and behavioral work may result in the use of animals which have been exposed to behavioral testing or have become familiar with repeated handling. Rats that have been exposed to extensive behavioral testing have been shown to have an endocrine profile that differs from that of naive animals. Prolactin is depressed in the serum of tested animals while corticosterone is elevated in male rats that have been tested (Uphouse et al., 1983). This reflects a different status of the hypothalamo-hypophyseal axis in the two groups of rats. It has been shown that the rate of recovery from kainic-acid induced hippocampal damage can be dramatically accelerated by behavioral training (Handleman et al., 1983).

The response to a toxic agent is likely to be altered in rats after behavioral testing. For example, treatment with acrylamide results in a significant reduction of plasma prolactin in naive rats. However this effect is lost in animals that have been handled for only three minutes a day for a week (Uphouse et al., 1982a). Such minor familiarity with handling is sufficient to alter the basal circulating levels of prolactin and corticosterone in rats otherwise receiving no treatment. These changes are probably related to stress. An animal familiar with handling has low intrinsic levels of prolactin but this hormone can rise very rapidly during the short handling prior to decapitation. Male rats subjected to extensive behavioral testing involving pain have an intrinsically higher level of corticosterone than untreated rats (Uphouse et al., 1983). Prolactin levels respond to acute stress while the slower responding levels of corticosterone may reflect a more chronically stressful state.

The example of acrylamide given above illustrates a response to a neurotoxicant that is only apparent together with a stressful state (handling for the first time). Acrylamide treatment appears to prevent a normal stress-induced elevation of prolactin but this is not seen in the absence of stress (familiarity with handling). Another example of the appearance of a change induced by a neurotoxic agent in conjunction with stress is seen after repeated daily injections of manganese chloride ($MnCl_2$). In this study, three groups of rats were used; $MnCl_2$-injected, saline-injected and an uninjected control. Dosing involved six weeks of daily intraperitoneal injections. Striatal levels of monoamines and their metabolites were determined by high performance liquid chromatography (Hong et al., 1984). The only significant difference found, was between the manganese treated group and the uninjected controls (Table 1).

Saline-injected controls had an intermediate value, not significantly different from either other group. In a study of the interaction of treatment with a toxic agent (chlordecone) and a severe stress (inescapable foot shock), some stress-induced biochemical changes were blocked by the toxic agent while other stress-related changes were only apparent in chlordecone-treated rats (Rosecrans et al., 1982). Injection of neonatal animals prior to weaning poses another hazard in that the maternal response toward injected offspring is not normal (Martin and Moberg, 1981).

Table 1.
Levels of Biogenic Amines and Their Acid Metabolites in the Striatum of Rat Exposed to $MnCl_2$ for Six Weeks

	$MnCl_2$ injected	Saline injected	Uninjected
Dopamine	16.30 ± 1.3	13.60 ± 1.10	13.40 ± 1.10
Dihydroxy-phenylacetic acid	1.38 ± 0.14*	1.13 ± 0.08	0.96 ± 0.08
Serotonin	1.02 ± 0.11*	0.83 ± 0.08	0.74 ± 0.03
5-hydroxy-indolacetic acid	0.86 ± 0.08*	0.73 ± 0.05	0.64 ± 0.01
Homovanillic acid	0.65 ± 0.07*	0.58 ± 0.05	0.46 ± 0.01

Each value represents a mean from 6-8 animals ± S.E. Data are given as g/g tissue weight. Male rats were dosed daily with intraperitoneal injections of manganese chloride (15 mg/kg body weight) or isotonic saline.
* $P < 0.05$ that value differ from <u>uninjected</u> group. In no case did values from the saline-injected group differ significantly from corresponding values in the other two groups (taken from Hong et al., 1984).

b) <u>The nature of the vehicle used</u>

Other stress-related phenomena may obscure rather than enhance the effect of a neurotoxicant. Dimethylsulfoxide (DMSO) is a widely used vehicle because of its ability to promote penetration of chemicals. A three-animal-group design was used in a chlordecone study; chlordecone in DMSO, DMSO alone, and a water injected group. Injections of DMSO or DMSO plus chlordecone, both depressed serum prolactin levels relative to the water-injected group (Uphouse et al., 1982b). On the other hand, hypothalamic weight was depressed in animals exposed to chlordecone + DMSO but not in the DMSO-alone group. Thus chlordecone caused a significant loss of hypothalamic weight but any possible influence of this compound on prolactin levels was obscured by the potent effect of DMSO on this hormone. This example illustrates the danger of inadvertantly studying irrelevant factors, and of the potential value of using more than two groups of animals in neurotoxicological studies. Stress of different types may produce differing endocrine responses so that potential chemical and physical stressors have to be separately taken into account (Gibbs, 1984).

c) Specific versus non-specific effects

It is likely that all neurotoxic agents are stressful to some extent, irrespective of their precise means of action. Thus the biochemical changes that are observed following treatment with a damaging agent may in part relate to general stress and in part to the specific effects of the toxic agent. This idea is substantiated by the fact that many toxic agents can cause similar biological lesions despite having a wide variety of suspected sites of action. Thus, testosterone levels are reduced following exposure to a whole series of agents (see previous section). A common response to stress may be the neuroendocrine shutdown of gonads which are, after all, not immediately essential for survival. Depressed testosterone levels should result in behavioral changes that are common to many neurotoxicants.

In a parallel manner, cerebral levels of the serotonin metabolite, 5-hydroxytryptamine indole acetic acid are elevated by a wide range of chemicals including manganese (Hong et al., 1984, Table 1), chlordecone (Rosecrans et al., 1982), acrylamide (Ali et al., 1983), trimethyl tin (De Haven et al., 1984), and organophosphates (Prioux-Guyonneau et al., 1982). This may reflect an activation of serotonergic circuits as a response to several kinds of toxic damage. Separation of specific and non-specific chemical changes is necessary in order to delineate the biochemical basis of the characteristic behavioral changes of a neurotoxic chemical.

ii) The relation of biochemical changes to altered behavior

Many behavioral changes caused by a neurotoxic agent are

rather non-specific and could be accounted for by a variety of changes of neuronal function. These changes include tremor, convulsions, paralysis and altered states of arousal or mentation. The biochemical steps penultimate to, and most closely related to behavior, are neurotransmission-related. In view of the broad range of potentially disturbed neuronal circuits, a preliminary objective survey of several pathways is desirable. This can be conveniently carried out by analysis of neurotransmitter receptor species. Since a series of these can be readily carried out, evaluation of receptors can be used in an impartial survey of the status of a variety of nerve tracts (Bondy, 1982). Such a survey takes advantage of the adaptive capacity of the brain. Postsynaptic receptors tend to up- or down-regulate in a manner inverse to the rate of firing of the presynaptic input (Yamamura et al., 1978). These receptor responses seem to represent an attempt to maintain homeostasis and may be instrumental in the maintenance of relatively normal behavior at moderate levels of CNS damage. For instance, near total degeneration of the nigrostriatal bundle must be effected before the expression of neurological symptoms in experimental animals (Zigmond and Stricker, 1984). The adaptive capacity of receptors has been widely used to enlarge understanding of many neurological and psychiatric disorders including Huntingdon's Disease, schizophrenia, epilepsy and myasthenia gravis (Melnechuk, 1978). While pharmacologists have exploited receptor characteristics in drug design and in furthering the understanding of neural mechanism (Snyder, 1983) this methodology has been somewhat neglected by toxicologists. Since many neurotoxic chemicals may alter neuronal activity patterns by varied means, analysis of receptor high affinity binding sites offers a convenient means of checking on the condition of various neural circuits. The availability of an increasing number of radiolabeled ligands provides a greater resolving power of receptor studies. These labeled pharmacological agents generally have a greater specificity, a greater affinity for receptors, and a greater stability than endogenous neurotransmitters.

Initial studies in our laboratory involved the use of neurotoxic chemicals whose mechanism of action was already partially understood. Triorthocresyl phosphate (TOCP) is known to have an inhibitory effect on acetylcholinesterase and thus causes cholinergic hyperactivity (Davis and Richardson, 1980; Abou-Donia, 1981). Avian species are especially vulnerable to this industrial product, and we have assayed receptor binding intensity in the forebrains of TOCP-treated hens (Ali et al., 1984). The muscarinic cholinergic receptor binding capacity was depressed in treated hens while no change was detected in six other receptor species. This implied that the firing rate of the muscarinic neurons was elevated, and probably due to a reduced rate of acetylcholine catabolism in the synaptic cleft. If less were known about TOCP, such data would immediately suggest acetylcholine systems as a target of this toxic agent, and this would lead to a closer examination of the cause of such cholinergic hyperactivity.

Another neurotoxic agent whose locus of damage is somewhat understood is manganese. This metal appears to selectively damage dopaminergic circuitry of treated animals (Donaldson et al., 1981). Exposure of humans to excessive amounts of this element results initially in a reversible, schizophrenia-like state, and later in a permanent Parkinsonian-like condition (Cook et al., 1974). This suggests an initially high level of dopaminergic activity followed by death of dopamine neurons (Cotzias et al., 1974). Various receptor species were examined in brain regions of rats repeatedly dosed with manganese (Seth et al., 1981a). Striatal spiroperidol binding was elevated in exposed rats and this was attributed to damaged dopamine neurons causing an upregulation of post-synaptic receptors. Cerebellar GABA receptors showed increased binding capacity, perhaps reflecting activation of inhibitory neurons in response to reduced dopaminergic activity. High pressure liquid chromatography of serotonin, dopamine and their metabolites suggested increased turnover of these monoamines in exposed rats (Hong et al., 1984). The apparent contradiction between dopamine and serotonin metabolite concentrations (suggesting increased neuronal activity) and receptor binding data (suggesting decreased activity) has a parallel in haloperidol-treated rats. Under certain conditions, the dopamine receptors can be elevated in rats while behavioral tests indicate dopaminergic hyperactivity (Fuxe et al., 1980).

There are several possible reasons that may account for apparent discrepancies of this nature. 1) If a proportion of a neuronal group is damaged or destroyed, the surviving neurons may compensate by becoming excessively active. Thus, levels of receptors and metabolites of neurotransmitters may not always be altered in a consonant manner. 2) The direction in which presynaptic receptor levels respond to altered rates of neuronal firing is generally opposite to that of postsynaptic responses (Lee et al., 1983). Presynaptic receptors are involved in release of neurotransmitters. Therefore, their downregulation in a circuit with unusually low activity decreases the reuptake rate of transmitters within the synaptic cleft and thus potentiates postsynaptic effects. Thus, the regulation of both pre- and postsynaptic receptors is in a direction tending to maintain homeostasis. 3) Many biological responses are multiphasic and overlapping. Thus patients chronically treated with neuroleptics may simultaneously present tardive dyskinesia and stereotypy (implying dopaminergic hyperactivity) and Parkinsonian symptoms (implying abnormally reduced activity of dopamine neurons) (Barnes et al., 1980). These complications can make the transmitter species affected by a toxic agent more readily detectable than the directionality of changes.

A widely used chemical that is damaging to peripheral nerve tissue is acrylamide. This chemical has been found to cause behavioral changes that also suggest involvement of the central nervous system (Schaumberg and Spencer, 1978). There was, however, no clear indication of which transmitter system might be modulated by acrylamide. For this reason, a broad survey of receptor status in acrylamide-treated rats was carried out (Bondy et al., 1981; Agrawal et al., 1981). At the lowest acrylamide dose used, striatal dopamine receptor binding was elevated, suggesting selective damage to, or suppression of, amine neurons (Table 2). At higher doses or repeated doses of acrylamide, an increasing number of receptor species appeared to be elevated. This may have been due to a broadening involvement of, and damage to, other nerve pathways.

Table 2.

Neurotransmitter Receptor Binding In Rats Receiving Acrylamide

		Acrylamide dose (mg/kg body wt/day)							
		24-hr exposure after a single dose				10 doses over 14 days			
Regions	Receptor species	0	25	50	100	0	5	10	20
Striatum	Dopamine	334 ± 13	413 ± 11*	417 ± 11*	481 ± 32*	237 ± 15	371 ± 15*	314 ± 17*	366 ± 11*
	Acetylcholine (muscarinic)	527 ± 26	490 ± 25	479 ± 21	549 ± 55	472 ± 22	591 ± 30*	594 ± 26*	618 ± 16
Frontal Cortex	Benzodiazepine	76 ± 6	79 ± 6	63 ± 5	80 ± 4	43 ± 6	43 ± 5	34 ± 2	40 ± 4
	Serotonin	66 ± 5	72 ± 5	70 ± 4	84 ± 7*	65 ± 3	76 ± 6	69 ± 6	97 ± 5*
Medulla	Glycine	558 ± 96	636 ± 24	654 ± 42	690 ± 35*	420 ± 18	456 ± 12	450 ± 18	492 ± 36*
Cerebellum	GABA	640 ± 64	768 ± 48	576 ± 48	544 ± 32	280 ± 24	312 ± 24	280 ± 16	440 ± 24*

Note: Binding expressed as pmol/g protein ± SE.
* Differs from zero-dose ($p<0.05$). Zero-dose animals received corresponding injections of water.

Further work showed that the elevation in dopamine receptors was a) reversible, b) attributable to post- rather than presynaptic receptors (Hong et al., 1982), and c) blocked by pretreatment of rats with SKF 525a, a mixed function oxidase inhibitor (Agrawal et al., 1981). This latter finding implied that observed changes in dopamine receptors were mediated by a metabolite of acrylamide. The behavioral response induced by apomorphine (increased motility, stereotypy) was suppressed in acrylamide-tested rats, further suggesting damage to the dopamine neurons of the nigrostriatal pathway. The inhibition of reinforced bar pressing by clonidine and chlordiazepoxide was unchanged after acrylamide treatment but the corresponding apomorphine depression was exacerbated (Tilson and Squibb, 1982), revealing a degree of specificity of dopaminergic changes.

Exposure of developing rats has been compared to similar exposure of adults using chlordecone and acrylamide as representative agents. In the adult male, chlordecone decreases striatal spiroperidol binding while this binding is increased by acrylamide. This situation is reversed after gestational and neonatal exposure of immature male rats (Agrawal and Squibb, 1981; Seth et al., 1981b). In this case acrylamide causes a depression and chlordecone an elevation of spiroperidol binding sites (Figure 4). This may be due to the differing response of postsynaptic receptors after adult denervation in comparison to failure of innervation in the immature animal. Damage to afferent neurons before axons reach their targets may cause failure of receptor development rather than supersensitivity in target cells.

Conversely, a high level of activity could play an inductive role during ontogenesis rather than effecting receptor downregulation. In addition to the data on acrylamide and chlordecone reported here, exposure of neonatal animals to neuroleptics or manganese has also been shown to cause receptor changes in a direction opposite to those found in mature animals (Rosengarten and Friedhoff, 1979; Seth and Chandra, 1984). Information gained from receptor data in developmental studies has therefore to be interpreted with this possibility in mind.

D. Conclusion

Longer exposure to a toxic agent potentially increases the complexity of the adaptive reaction. Such adaptation can be

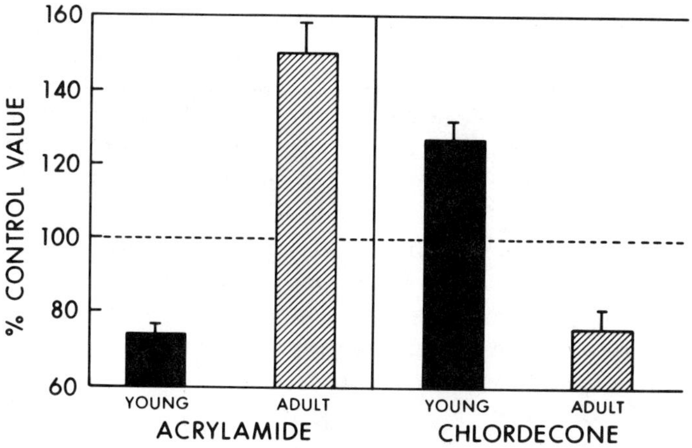

Figure 4
Spiroperidol binding to striatal membranes of male rats exposed to toxic agents. Chlordecone was given in the diet (6 ppm) of dams for 60 days prior to mating throughout gestation and lactation. At 12 days of age, offspring were maintained on a normal diet before being killed at 30 days. In adult studies, dietary chlordecone was (30 ppm) given for 90 days preceding sacrifice. Acrylamide was given to dams orally (20 mg/kg body weight) daily while gestational age was 7-17 days. Offspring were killed 14 days postnatally. For adult rats, 20 mg/kg acrylamide was given daily for 10 of the 14 days preceding sacrifice.

extremely successful if allowed to occur over an extended period. The astonishing compensatory capacity of the young brain is exemplified by the fortuitous discovery of a case of hydrocephalus in a young man whose final brain weight was around 10% of the normal. This man had obtained a mathematics degree and showed no obvious neurological abnormality (Lewin, 1980).

The receptor changes found in animals exposed to neurotoxic agents often represent homeostatic adaptive responses. These responses may be especially relevant to chronic exposure to lower levels of harmful agents. Acute poisoning of an animal may not allow time for such changes or may render the animal incapable of such modulating responses. The receptor-oriented type of interpretation of the action of substances harmful to the nervous system may have practical application in furthering the understanding of various hazardous industrial and environmental chemicals. Knowledge concerning damage to defined nerve circuits may also assist in the development of therapeutic strategies following exposure to neurotoxic chemicals.

A rather general disruption of membrane stability or inhibition of an ubiquitous enzyme might ultimately find expression by disturbance of a particularly vulnerable nerve pathway. This apparent selectivity does not imply that the primary locus of action of a toxic agent is confined to that neuronal species. For example, catecholamine neurons may be especially sensitive to oxidative conditions because of the susceptibility of several monoamines to oxidation (Balentine, 1968). An enzyme that is very readily damaged by oxygen is glutamate decarboxylase (Tunnicliff and Wood, 1974) and thus oxidizing conditions may cause an elevation of the excitatory transmitter glutamate, and depression of levels of its decarboxylated product, GABA, an inhibitory transmitter. This imbalance may lead to convulsions and brain damage. This may, in part, account for the susceptibility of the developing retina to hyperbaric concentrations of oxygen. Failure of oxygen supply may also damage distinct areas of the brain (Daughtrey and Norton, 1982).

A limitation of receptor evaluation is that this approach does not automatically throw light on the series of biochemical steps leading to these adaptive changes. Mechanisms of action at the molecular level can only be reached by working backwards toward the initial targets of a toxic agent. The 'mechanism of action' of a neurotoxic agent can only be defined when all intermediate steps are delineated. In view of the multifocal assault of many toxic agents, it may be wise to define a more limited and concise research goal. It is important, however, to be aware of the complex sequence of events that lead to the expression of neurotoxicity.

E. References

Abou-Donia, M.B., 1981, Organophosphorus ester-induced delayed neurotoxicity, Pharmacol.Toxicol., 21:511.

Agrawal, A.K., Seth, P.K., Squibb, R.E., Tilson, H.A., Uphouse, L.L. and Bondy, S.C., 1981, Neurotransmitter receptors in brain regions of acrylamide treated rats. I. Effects of a single exposure to acrylamide, Pharmacol.Biochem.Behav., 14:527.

Agrawal, A.K. and Squibb, R.E., 1981, Effects of acrylamide given during gestation on dopamine receptors binding in pups, Toxicol.Letters, 7:233.

Aldridge, W.N., 1978, The biological properties of organo-germanium, tin and lead compounds, in: "The Organometallic and Coordination Chemistry of Germanium, Tin and Lead", M. Geilen and P.G. Harrison, eds., Georgi Publishing, St.Saphorin, Switzerland.

Aldridge, W.N. and Rose, M.S., 1969, The mechanism of oxidative phosphorylation. A hypothesis derived from studies of tri-methyl tin and triethyl tin compounds, FEBS Letters, 4:61.

Ali, S.F., Hong, J.S., Wilson, W.E., Uphouse, L.L. and Bondy, S.C., 1983, Effect of acrylamide on neurotransmitter metabolism and neuropeptide levels in several brain regions and upon circulating hormones, Arch.Toxicol., 52:35.

Ali, S.F., Abou-Donia, M.B. and Bondy, S.C., 1984, Modulation of avian muscarinic cholinergic high affinity binding sites by a neurotoxic organophosphate, Neurochem.Pathol., 2:267.

Balentine, J.E., 1968, Pathogenesis of central nervous system lesions induced by exposure to hyperbaric oxygen, Am.J.Pathol., 53:1097.

Barnes, T.R.E., Kidger, T., Trauer, T. and Taylor, P., 1980, reclassification of the Tarditive Dyskinesia Syndrome, Adv. Biochem.Psychopharm., 24:565.

Bass, N.H., 1968, Pathogenesis of myelin lesions in experimental cyanide encephalopathy, Neurology, 18:167.

Blaker, W.D., Krigman, M.R., Thomas, D.J., Mushak, P. and Morell, P., 1981, Effect of triethyl tin on myelination in the developing rat, J.Neurochem., 36:44.

Bondy, S.C., 1982, Neurotransmitter binding interactions as a screen for neurotoxicity, in: "Mechanisms of Actions of Neurotoxic Substances", K.N. Prasad and A. Vernadakis, eds., Raven Press, New York.

Bondy, S.C., Tilson, H.A. and Agrawal, A.K., 1981, Neurotrans-mitter receptors in brain regions of acrylamide treated rats. II. Effect of extended exposure to acrylamide, Pharmacol.Biochem.Behav., 14:533.

Bulger, W.H., Muccitelli, R.M. and Kupfer, D., 1978, Interactions of chlorinated hydrocarbon pesticides with the 8S estrogen binding protein in rat testes, Steroids, 32:165.

Chang, L.W., Tiemeyer, T.M., Wenger, G.R., McMillan, D.E. and Reuhl, K.R., 1982, Neuropathology of trimethyl tin intoxication. I. Light microscopy study, Environ.Res., 29:435.

Clingbine, N., 1977, Effect of colchicine and lumicolchicine on learning in goldfish, Br.J.Pharmacol., 59:449.

Cook, D.G., Fahn, S. and Brout, K.A., 1974, Chronic manganese intoxication, Arch.Neurol., 30:59.

Cook, L.L., Stine, K.E. and Reiter, L.W., 1984, Tin distribution in adult rat tissues following exposure to trimethyl tin and triethyl tin, Toxicol.Apl.Pharmacol., 76:344.

Cotzias, G.C., Papavasiliou, P.S., Mena, I., Tang, L.C. and Miller, S.T., 1974, Manganese and catecholamines, Adv.Neurol., 5:235.

Cremer, J.E. and Callaway, S., 1961, Further studies on the toxicity of some tetra and trialkyl lead derivatives, Br.J.Indust.Med., 18:277.

Daughtrey, W.C. and Norton, S., 1982, Morphological damage to the premature fetal rat brain after acute carbon monoxide exposure, Exp.Neurol., 78:26.

Davies, P.W. and Bronk, D.W., 1957, Oxygen tension in mammalian brain, Fed.Proc., 16:689.

Davis, C.S. and Richardson, R.J., 1980, Organophosphorous compounds, in: "Experimental and Clinical Neurotoxicology, P.S. Spencer and H.H. Schaumberg, eds., Williams and Williams, Baltimore.

Davis, R.E., Schlumpf, B.E. and Klinger, P.D., 1984, Systemic colchicine inhibits goldfish optic nerve regeneration, Toxicol.Appl.Pharmacol., 73:268.

De Haven, D.L., Walsh, T.J. and Mailman, R.B., 1984, Effects of trimethyl tin on dopaminergic and serotonergic function in the central nervous system, Toxicol.Appl.Pharmacol., 75:182.

Diemer, H.N., 1976, Glial and neuronal alterations in the corpus striatum of rats with CCl_4-induced liver disease, Acta Neurol.Scand., 55:16.

Donaldson, J., LaBella, F.S. and Gesser, D., 1981, Enhanced auto-oxidation of dopamine as a possible basis of manganese neurotoxicity, Neurotoxicology, 2:53.

Fuxe, K., Orgren, S.O., Hall, H., Agnati, F.F., Andersson, K., Kohler, C. and Schwarcz, R., 1980, Effects of chronic treatment with l-sulpiride and haloperidol on central monoaminergic mechanisms, Adv.Biochem.Psychopharm., 24:193.

Gibbs, D.M., 1984, Dissociation of oxytocin, vasopressin and corticotropin secretion during different types of stress, Life Sci., 35:487.

Guzelian, P.S., 1982, Comparative toxicology of chlordecone

(kepone) in humans and experimental animals, Ann.Rev. Pharmacol.Toxicol., 22:89.

Hammond, G., Katzenellenbogen, B.S., Krauthammer, N. and McConnell, J., 1979, Estrogenic activity of the insecticide chlordecone (kepone) and interaction with uterine estrogen receptors, Proc.Natl.Acad.Sci.USA, 76:6641.

Handleman, G.E., Alton, D.S., O'Donohue, T.L., Beinfeld, M.C., Jacobowitz, D.M. and Cummins, C.J., 1983, Effects of time and experience on hippocampal neurochemistry after damage to the CA3 subfield, Pharmacol.Biochem.Behav., 18:551.

Hong, J.S., Hung, C.R., Seth, P.K., Mason, G. and Bondy, S.C., 1984, The results of manganese treatment on the levels of neurotransmitters, hormones, and neuropeptides: Interaction of stress with such effects, Environ.Res., 34:242.

Hong, J.S., Tilson, H.A., Agrawal, A.K., Karoum, F. and Bondy, S.C., 1982, Postsynaptic location of acrylamide-induced modulation of striated ^{3}H-spiroperidol binding, Neurotoxicology, 3:108.

Imam, Z. and Chandra, S.V., 1975, Histochemical alterations in rabbit testes produced by manganese chloride, Toxicol.Appl. Pharmacol., 22:534.

Lee, C.M., Javitch, J.A. and Snyder, S.H., 1983, Recognition sites for norepinephrine uptake: Regulation by neurotransmitter, Science, 220:1232.

Lewin, R., 1980, Is your brain really necessary?, Science, 210:1232.

Mactutus, C.F. and Fechter, L.D., 1984, Prenatal exposure to carbon monoxide: Learning and memory deficits, Science, 223:409.

Martin, S.M. and Moberg, G.P., 1981, Developmental effects of intraperitoneal saline injection in neonatal rats, Life Sci., 29:143.

Matsutani, T., Tamaru, M., Nagayoshi, M., Hayakawa, Y., Nakara, T. and Tsukada, Y., 1983, Neurochemical studies on the developmental impairment of the brain by the administration of cytosine arabinoside in the fetal or neonatal periods of rats, Neurochem.Res., 8:1295.

McLean, G., 1984, Neurotoxicity and axonal transport, Trends Pharmacol.Sci., 5:243.

Melnechuk, T., 1978, Cell Receptor Disorders, Western Behavioral Sciences Institute, La Jolla, CA.

Monjan, A.A. and Collector, M.I., 1977, Stress-induced modulation of the immune response, Science, 196:307.

Neibuhr, E. and Wulf, H.C., 1984, Genotoxic effects, in: "Biological Effects of Organolead Compounds", P. Grandjean and E. J. Grandjean, eds., CRC Press, Boca Raton FL.

Nemeroff, C.B., Lamartiniere, C.A., Mason, G.A., Squibb, R.E., Hong, J.S. and Bondy, S.C., 1981, Marked reduction in gonadal steroid hormone levels in rats treated neonatally with monosodium glutamate: further evidence for disruption of hypothalamus-pituitary-gonadal axis regulation, Neuroendocrinology, 33:265.

Olney, J.W., 1971, Glutamate-induced neuronal necrosis in the infant mouse hypothalamus, J.Neuropath.Exp.Neurol., 30:75.

Petrovic, S.L., McDonald, J.K., Snyder, G.D. and McCann, S.M., 1984, Testosterone control of brain and interior pituitary adrenergic receptors, Life Sci., 34:2399.

Prioux-Guyonneau,M., Coudray-Lukas, C., Cog, H.M., Cohen, Y. and Wepierre, J., 1982, Modification of rat brain 5-hydroxytryptamine by sublethal doses of organophosphate agents, Acta Pharmacol.Toxicol., 51:278.

Rosencrans, J.A., Hong, J.S., Squibb, R.E., Johnson, J.H., Tilson, H.A., Wilson, W.E., 1982, Effects of perinatal exposure to chlordecone (kepone) on neuroendocrine and neurochemical responsiveness to environmental challenges, Neurotoxicol., 3:131.

Rosengarten, H. and Friedhoff, A.J., 1979, Enduring changes in dopamine receptor cells of pups from drugs administered to pregnant and nursing rats, Science, 203:1133.

Schaumberg, H.H. and Spencer, P.S., 1978, Environmental hydrocarbons produce degeneration in cat hypothalamus and optic tract, Science, 199:199.

Seawright, A.A., Brown, A.W., Ng, J.C. and Hrdlicka, J., 1984, Experimental pathology of short-chain alkyl lead compounds, in: "Biological Effects of Organolead Compounds", P. Grandjean and E.J. Grandjean, eds., CRC Press, Boca Raton Fl.

Seth, P.K., Hong, J.S., Kilts, K. and Bondy, S.C., 1981a, Alteration of cerebral high affinity binding sites by exposure of rats to manganese, Toxicol.Letters, 9:247.

Seth, P.K., Agrawal, A.K. and Bondy, S.C., 1981b, Biochemical changes in the brain consequent to dietary exposure of developing and mature rats to chlordecone, Toxicol.Appl. Pharmacol. 59:262.

Seth, P.K. and Chandra, S.V., 1984, Neurotransmitters and neurotransmitter receptors in developing and adult rats during manganese poisoning, Neurotoxicol., 5:67.

Sklar, L.S. and Anisman, H., 1979, Stress and coping factors influence tumor growth, Science, 205:513.

Snyder, S.H., 1983, Neurotransmitter receptor binding and drug discovery, J.Med.Chem., 26:1667.

Stein, M., Schiavi, R.C. and Camerino, M., 1976, Influence of brain and behavior on the immune system, Science, 191:435.

Tilson, H.A. and Mactutus, C.F., 1982, Chlordecone neurotoxicity: a brief overview, Neurotoxicol., 3:1.

Tilson, H.A. and Squibb, R.E., 1982, The effects of acrylamide on the behavioral suppression produced by psychoactive agents, Neurotoxicol., 3:113.

Tomiwa, K., Hazama, F. and Mikawa, H., 1983, Neurotoxicity of vincristine after the osmotic opening of the blood-brain barrier, Neuropath.Appl.Neurobiol., 9:345.

Tunnicliff, G. and Wood, J.D., 1974, Influence of hyperbaric oxygen upon transmitter enzymes of the chick brain, Int. J.Biochem., 5:555.

Uphouse, L.L., Tilson, H. and Mitchell, C.L., 1983, Long term effects of behavioral testing on serum hormones and brain weight, Life Sci., 33:1395.

Uphouse, L.L., Nemeroff, C.B., Mason, G. and Bondy, S.C., 1982a, Interactions between "handling" and acrylamide on endocrine responses in rats, Neurotoxicol., 3:121.

Uphouse, L.L., Mason, G. and Bondy, S.C., 1982b, Comments concerning the use of dimethylsulfoxide as a solvent for studies of chlordecone neurotoxicity, Neurotoxicol., 3:149.

VanRee, J.M., Bohus, B., Versteeg, D.H.G. and DeWeid, D., 1978, Neurohypophyseal principles and memory process, Biochem. Pharmacol., 27:1793.

Walsh, T.J., Miller, D.B. and Dyer, R.S., 1982, Trimethyl tin, a selective limbic system neurotoxicant impairs radial arm performance, Neurobehav.Toxicol.Teratol., 4:177.

Wilson, W.E., Hudson, P.N., Kawamatsu, T., Walsh, T.J., Tilson, H.A. and Hong, J.S., 1984, Studies on the neurotoxicity of trimethyl tin (TMT). Evidence that the 'TMT syndrome' reflects a TMT-dependent hyperammonemia, in preparation.

Yamamura, H.I., Enna, S.J. and Kuhar, M.J., 1978, Neurotransmitter receptor binding, Raven Press, New York.

Zigmond, M.J. and Stricker, E.M., 1984, Parkinson's disease: studies with an animal model, Life Sci., 35:5.

METABOLIC ACTIVATION OF NEUROTOXICANTS

Emilio Perucca and Luigi Manzo

Institute of Pharmacology
University of Pavia, School of Medicine
Piazza Botta 10, 27100 Pavia, Italy

INTRODUCTION

The fact that drugs, food additives, industrial chemicals and environmental contaminants can be activated in the living organism to toxic metabolites is a well established concept in general pharmacology. As the liver is usually the predominant site of biotransformation, tissue damage by metabolites most frequently involves hepatotoxic reactions. Well known examples of drugs converted to hepatotoxic metabolites include paracetamol and isoniazid (Perucca and Richens, 1980).

The possibility of toxic metabolites affecting organs other than the liver is also widely appreciated. Examples include the myelotoxicity of benzene, the methemoglobinemia caused by aniline and the pulmonary necrosis induced by bromobenzene and 4-ipomeanol (Mitchell and Jollows, 1975; Boyd and Stratham, 1983).

Although metabolic activation resulting in neurotoxicity has been less extensively investigated, evidence is accumulating that this may be an important mechanism of nervous system damage by a variety of xenobiotics. The present article will provide a general overview of the role of metabolic activation in the pathogenesis of neurotoxic reactions, with a discussion of selected examples particularly relevant to clinical medicine.

METABOLIC ACTIVATION AS A MECHANISM OF NEUROTOXICITY

Once the neurotoxic potential of a given substrate has been established, an important question that arises is whether the toxicity is caused by the parent compound or by one or more of its metabolites. Characterization of all relevant metabolic pathways in the affected species is obviously the first step that must be taken to answer this question. It should be pointed out, however, that demonstration of a toxic metabolite being formed can not be regarded as proof that this metabolite is responsible for the observed effect. A highly toxic metabolite formed in the liver, for example, may be too short-lived to leave the hepatocyte and to cause tissue damage in the nervous system. The presence of the blood-brain barrier may further complicate the tissue availability of peripherally formed metabolites. Ultimately, therefore, demonstration of a cause-effect relationship must rest on the evidence that the metabolite is produced in the affected tissue (or reaches the affected tissue) at concentrations sufficient to induce the toxic effect.

The contribution of the parent compound and/or other metabolites also needs to be assessed. As a general rule, this information can be obtained by relating the concentration of the parent xenobiotic and its metabolite(s) in biological fluids and tissues to the magnitude of biological (toxic) effect. If the metabolite is chemically stable, these studies are usually relatively simple and can be supplemented by characterizing the effect induced by exogenous administration of the metabolite itself. When the metabolite is unstable and/or chemically reactive, the experimental evaluation is obviously more complicated and may require a complex integrated approach relating the kinetics of individual metabolites and/or degree of covalent binding with available parameters of toxicological damage (Mitchell and Jollow, 1975; Gillette, 1982).

Assessment of Metabolic Activation: Experimental Models and Methodological Problems

Experimental models to study metabolic activation can be distinguished into *in vitro* and *in vivo* systems. *In vitro* systems have the advantage of easy standardization of experimental variables. Under these conditions, it is generally possible to characterize specific metabolic pathways, identify relatively unstable intermediates and compare the relative ability of isolated organs and tissues in operating a given metabolic reaction. In particular, *in vitro* systems may allow detection of covalent binding by reactive intermediates, assessment of the stability of individual metabolites and identification of the enzyme system responsible for the activation process.

In several laboratories, elegant *in vitro* systems have been developed which allow the investigation of particular neurotoxic events. Organotypic cultures (cord-ganglia-muscle cultures), for example, have been usefully employed to investigate the pathogenesis of methyl n-butyl ketone (MnBK) neuropathy and to establish the role of 2,5-hexandione as a primary neurotoxin (Veronesi et al., 1980).

Although in vitro studies do allow some prediction of the kinetics of individual metabolites in the living organism, these data need to be supplemented by in vivo experiments. An integrated approach is necessary in order to correlate the formation of given metabolites with the incidence, type and severity of tissue damage by xenobiotics. If tissue damage is caused by very unstable reactive metabolites, rarely can the relationship between the level of the metabolite in biological fluids and the severity of the lesion be determined.

As discussed below, certain short-lived metabolites may not even leave the cell in which they are formed. Frequently (but not invariably) these metabolites cause tissue damage by binding covalently to cell macromolecules. In this case one experimental approach would be to determine whether administration of the parent xenobiotic in a wide dose range to laboratory animals results in the formation of metabolites which bind covalently in the tissues that subsequently become necrotic (Mitchell and Jollows, 1975). It is clear, however, that the incidence or severity of a toxic effect can not be predicted from the total amount of chemically reactive metabolite covalently bound to proteins. Indeed, most of the covalently bound metabolite is usually associated with non-target proteins and other macromolecules (Gillette, 1982). Moreover, large amounts of reactive metabolites may bind covalently to tissues without causing detectable damage (Caldwell, 1982). As pointed out by Gillette (1982), "it is the effect of various treatments in changing the covalent binding of the reactive metabolite and the incidence of toxicity that establishes the relationship between the chemically reactive metabolite and the toxicity, and not the magnitude of covalent binding per se".

Irrespective of whether the toxic metabolite acts by covalent binding or by other mechanisms the most widely used experimental approach to the study of metabolic activation in vivo is based on diet manipulation and various pre-treatments aimed at modifying metabolizing enzyme activities and/or availability of endogenous substrates. Phase II substrates such as glutathione and anti-oxidants such as vitamin E, for example, are known to protect the cell against toxicity induced by certain types of chemically reactive metabolites (Hill and Burk, 1984). As a result, depletion and/or repletion of these and other endogenous substrates have provided a most useful approach to the assessment of the mechanism of tissue damage (see Mitchell et al., 1982 for details and examples).

Inducers and inhibitors of metabolism have also been invaluable tools in determining whether a compound causes toxicity by itself or through an active metabolite. Enzyme inducers and enzyme inhibitors have been used not only to assess the mechanism(s) of tissue damage but also to better characterize the stability of toxic intermediates (a most important factor in assessing whether a given neurotoxic effect is caused by metabolites formed locally and/or at distant organs such as the liver). If a metabolite is long-lived, pre-treatment of animals with an inducer that selectively stimulates metabolic activation in the liver but not in extrahepatic tissues should result in potentiation of toxicity both in the liver and extrahepatic sites; by contrast, if the metabolite is short-lived, selective induction of the hepatic metabolism will be expected to decrease toxicity in extrahepatic organs (Gillette, 1982). In a similar way, substances that specifically inhibit the extrahepatic enzymes would also be expected to decrease extrahepatic toxicity (Mitchell and Jollows, 1975).

It should be noted, however, that prediction and evaluation of the *in vivo* effect of a particular agent is complicated by a number of factors:

(1) The effect of a given pre-treatment may vary among different organs and tissues. Certain enzyme inhibitors, for instance, do not cross readily the blood-brain barrier and therefore cause differential metabolic effects in the periphery and in the central nervous system. A representative example is provided by carbidopa and benserazide which potentiate the therapeutic and neurotoxic effects of L-DOPA by blocking its metabolic activation to dopamine in peripheral tissues but not in the brain. Inducers and inhibitors may even change the location of the lesion within an organ or from one organ to another. Frusemide, for example, causes renal but not hepatic necrosis in untreated rats and hepatic rather than renal necrosis in 3-methylcholanthrene-treated animals.

(2) Most inducers and inhibitors are relatively non selective. Since the toxicological potential may depend on a balance between simultaneously occurring toxification and detoxification processes, the final effect will depend on the relative stimulation/inhibition of several pathways characterized by opposed biological significance. For example, phenobarbital pre-treatment decreases the hepatic

damage produced by paracetamol in hamsters by stimulating detoxifying pathways more than toxifying ones (Mitchell and Jollow, 1975).

(3) The pattern of metabolic activation/inactivation may vary from one species to another and, within the same species, may be markedly influenced by genetic and environmental factors. The response to inducers and inhibitors is also subject to a similar variation. In many cases, species-related differences in metabolic patterns can be usefully exploited to test the contribution of given pathways to the toxicological potential. Toxic damage, for example, may not be reproduced in those species showing a defective activation pathway.

SITES AND MECHANISMS OF METABOLIC ACTIVATION

Sites of Metabolic Activation

Identification of the site(s) of metabolic activation is obviously most important not only for a proper understanding of the factors affecting the neurotoxic potential but also to allow the design of adequate preventive and/or therapeutic interventions.

Neurotoxicants may undergo metabolic activation at various levels in the biosphere or in the body. From a general point of view, a distinction can be made between bioactivation reactions taking place at the site of toxicity (i.e. within the nervous system), those taking place in other organs and those taking place outside the living organism. Of course, bioactivation may occur at a combination of these sites (Table 1).

Metabolism outside the nervous system is important when the toxic metabolite (i) penetrates to a significant extent the blood-brain barrier (for neurotoxic reactions in the relevant brain areas) and (ii) is sufficiently stable to reach the nervous system via the blood stream. Certain toxic metabolites are so unstable that they never leave the enzyme that catalyzes their formation. These "suicide enzyme inhibitors" may only damage the specific tissue within which they are formed. Conversely, other metabolites are sufficiently stable to leave not only the enzyme but also the cell and the organ where they are formed. For well perfused organs, equilibration processes between extracellular fluids may occur within 1-2 minutes. Therefore, any reactive metabolite formed in the liver and having a half-life longer than 1-2 minutes can be considered a long-lived metabolite in this context (Gillette, 1982).

Table 1. Sites of Metabolic Activation of Neurotoxicants

Site	Comment	Examples
Nervous System	toxicity usually limited to site of metabolism	methanol, meperidine
Liver, Kidney, Other Organs	toxic metabolites must be sufficiently stable to allow delivery to the nervous system via the circulation. Metabolizing organs may also be affected by the toxicity	isoniazid
Gut Micro-organisms	toxic metabolites must be sufficiently stable to allow delivery to the target tissue. Toxicity may affect multiple systems	cyanogenetic agents
Environment	as above	mercury

Mechanisms of Metabolic Activation

Since any type of metabolic reaction can result in activation, a detailed discussion of the mechanism involved will ultimately identify with a description of the processes of biotransformation. Although this is clearly beyond the purpose of the present article, a few relevant generalizations can be made:

(1) Active metabolites are more frequently produced by phase I reactions (oxidation, reduction, hydrolysis) than by phase II reactions (conjugations). The best documented activation pathways are those involving oxidation via the microsomal cytochrome P-450 enzyme system (mixed function oxidase). This system, which is present in both liver and extrahepatic organs, exists in different forms, each characterized by its own substrate specificities and differential response to enzyme inducers and enzyme inhibitors. For a detailed description of the role of the mixed function

oxidase in metabolic activation the reader is referred elsewhere (Schenkman and Kupfer, 1982).

(2) Conjugation reactions usually lead to detoxification. Examples include the conjugation of phenolic compounds with glucuronic acid (or sulfate) and the conjugation of electrophile reactive toxic intermediates with glutathione. Impairment of detoxification pathways, by saturation or by depletion of endogenous substrates, may play a major role in modulating the toxicological potential of active metabolites.

(3) Conjugation reactions leading to activation of a xenobiotic are less common but well documented (Caldwell, 1982). Activation by this mechanism can lead to (i) chemically stable conjugates with biological activity (e.g. morphine glucuronide, which is a potent analgesic), (ii) formation of reactive metabolites (e.g. conjugation of dihaloalkanes with glutathione resulting in the formation of compounds acting as sulfur mustards), and (iii) formation of conjugates active after further metabolism (e.g. conversion of isoniazid to N-acetylhydrazine, whose cleavage is the first step towards production of hepatotoxic metabolites).

It should be noted that while conjugation reactions usually do not cause metabolic activation *per se*, they often play a primary role in the pathogenesis of tissue damage by phase I metabolites. The binding of reactive metabolites to proteins, lipids and nucleic acids has in fact been regarded as a conjugation process. Although many of these conjugations with macromolecules occur spontaneously, some may involve enzymatic catalysis (Caldwell, 1982).

PATHOGENESIS OF TOXICITY INDUCED BY ACTIVE METABOLITES

A useful classification of the mechanisms of toxicity mediated by metabolic activation can be based on the reactivity pattern of the relevant metabolite(s).

Metabolites can induce toxic effects (i) by combining reversibly with receptor systems; (ii) by more or less specific irreversible binding to macromolecules (enzymes, lipids, nucleic acids etc.), whose altered function results in tissue damage or dysfunction; (iii) by reacting with lipids or DNA to form a stable metabolite and a chemically reactive lipid or DNA, which in turn results in toxicity; (iv) by interacting with vitally important tissue components of low molecular weight such as nucleotides; (v) by reacting with oxygen to form singlet oxygen, superoxide, hydrogen peroxide or hydroxyl free radicals which, in turn, cause toxicity; (vi) by a combination of the above mechanisms (Gillette, 1982).

Nervous system (especially CNS) toxicity caused by stable reversibly acting metabolites (mechanism i) is relatively common in clinical practice. Most adverse reactions caused by exaggeration of the normal (usually desired) pharmacological effect of biologically active metabolites are due to this mechanism. Examples include dopamine-mediated psychotic reactions in Parkinsonian patients treated with L-DOPA or the prolonged sedation induced by active metabolites of rapidly metabolized benzodiazepines (e.g. flurazepam). Of perhaps greater toxicological interest is the possibility of tissue damage by reactive, irreversibly acting metabolites (mechanisms ii-v). Much information of the mode of action of these metabolites (usually phase I intermediates) derives from studies with hepatotoxic compounds such as paracetamol, halothane and nitrofurantoin.

As outlined above, a primary mechanism of tissue damage by reactive metabolites is covalent binding with macromolecules (Trush et al., 1982). At least three major submechanisms of covalent binding have been identified (Mitchell et al., 1982): (i) alkylation of proteins and nucleic acids by electrophilic intermediates showing significant glutathione conjugation in vivo and potentiation by prior depletion of glutathione (e.g. bromobenzene, paracetamol); (ii) alkylation of proteins and nucleic acids by electrophiles not showing glutathione conjugation in vivo or potentiation by glutathione depletion (e.g. frusemide); (iii) alkylation of proteins, nucleic acids and lipids by organic free radicals, whose toxicity is little affected by glutathione or vitamin E depletion. It appears that the principal sites for covalent binding of reactive metabolites to protein are the -OH group of serine residues, the -SH of cysteine and the -NHs of histidine and lysine. C=C bonds of lipids are also likely targets for covalent binding. Chemically reactive metabolites may also cause toxicity by mechanisms in which they do not covalently bind to target macromolecules. Non-alkylating metabolites may generate oxygen intermediates causing tissue peroxidation, a mechanism which is markedly potentiated in animal models by glutathione depletion of vitamin E deficient diets. For a comprehensive discussion of the actions of chemically reactive metabolites and their relationship with tissue peroxidation the reader is referred elsewhere (Gillette, 1982; Mitchell et al., 1982).

Examples of compounds that may exert neurotoxic effects by

way of chemically reactive intermediates include organophosphorous insecticides, acrylamide and carbon disulfide. It should be noted that the biological implications of reactive metabolites may be greater in the nervous system than in other organs, for a number of reasons:

(i) On a tissue-weight basis, the energy requirements of nervous tissue are greater than those of other organs, resulting in higher vulnerability to reactive toxicants affecting energy-producing or energy-transforming pathways. Since nervous tissue is exclusively dependent on glucose as a source of ATP, inhibition of the enzymes of the glycolytic pathway may prove particularly detrimental to neuronal function and integrity;

(ii) The morphological structure of the neuronal cell (a long axon dependent on the soma for metabolic support) provides a large surface area open to toxic attack with little defense capabilities. For example, if a glycolytic enzyme along the axon is inactivated by a reactive neurotoxin, restoration of adequate energy production will be dependent on supply of newly synthetized enzyme from the distant neuronal soma. Under these conditions, the level of enzyme transport may be sufficient to meet the increased demand in the proximal segment but not in the distal part of the axon, where impaired energy production will eventually lead to degeneration. This hypothetical mechanism may explain the distal neuropathy caused by various chemically reactive neurotoxicants (Sabri and Spencer, 1980; Spencer et al., 1980; Cavanagh, 1985);

(iii) The functional integrity of the nervous system is dependent on a delicate balance between neurotransmitter's synthesis and breakdown. Molecular interactions disrupting these processes can easily result in toxicity;

(iv) the nervous tissue may be relatively inefficient in detoxifying certain reactive intermediates. It has been speculated, for example, that the neurotoxicity of acrylamide is related to inadequate detoxification of a reactive epoxide-metabolite by glutathione epoxide transferase.

FACTORS AFFECTING THE RESPONSE TO METABOLICALLY ACTIVATED NEUROTOXICANTS

A list of factors that may influence the response to metabolically activated toxicants is shown in Table 2.

The pattern of exposure (dose, continuous vs. acute exposure,

Table 2. Factors Affecting the Response to Metabolically Activated Neurotoxicants

Type of Exposure
Dose
Duration of exposure (single, multiple, chronic)
Route of administration
Degree of Metabolic Activation/Inactivation
Genetic factors (species, ethnic origin, etc.)
Physiological factors (age, diet, pregnancy, etc.)
Disease
Interactions with other xenobiotics (enzyme induction or inhibition)
Toxicant Availability at the Site of Action
Integrity of the blood-brain barrier
Cellular uptake
End Organ Responsiveness
Genetic factors
Environmental factors
Pathological factors

accumulation, etc.) is obviously a most important determinant and can be particularly critical for compounds subject to saturable detoxification mechanisms. If these require the intervention of "protective" substrates (glutathione, vitamin E, selenium, etc.), the availability of the latter may also play an important role in determining the toxicological potential. The mode of exposure (inhalation, ingestion, etc.) should also be considered since it may influence not only the degree of absorption, but also the extent and the pattern of metabolic activation by the gut microflora or first-pass metabolism in the gastrointestinal tract or the liver.

Although a discussion of the factors affecting the variation in metabolizing enzyme activities is beyond the purpose of this article, its relevance to metabolic activation is obvious. Changes in metabolic capacity due to genetic or environmental factors are a major determinant of the response to neurotoxic agents. For example, evidence has been provided that the incidence of central nervous system reactions to pethidine is increased in enzyme-induced patients, probably due to accumulation of the desmethylated neurotoxic metabolite norpethidine (Stambaugh et al., 1977).

Pharmacokinetic factors and changes in end-organ responsiveness may further complicate individual responses to a given concentration of the active metabolite. There is evidence, for example, that the developing nervous system is particularly susceptible to damage by several neurotoxicants (Suzuki, 1980). This can not always be explained by immaturity of the blood-brain barrier.

SELECTED EXAMPLES

Acrylamide

Acrylamide is an important neurotoxicant, whose best known clinical effect is a sensimotor distal neuropathy (see the chapter by Dr. Spencer in this volume). Schoental and Cavanagh (1977) suggested that acrylamide is oxidized to a chemically reactive epoxide which is dependent on glutathione epoxide transferase for detoxification. The low levels of the enzyme in the nervous tissue would result in inadequate inactivation of the epoxide, which would then react with thiol-groups (including those of coenzyme A) to form nonfunctional alkylated derivatives. This hypothesis is largely speculative. Enzyme inducers appear to decrease rather than potentiate the toxicity of acrylamide in animal models (Kaplan et al., 1973).

Spencer et al. (1980,1980a) noted that the distal axonopathy caused by acrylamide is similar to that seen with carbon disulfide and 2,5-hexanedione, and suggested that these chemically unrelated compounds may share common neurotoxic mechanisms. Indeed, acrylamide, carbon disulfide and 2,5-hexanedione have all been shown to inhibit glycolytic enzymes such as glyceraldehyde-3-phosphate dehydrogenase and phosphofructokinase. This would impair the utilization of glucose in the nerve fibre with consequent axonal degeneration.

Morphological findings in acrylamide neuropathy (Cavanagh, 1985) indicate that this agent gravely disturbs the metabolism of the whole cell. Whether the neural damage results from a general metabolic lesion or from some local defect in the axon with secondary repercussions throughout the cell remains to be clarified.

Organophosphorous Compounds

Intoxication by organophosphorous compounds may occur as a result of accidental or occupational exposure (inhalation or skin contact with insecticides, petroleum additives, plasticizers, ingestion of contaminated food, etc.). The acute toxicity consists of a cholinergic syndrome related to inhibition (phosphorylation) of acetylcholinesterase in the central and peripheral nervous system (Abou-Donia, 1985). Certain organophosphorous compounds can induce acute neurotoxic symptoms independent of acetylcholinesterase blockade (Bellet and Casida, 1973). After a single-dose absorption, many organophosphorous compounds can also cause a delayed neuropathy with symmetrical distal axonal degeneration in the central and peripheral nervous system. This neuropathy is not related to acetylcholinesterase inhibition but rather to inhibition (phosphorylation) of another esterase (neurotoxicity target esterase), as described elsewhere in this volume.

Biotransformation, usually oxidation, represents an important activation step of many organophosphorous compounds. At least three activation reactions have been identified: (i) Oxidative desulfuration of the thiophosphoryl group:

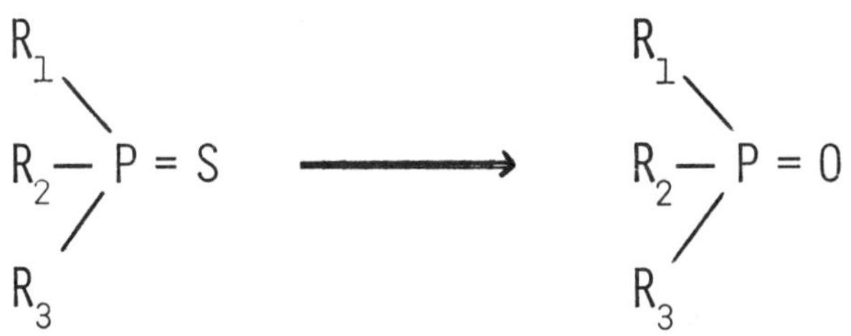

The resulting phosphoryl group increases the hydrolyzability and phosphorylating activity of the ester accounting, for example, for the delayed neurotoxicity of various phosphothionates (Johnson, 1975). (ii) Oxidation of the thioether moiety to sulfoxide and sulfone:

$$-S- \longrightarrow -SO- \longrightarrow -SO_2$$

This reaction is important in the acute toxicity of certain insecticides. (iii) Side-chain alpha-hydroxylation of triarylphosphate (Fig. 1). If the side chain is in the ortho position, the reaction results in generation of cyclic phosphate esters (A), many of which are very potent inducers of delayed neurotoxicity. If the side chain is in the meta or para position, cyclization does not occur. If the hydroxylated alpha carbon contains only one hydrogen, further

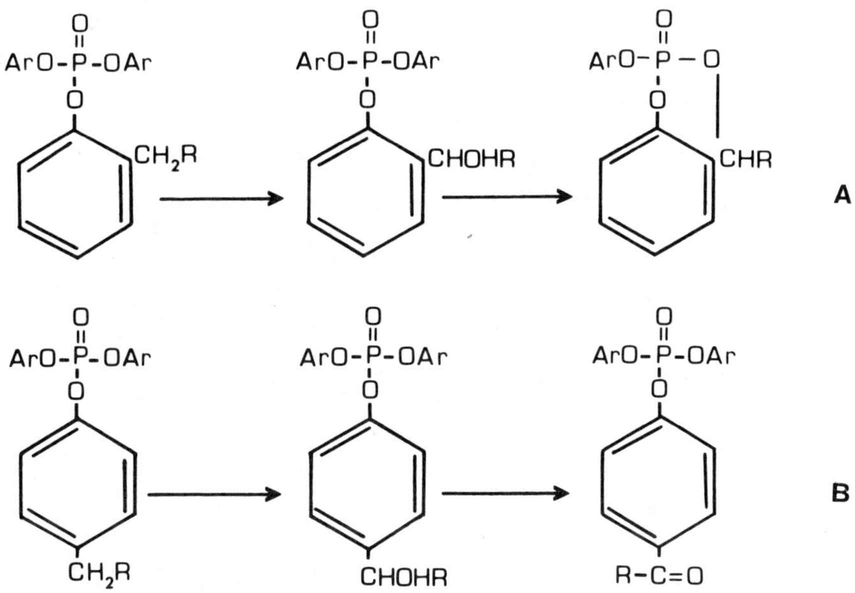

Fig. 1. Bioactivation of triarylphosphates to neurotoxic metabolites

oxidation can not take place and there is no delayed neurotoxicity. If the alpha chain has two hydrogens, further oxidation to an oxo- group occurs (B). If this group is in the <u>para</u> position, the metabolite has potent neurotoxic and phosphorylating activity even though this is generally lower than that of the cyclic esters (Johnson, 1975). If the alpha oxo- group is in the <u>meta</u> position, the neurotoxic potential is absent or low.

Detoxification of organophosphorous compounds also involves metabolic biotransformations. In general, detoxification requires cleavage of a phospho-ester bond with or without conjugation of the hydrolytic products. An important hydrolytic reaction is the oxidative dearylation catalyzed by a microsomal mixed function oxidase system distinct from that catalyzing the activating oxidative desulfuration of the thiophosphoryl group (Neal, 1967).

n-Hexane and Methyl n-Butyl Ketone (MnBK)

In 1973, an outbreak of peripheral neuropathy was noted among workers exposed to a variety of solvents in an industrial plant in Ohio. Careful investigations led to identifying MnBK as the causative agent (Allen et al., 1975). The fact that other commonly used aliphatic ketones had not been reported to be neurotoxic suggested that MnBK toxicity could be related to a metabolite rather than to the compound itself.

Two major pathways of MnBK metabolism have been identified (Di Vincenzo et al., 1977,1980): (i) -oxidation via 5-hydroxy-2--hexanone to 2,5-hexanedione (2,5-HD), and (ii) reduction to 2-hexanol, which can be further converted to MnBK itself, 2,5-HD and 2,5-hexanediol. Although many other metabolites have been identified, attention has focused on 2,5-HD because of its key role in MnBK biotransformation and because of its long serum residence time.

Subchronic peritoneal administration of 2,5-HD was found to induce in animal models a neuropathy indistinguishable from that produced by MnBK. Although other MnBK metabolites such as 5-hydroxy--2-hexanone, 2-hexanol and 2,5-hexanediol produce a similar neuropathy, they are all converted <u>in vivo</u> to 2,5-HD (Spencer et al., 1980a).

Of extreme interest is the fact that another solvent, n-hexane, is oxidized by the microsomal enzymes to 2,5-HD, MnBK itself and other MnBK metabolites. n-Hexane is widely known as a major cause of neuropathy among individuals who deliberately inhale vapours from solvents, lacquers and glue-thinners (Schaumburg, 1980). Since n-hexane neuropathy is remarkably similar to that caused by MnBK, the suggestion has been made that there may be a common metabolic basis for the toxicity of these compounds. This hypothesis has been tested by assessing the comparative neurotoxicity of MnBK, n-hexane and various common metabolites in animal models. An inverse relationship was found between peak serum 2,5-HD levels and the time required for severe neuropathy to develop, e.g. the higher level of 2,5-HD the more rapid was the development of neuropathy (Krasavage et al., 1980). The relative neurotoxicity of the compounds tested was 2,5-HD > 5-hydroxy-2-hexanone > 2,5-hexanediol > MnBK > 2-hexanol > n-hexane. These findings provide strong evidence that 2,5-HD is the active agent responsible for n-hexane and MnBK toxicity.

$CH_3CH_2CH_2CH_2CH_2CH_3$ (n-Hexane)

$CH_3COCH_2CH_2CH_2CH_2CH_3$ (Methyl n-Butyl Ketone)

$CH_3COCH_2CH_2COCH_3$ (2,5-Hexanedione)

Other gamma-diketones such as 2,5-heptanedione and 3,6-octanedione cause neuropathy (O'Donoghue and Krasavage, 1979, 1979a), while related compounds (2,4-hexanedione, 2,3-hexanedione and 2,6-heptanedione which lack the 1,4 spacing on the carboxyl groups are inactive in this respect (Spencer et al., 1980a).

Surprisingly little information is available on the effect of changes in microsomal enzyme activity in hexacarbon toxicity. It is of interest that methyl ethyl ketone (MEK), a solvent sometimes present in mixtures with MnBK and n-hexane, is itself devoid of neurotoxic activity (Spencer and Schaumburg, 1976) but accelerates the development of hexacarbon toxicity in animal models (Abdel-Rahman et al., 1976; Saida et al., 1976; Altenkirch et al., 1977). This may be related to the enzyme inducing properties of MEK (Couri et al., 1977) enhancing the formation of neurotoxic 2,5-HD. Phenobarbitone, another enzyme inducer, not only fails to potentiate MnBK and n-hexane neurotoxicity but may actually slow its onset (Spencer et al., 1980). One explanation would be that this drug not only stimulates 2,5-HD formation but also 2,5-HD detoxification via the alpha oxidative pathway. Studies are also required to clarify the relative importance of the various sites at which metabolic activation may occur. It is of interest, in this respect, that conversion of n-hexane, MnBK and various other metabolites to 2,5-HD has been observed in cultured explants of spinal cord and attached dorsal root ganglia coupled with striatal muscle (Veronesi et al., 1980).

While the role of 2,5-HD as a mediator of hexacarbon toxicity is well established, the molecular mechanism of the interaction between the toxin and its target(s) is still incompletely understood. Morphological studies of the damaged nerve fibres have documented the development of multiple proximal paranodal swellings with accumulation of neurofilaments, followed by Wallerian-like degeneration. This pattern resembles that seen in the neuropathy by acrylamide and carbon disulfide. Alike the latter compounds, 2,5-HD may irreversibly inhibit glyceraldehyde-3-phosphate dehydrogenase by reacting with amino groups of the protein (Sabri and Spencer, 1980; Spencer et al., 1980). Recently, evidence has been provided that 2,5-HD reacts with protein lysyl groups in axonal neurofilaments resulting in pyrrolic derivatization and subsequent formation of cross-linked aggregates of neurofilaments during the distal flow of axoplasm (De Caprio et al., 1982; Graham et al., 1982; Anthony et al., 1983). The growing mass of covalently cross-linked neurofilaments would then result in obstruction of axonal transport at the nodes of Ranvier of large myelinated axons, with subsequent distal degeneration (Anthony et al., 1983).

Disulfiram and Carbon Disulfide

Rainey (1977) compared the clinical, biochemical and pathological neurotoxic effects of disulfiram and found them to be strikingly similar to those of carbon disulfide. Both disulfiram and carbon disulfide induce depression, lethargy, loss of libido, psychosis, variable and fluctuating neurological signs, ataxia, incoordination and peripheral neuropathy. There is evidence that disulfiram and carbon disulfide cause neurotoxicity at least in part by a common mechanism which involves sequential biotransformation steps (Haley, 1979).

In man, disulfiram is very rapidly converted to diethyldithiocarbamate (DDC) by a reductive pathway taking place in the erythrocytes and probably also in the liver. In a subsequent step DDC, which is the predominant compound found in blood after absorption of disulfiram, is converted primarily in the liver to several metabolites, including carbon disulfide.

Following ingestion of disulfiram by alcoholics, carbon disulfide has been detected in both plasma and expired air. In some subjects, the hepatic enzymes catalyzing the conversion of DDC to carbon disulfide have high activity so that this reaction becomes the principal metabolic pathway (Brien and Loomis, 1983). Although other disulfiram metabolites, notably DDC and diethylamine, can have independent neurotoxic activity (Rainey, 1977), a comparison of the neurological and behavioral symptoms caused by disulfiram and carbon disulfide suggests that the latter compound play a key role in the pathogenetic event.

The toxicity of carbon disulfide is, at least in part, also mediated by metabolic activation (Ziegler, 1984). The metabolism takes place in two steps: oxidative desulfuration (a), followed by hydration and decomposition of the intermediate carbonyl sulfide (b).

$$\text{(a)} \quad CS_2 \xrightarrow[O_2]{\text{NADPH}} S{=}C{=}O + S$$

$$\text{(b)} \quad S{=}C{=}O + H_2O \underset{\text{carbonic anhydrase}}{\rightleftharpoons} H_2CO_2S \longrightarrow H_2S + CO_2$$

The oxidative desulfuration, catalyzed by cytochrome P-450, yeilds, in addition to carbonyl sulfide, elemental sulfur which in turn is reduced to hydrogen disulfide (H_2S) in the strong reducing environment within the cell. Additional H_2S is formed by decomposition of monothiocarbonic acid (H_2CO_2S) produced by hydration of carbonyl sulfide. Hydrogen sulfide is a well known neurotoxin and is no doubt responsible for at least part of carbon disulfide toxicity (Ziegler, 1984). Dithiocarbamates formed as metabolites of carbon disulfide may also contribute to toxicity, possibly by interfering with distribution of essential metals (see Danielsson et al., 1984 for a list of references).

Other Compounds

Many other compounds, including methanol, cyanide, cyanogenetic agents and several metals, are known to induce neurotoxic effects after bioactivation. An exhaustive review on this topic is beyond the purpose of the present article.

REFERENCES

Abdel-Rahman, M., Hetland, L., and Couri, D., 1976, Toxicity and metabolism of methyl-n-butyl ketone, Am.Ind.Hyg.Ass.J., 37:95.

Abou-Donia, M.B., 1985, Biochemical toxicology of organophosphorous compounds, in "Neurotoxicology", K. Blum and L. Manzo, eds., Dekker, New York, p.423.

Allen, N., Mendell, J.R., Billmaier, D.J., Fontaine, R.E., and O'Neill, J., 1975, Toxic polyneuropathy due to methyl n-butyl ketone, Arch.Neurol., 32:209.

Altenkirch, H., Mager, J., Stoltenburg, G., and Helmbrecht, J., 1977, Toxic polyneuropathies after sniffing a glue thinner, J. Neurol., 214:152.

Anthony, D.C., Boekelheide, K., and Graham, D.G., 1983, The effect of 3,4-dimethyl substitution on the neurotoxicity of 2,5-hexandione, Toxicol.Appl.Pharmacol., 71:362.

Bellet, E.M., and Casida, J.E., 1973, Bicyclic phosphorous esters: high toxicity without cholinesterase inhibition, Science, 182:1135.

Boyd, M.R. and Stratham, C.N., 1983, The effect of hepatic metabolism on the production and toxicity of reactive metabolites in extrahepatic organs, Drug Metab.Rev., 14:35.

Brien, J.F., and Loomis, C.W., 1983, Disposition and pharmacokinetics of disulfiram and calcium carbimide (calcium cyanamide), Drug Metab.Rev., 14:113.

Caldwell, J., 1982, Conjugation reactions in foreign-compound metabolism: definition, consequences and species variations, Drug Metab.Rev., 13:745.

Cavanagh, J.B., 1985, Peripheral nervous system toxicity: a morphological approach, in: "Neurotoxicology", K. Blum and L. Manzo, eds., Dekker, New York, p.1.

Couri, D., Hetland, L.B., Abdel-Rahman, M., and Weiss, H., 1977, The influence of inhaled ketone solvent vapors on hepatic microsomal biotransformation activities, Toxicol.Appl. Pharmacol., 41:285.

Danielsson, B.R.G., Bergman, K., and D'Argy, R., 1984, Tissue disposition of carbon disulfide. II. Whole body autoradiography of ^{35}S- and ^{14}C-labelled carbon disulfide in pregnant mice, Acta Pharmacol.Toxicol., 54:223.

De Caprio, A.P., Weber, P., and Abraham, R., 1982, Covalent binding of a neurotoxic n-hexane metabolite: conversion of primary amines to substitute pyrrole adducts by 2,5-hexandione, Toxicol.Appl.Pharmacol., 65:440.

Di Vincenzo, G.D., Hamilton, M.L., Kaplan, C.J., and Dedinas, J., 1977, Metabolic fate and disposition of ^{14}C-labelled MnBK in the rat, Toxicol.Appl.Pharmacol., 41:547.

Di Vincenzo, G.D., Hamilton, M.L., Kaplan, C.J., and Dedinas, J., 1980, Characterization of metabolites of methyl n-butyl ketone, in: "Experimental and Clinical Neurotoxicology", P.S. Spencer and H.H. Schaumburg, eds., Williams and Wilkins, Baltimore, p.846.

Gillette, J.R., 1982, The problem of chemically reactive metabolites, Drug Metab.Rev., 13:941.

Graham, D.G., Anthony, D.C., Boekelheide, K., Maschmann, N.A., Richards, R.G., Wolfram, J.W., and Shaw, B.R., 1982, Studies of the molecular pathogenesis of hexane neuropathy. II. Evidence that pyrrole derivatization of lysyl residues leads to protein cross-linking, Toxicol.Appl.Pharmacol., 64:405.

Haley, T.J., 1979, Disulfiram (tetraethylthioperoxydicarbonic diamide): a reappraisal of its toxicity and therapeutic application, Drug Metab.Rev., 9:319.

Hill, K.E., and Burk, R.F., 1984, Influence of Vitamin E and selenium on glutathione-dependent protection against microsomal lipid peroxidation, Biochem.Pharmacol., 33:1065.

Johnson, M.K., 1975, Organophosphorous esters causing delayed neurotoxic effects, Arch.Toxicol., 34:259.

Kaplan, M.L., Murphy, S.D., and Gilles, F.H., 1973, Modification of acrylamide neuropathy in rats by selected factors, Toxicol. Appl.Pharmacol., 24:564.

Krasavage, W.J., O'Donoghue, J.L., Di Vincenzo, G.D., and Terhaar, C.J., 1980, The relative neurotoxicity of methyl n-butyl ketone, n-hexane and their metabolites, Toxicol.Appl.Pharmacol., 52:433.

Mitchell, J.R., Hughes, H., Canterbury, B.H., and Smith, C.V., 1982, Chemical nature of reactive intermediates as determinants of toxicologic responses, Drug.Metab.Rev., 13:539.

Mitchell, J.R., and Jollows, D.L., 1975, Metabolic activation of drugs to toxic substances, Gastroenterology, 68:392.

Neal, R.A., 1967, Studies on the metabolism of diethyl 4-nitrophenyl phosphorothionate (parathion) in vitro, Biochem.J., 103:183.

O'Donoghue, J.L., and Krasavage, W.J., 1979, The structure-activity relationship of aliphatic diketones and their potential neurotoxicity, Toxicol.Appl.Pharmacol., 48:A55.

O'Donoghue, J.L., and Krasavage, W.J., 1979a, Hexacarbon neuropathy: a gamma-diketone neuropathy ? J.Neuropathol.exper.Neurol., 38:333.

Perucca, E., and Richens, A., 1980, The pathophysiological basis of drug toxicity, in: "Drug-Induced Toxicity", Current Topics in Pathology, Vol. 69, E. Grundmann, ed., Springer Verlag, Berlin, p. 17.

Rainey, J.M., 1977, Disulfiram toxicity and carbon disulfide poisoning, Am.J.Psychiat., 134:371.

Sabri, M.I., and Spencer, P.S., 1980, Toxic distal axonopathy: biochemical studies and hypothetical mechanisms, in: "Experimental and Clinical Neurotoxicology", P.S. Spencer and H.H. Schaumburg eds, Williams and Wilkins, Baltimore, p.206.

Saida, K., Mendell, J.R., and Weiss, H., 1976, Peripheral nerve changes induced by methyl n-butyl ketone and potentiation by methyl ethyl ketone, J.Neuropathol.exper.Neurol., 35:207.

Schaumburg, H.H., 1980, Chronic hexacarbon intoxication in man, in: "Advances in Neurotoxicology", L.Manzo, ed., Pergamon Press, Oxford, p. 187.

Schenkman, J.B., and Kupfer (eds), 1982,"Hepatic cytochrome P-450 monooxygenase system",Pergamon Press, Oxford.

Schoental, R., and Cavanagh, J.B., 1977, Mechanisms involved in the "dying-back" process - an hypothesis implicating coenzymes, Neuropathol.Appl.Neurobiol., 3:135.

Spencer, P.S., Couri, D., and Schaumburg, H.H., 1980, n-Hexane and methyl n-butyl ketone, in: "Experimental and Clinical Neurotoxicology", P.S. Spencer and H.H. Schaumburg, eds., Williams and Wilkins, Baltimore, p.456.

Spencer, P.S., Sabri, M.I., and Politis, M., 1980a, Methyl n-butyl ketone, carbon disulfide and acrylamide. Putative mechanisms of neurotoxic damage, in: "Advances in Neurotoxicology", L. Manzo, ed., Pergamon Press, Oxford, p. 173.

Spencer, P.S., and Schaumburg, H.H., 1976, Feline nervous system response to chronic intoxication with commercial grades of methyl n-butyl ketone, methyl isobutyl ketone and methyl ethyl ketone, Toxicol.Appl.Pharmacol., 37:301.

Stambaugh, J.E., Wainer, I.W., Hemphill, D.M., and Schwartz, I., 1977, A potentially toxic drug interaction between pethidine (meperidine) and phenobarbitone, Lancet, i:398.

Suzuki, K., 1980, Special vulnerabilities of the developing nervous system to toxic substances, in: "Experimental and Clinical Neurotoxicology", P.S. Spencer and H.H. Schaumburg, eds., Williams and Wilkins, Baltimore, p. 48.

Trush, M.A., Mimnaugh, E.G., and Gram, T.E., 1982, Activation of pharmacological agents to radical intermediates, Biochem. Pharmacol., 31:3335.

Veronesi, B., Peterson, E.R., and Spencer, P.S., 1980, Reproduction and analysis of methyl n-butyl ketone neuropathy in organotypic tissue culture, in: "Experimental and Clinical Neurotoxicology", P.S. Spencer and H.H. Schaumburg, eds., Williams and Wilkins, Baltimore, p.863.

Ziegler, D.M., 1984, Metabolic oxygenation of organic nitrogen and sulfur compounds, in: "Drug Metabolism and Drug Toxicity", Raven Press, New York, p.33.

MEMBRANE EFFECTS OF NEUROTOXIC CHEMICALS

Joep van den Bercken

Department of Veterinary Pharmacology, Pharmacy and Toxicology, University of Utrecht, P.O. Box 80.176
3508 TD Utrecht, The Netherlands

The most characteristic feature of the nerve membrane is its electrical excitability. The basis for excitation lies in the ionic concentration gradients across the membrane (low sodium and high potassium at the inside, high sodium and low potassium at the outside), in combination with the selective permeability characteristics of the membrane for these ions. The ion gradients which are maintained by the sodium/potassium pump, result in an electrical polarization of the nerve membrane; the potential at the inside being negative by 60-80 mV with respect to the outside. A nervous impulse is brought about by a rapid, transient increase in the permeability of the membrane for sodium, resulting in an inward sodium current, followed by an increase in the potassium permeability, resulting in an outward potassium current. As a result, the membrane potential temporarily reverses sign and an action potential is conducted along the nerve fibre.

The nerve membrane permeability changes can be studied in detail by a method called the voltage clamp technique. With this technique, which was originally developed for the giant axon of the squid, it is possible to control the voltage across the membrane and to measure the ionic currents through the membrane. The voltage clamp technique has since been adapted for other excitable tissues, e.g., single myelinated nerve fibres and, more recently, the nerve cell soma.

The changes in nerve membrane ionic permeability are mediated by discrete molecular structures, called sodium and potassium channels, respectively. These are large, integral membrane proteins imbedded in the lipid matrix of the membrane, which undergo conformational changes under the influence of the electric field across the membrane and thus become selectively permeable for either sodium or potassium. The transient opening of the sodium channel can be described by two, largely independent gating mechanisms, the activation and the inactivation gate, which are oppositely dependent on membrane potential. The opening of the potassium channel is governed by only one gating mechanism.

Numerous chemicals owe their neurotoxicity to the ability to interfere with the functioning of the ion channels in the nerve membrane. Many organic solvents, like the alcohols and other lipophilic compounds, have an anesthetic action and block both types of channels. These compounds dissolve in the lipid matrix of the membrane and hinder the conformational changes of the channel proteins. Other compounds, however, mostly of biological origin, specifically affect the sodium channels in the nerve membrane. Tetrodotoxin and the closely related saxitoxin completely block the sodium channel in a highly selective manner; one toxin molecule blocking one channel. Other neurotoxins, like batrachotoxin, grayanotoxin, aconitine and veratridine interfere with the gating mechanism of the sodium channel. They keep the sodium channel open for a much longer time than is normal or even prevent its closure. Sea anemone toxins and several scorpion toxins selectively delay the closing of the sodium channel inactivation gate. The proteolytic enzyme pronase as well as some protein reagents completely destroy sodium inactivation, indicating that the inactivation gate is a separate molecular entity.

The sodium channel is also the primary target site of the insecticide DDT. Its excitatory action is caused by intense repetitive activity, notably in the sensory nervous system. DDT selectively delays the closing of the sodium channel activation gate resulting in a marked prolongation of the sodium current during excitation. The mode of action of pyrethroid insecticides, which is treated in a separate chapter, is very similar to that of DDT and its analogs, despite marked differences in molecular structure between these two classes of insecticides.

The potassium channel is much less liable to selective pharmacological modification. Most chemicals that block the potassium channel also block the sodium channel. Only tetraethylammonium in rather high concentrations and aminopyridines, in particular 3,4 aminopyridine, selectively block the potassium channel. A few toxins, like sparteine, lupanine and a scorpion toxin, also rather selectively block the nerve membrane potassium channel.

Besides these sodium and potassium channels there are several other types of voltage-dependent ion channels, like calcium channels and calcium-dependent potassium channels. These and the neurotransmitter activated ion channels in the postsynaptic membrane fall outside the scope of the present paper.

REFERENCES

Adelman W.J. Jr. ed., 1971, "Biophysics and physiology of excitable membranes," Van Nostrand Reinhold Company, New York.

Armstrong C.M., 1975, Ionic pores, gates and gating currents, Q. Rev. Biophys., 7: 179.

Cahalan M., 1980, Molecular properties of sodium channels in excitable membranes, in, "The cell surface and neuronal function," C.W. Cotman et al. eds., Elsevier/North-Holland Biomedical Press, Amsterdam, p. 1.

Carbone E., Wanke E., Prestipino G., Possani L.D. and Maelicke A., 1982, Selective blockage of voltage-dependent potassium channels by a novel scorpion toxin, Nature, 296: 90.

Catterall W.A., 1980, Neurotoxins that act on voltage-sensitive sodium channels in excitable membranes, Ann. Rev. Pharmacol. Toxicol., 20: 15.

Hille B., 1984, "Ionic channels of excitable membranes," Sinauer Associates Inc., Sunderland, Mass., U.S.A.

Hodgkin A.L. and Huxley A.F., 1952, A quantitative description of membrane currents and its application to conduction and excitation in nerve, J. Physiol., 117: 500.

Kuffler S.W. and Nicholls J.G., 1984, "From neuron to brain," Sinauer Associates Inc., Sunderland, Mass., U.S.A.

Lazdunski M., Balerna M., Barhanin J., Chicheportiche M., Fosset M., Frelin C., Jacques Y., Pouyssegur J., Renaud J.F., Romey G., Schweitz H. and Vincent J.P., 1980, Molecular aspects of the structure and mechanism of the voltage-dependent sodium channel, Ann. N.Y. Acad. Sci., 358: 169.

Narahashi T., 1974, Chemicals as tools in the study of ecitable membranes, Physiol. Rev., 54: 813.

Noda M. et al., 1984, Primary structure of Electrophorus electricus sodium channel deduced from cDNA sequence, Nature, 312: 121.

Sakman B. and Neher E. eds., 1983, "Single channel recording," Plenum Press, New York.

Vijverberg H.P.M. and van den Bercken J., 1982, Action of pyrethroid insecticides on the vertebrate nervous system, Neuropathol. Appl. Neurobiol., 8: 421.

MODE OF ACTION OF PYRETHROID INSECTICIDES

Joep van den Bercken and Henk P.M. Vijverberg

Department of Veterinary Pharmacology, Pharmacy and Toxicology, University of Utrecht, P.O. Box 80.176
3508 TD Utrecht, The Netherlands

INTRODUCTION

The natural pyrethrins, also called pyrethrum, which are contained in the flowers of Chrysantemum cinerariaefolium, have been known for their insecticidal activity for a very long time. They have, however, never been used on large scale, because they are susceptible to rapid degradation in the environment. Around 1950 several derivatives of the pyrethrins have been synthesized, e.g. allethrin, but these compounds had little advantage over the natural product. It was not until the late 60's and early 70's that notably Elliott and coworkers in England and Fujimoto and others in Japan succeeded in synthesizing new pyrethroids, which not only are more active than the natural pyrethrins, but also are more stable under field conditions. A dramatic enhancement of insecticidal activity of the pyrethroids was achieved by the incorporation of a cyano group on the α-C atom of the 3-phenoxybenzyl alcohol moiety, as for instance in deltamethrin and cypermethrin. In recent years numerous new pyrethroids have been developed, some of which seem only remotely related to the natural compounds. Most major chemical companies are now marketing these new insecticides and their practical application is rapidly increasing. Structural formulas of pyrethrin I, the most active constituent of pyrethrum, and of some important synthetic pyrethroids are depicted in Fig. 1.

The pyrethroids combine a high insecticidal activity with a low oral toxicity to mammals and their insect to mammal toxicity ratio is much higher than for the other major classes of insecticides. They are readily metabolized and they do not accumulate in the biosphere. However, their i.v. toxicity to rodents and other mammals may approach the toxicity to insects. Symptoms of

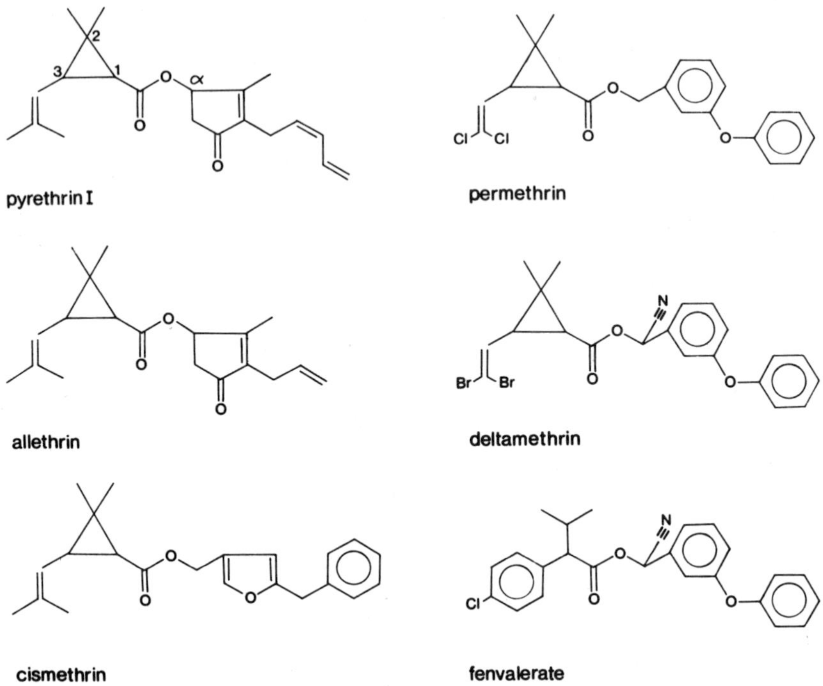

Fig. 1. Chemical structure of pyrethrin I and some important synthetic pyrethroids.

poisoning are characteristic for a strong excitatory action on the nervous system. Non-cyano pyrethroids cause hyperexcitation, tremor and convulsions. The cyano pyrethroids produce a quite different syndrome, which includes profuse salivation and choreoathetosis. It has been suggested that their mode of action differs from that of the non-cyano pyrethroids. In man occupational exposure, in particular to cyano pyrethroids may cause burning and itching sensations, especially of the facial skin, but other parts of the body which come into direct contact with pyrethroids may be affected as well. For detailed information on chemistry, insecticidal action, toxicity and practical application of pyrethroids the reader is refered to a number of recent reviews (Narahashi, 1976; Elliott, 1977; Elliott et al., 1978; Wouters and van den Bercken, 1978; Elliott and Janes, 1978; Casida, 1980; Naumann, 1981; Vijverberg and van den Bercken, 1982; Casida et al., 1983; Ruigt, 1985).

Our research of recent years has been directed toward elucidating the neurotoxic mode of action of pyrethroids down to the level of ion channels in the nerve membrane. The experiments were performed on excised preparations of the peripheral nervous system of the South African clawed frog, Xenopus laevis, using standard electrophysiological methods, including voltage clamp measurements on single myelinated nerve fibres. Pyrethroids were applied as a fine suspension in Ringer's solution at a nominal concentration of 1-20 µM. Further details on the experimental procedures can be found in the original research papers.

EFFECTS ON THE NERVOUS SYSTEM

Repetitive activity

The principal effect of pyrethroids is to induce repetitive activity in various parts of the frog peripheral nervous system, though the intensity of repetitive firing differs considerably for the various compounds, in particular between non-cyano and cyano pyrethroids.

After treatment with non-cyano pyrethroids the nerve action potential is followed by repetitive afterdischarges (Fig. 2A,B) which are usually superimposed on a depolarizing afterpotential. By using different nerve branches as well as the spinal roots it was shown that the repetitive activity induced by non-cyano pyrethroids is almost exclusively due to repetitive firing of sensory nerve fibres (van den Bercken et al., 1973; van den Bercken, 1977; Wouters et al., 1977; Vijverberg et al., 1982a). In contrast, cyano pyrethroids fail to induce repetitive activity in peripheral nerve branches. Instead, these compounds cause a progressive suppression of the action potential amplitude during train stimulation (Fig. 2C) (Vijverberg and van den Bercken, 1979; Vijverberg et al., 1982a). This was never observed after non-cyano pyrethroids under similar experimental conditions. Recordings from single myelinated nerve fibres show that this suppression is due to a gradual depolarization caused by summation of depolarizing afterpotentials following each action potential (Fig. 2D).

Non-cyano pyrethroids cause repetitive end-plate potentials at the neuromuscular junction, as illustrated in Fig. 2E,F (Evans, 1976; Wouters et al., 1977; Ruigt and van den Bercken, 1985). The multiple end-plate potentials originate from repetitive nerve impulses in the presynaptic nerve endings, whereas at the same time more proximal parts of the motor nerve do not show any sign of repetitive activity. Some cyano pyrethroids, e.g. fenpropathrin, fenvalerate and cyphenothrin, are also able to induce repetitive firing in frog motor nerve endings. In addition, some non-cyano pyrethroids and most cyano pyrethroids induce marked repetitive activity in the muscle fibre membrane (Ruigt and van den Bercken, 1985). So far we have found no evidence for a direct effect of pyrethroids on the chemical neurotransmission process in frog neuromuscular junction.

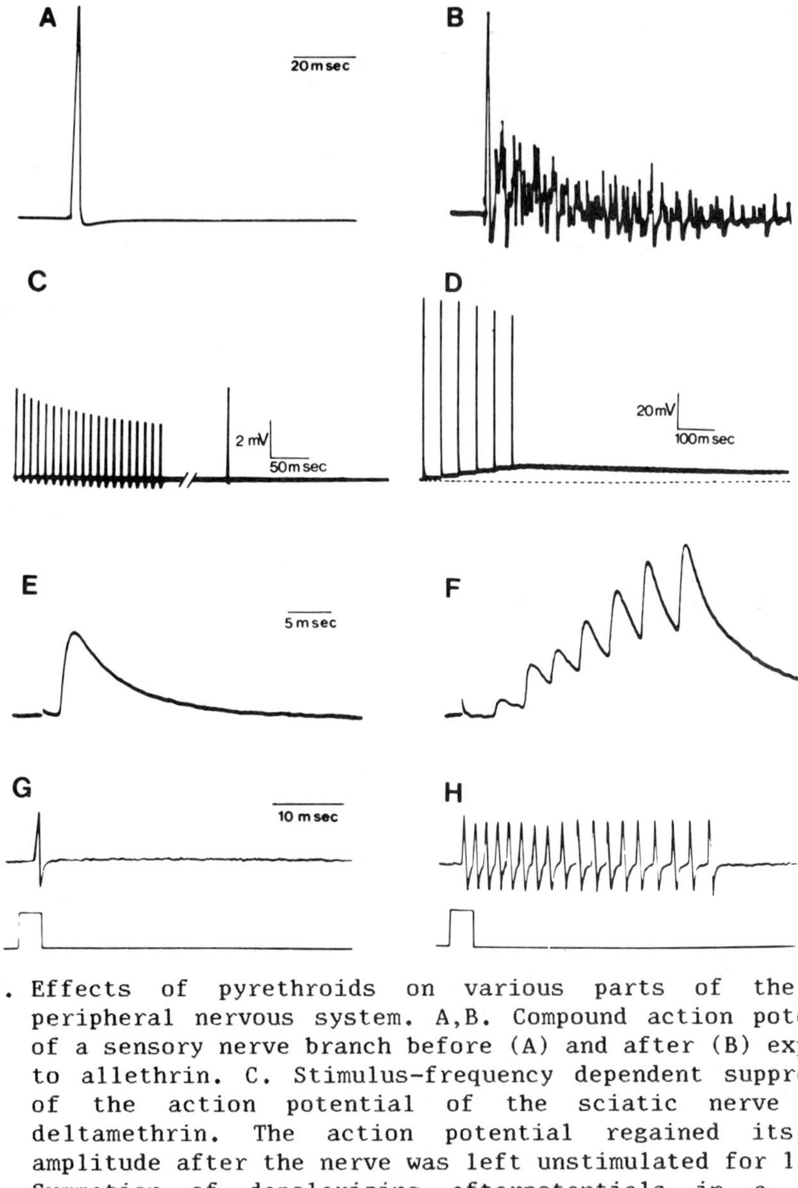

Fig. 2. Effects of pyrethroids on various parts of the frog peripheral nervous system. A,B. Compound action potential of a sensory nerve branch before (A) and after (B) exposure to allethrin. C. Stimulus-frequency dependent suppression of the action potential of the sciatic nerve after deltamethrin. The action potential regained its full amplitude after the nerve was left unstimulated for 1 s. D. Summation of depolarizing afterpotentials in a single myelinated nerve fibre treated with deltamethrin. E,F. Intracellular recorded end-plate potentials in the sartorius muscle, evoked by a single stimulus to the motor nerve before (E) and after (F) treatment with allethrin. G,H. Response of a cutaneous touch receptor to a brief mechanical stimulus before (G) and after (H) treatment with allethrin.

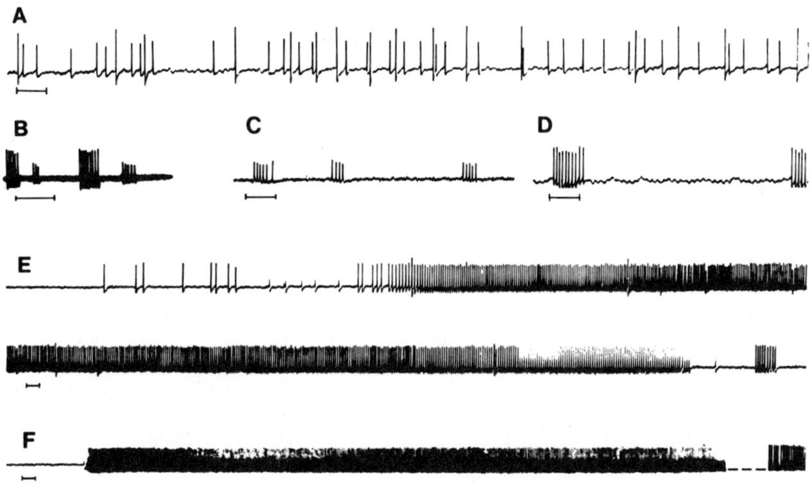

Fig. 3. Effects of various pyrethroids on the spontaneous activity of the lateral-line sense organ of Xenopus.
A. Control, B. allethrin, C. permethrin, D. cismethrin, E. cypermethrin and F. fenpropathrin. Time calibration: 100 ms/div. In (F) 8.3 s of the nerve impulse train have been omitted.

Sense organs appear to be most susceptible to the action of pyrethroids. In the cutaneous touch receptor (Fig. 2G,H) a brief, carefully adjusted mechanical stimulus evokes a single nerve impulse in one of the afferent nerve fibres. After treatment with allethrin the same stimulus invariably elicits a train of nerve impulses (Akkermans et al., 1975).

The lateral-line sense organ of Xenopus proved to be a very useful preparation to study the sensory effects of pyrethroids more quantitatively. This sense organ is located in the skin and its sensory hair cells are grouped together in so called stitches which are innervated by two afferent nerve fibres only. The lateral-line sense organ is spontaneously active and usually the two types of nerve impulses, each originating from one of the afferent nerve fibres, can be easily recognized by their difference in amplitude (Fig. 3A). The pyrethroids cause pronounced repetitive activity in the lateral-line sense organ and after treatment with the insecticides spontaneous trains of nerve impulses occur alternated by silent periods (van den Bercken et al., 1973; van den Bercken et al., 1979; van den Bercken and Vijverberg, 1980a; Vijverberg et al., 1982a).

The number of nerve impulses per train markedly varies for the different compounds and also strongly depends on temperature as described below. The non-cyano pyrethroids cause relatively short trains of nerve impulses, usually consisting of 5-15 impulses (Fig. 3B-D), whereas the cyano pyrethroids induce long-lasting impulse trains containing hundreds or even thousands of impulses (Fig. 3E,F). The results are summarized in Table 1. It is clear that there is a large difference in intensity of repetitive firing between non-cyano pyrethroids and cyano pyrethroids. Since permethrin and cypermethrin have identical chemical structures, except that cypermethrin contains a cyano group, it seems evident that this difference is solely due to the presence of the cyano group. Recently we have found that the pyrethroid fenfluthrin (NAK1901), which is an ester of permethrin acid with a pentafluorbenzyl alcohol, causes much longer impulse trains in the lateral-line sense organ than the other non-cyano pyrethroids, i.e., 100-200 impulses per train (J.R. de Weille, unpublished result). It is expected that in the future more pyrethroids will emerge that fill the gap between the non-cyano and the cyano compounds.

Effects of temperature

A very interesting characteristic of the repetitive activity induced by non-cyano as well as cyano pyrethroids in the lateral-line sense organ is its negative temperature coefficient. The number of impulses per train and train duration increase dramatically with cooling (van den Bercken et al., 1973; van den Bercken and Vijverberg, 1980a; Vijverberg et al., 1982a). This is illustrated for permethrin in Fig. 4A. This effect is readily reversed by raising the temperature and occasionally all repetitive activity disappears at temperatures above 22 ^{o}C. The relation between temperature and number of impulses per train, c.q. train duration for two non-cyano and two cyano pyrethroids is shown in

Table 1. Characteristics of repetitive activity in the lateral-line sense organ of *Xenopus* after various pyrethroids at 18 ^{o}C.

Compound	Average train duration (ms)	Number of impulses per train
allethrin	60	4 - 15
bioresmethrin	15	2 - 3
cismethrin	80	5 - 20
permethrin	40	5 - 15
cypermethrin	2000	50 - 500
deltamethrin	4500	100 - 3000
fenpropathrin	2500	50 - 2000
fenvalerate	2000	20 - 1000

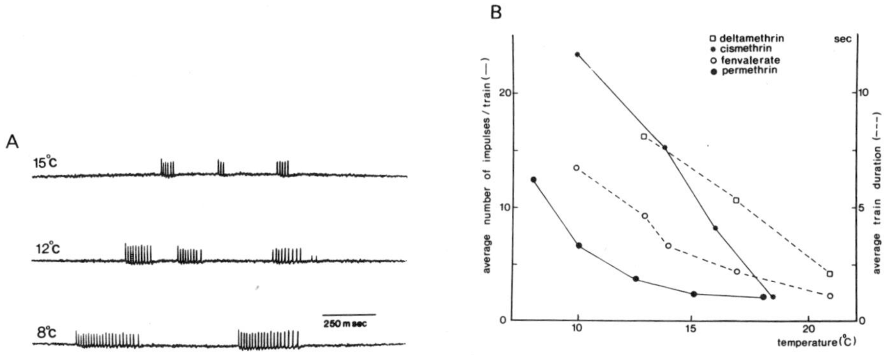

Fig. 4. Negative temperature coefficient of pyrethroid-induced repetitive activity in the lateral-line sense organ of Xenopus.
A. Repetitive activity after treatment with permethrin at the temperatures indicated.
B. Relation between temperature and average number of impulses per train (left axis) or average train duration (right axis) after treatment with four different pyrethroids.

Fig. 4B. A similar increase in repetitive activity after cooling occurs in motor nerve endings treated with allethrin (Wouters et al., 1977). In this context it is worth noting that pyrethroids also have a negative temperature coefficient of toxicity in insects (Harris and Kinoshita, 1977; Hirano 1979) and other poikilothermic animals (Mauck et al., 1976).

Effects on Na channel gating

Fig. 5A shows a typical inward Na current in an untreated myelinated nerve fibre evoked by a step depolarization under voltage clamp conditions. The Na current rapidly reaches its peak because of the fast opening of the activation gates and then gradually declines as the inactivation gates close. Na channels that are still open at the end of the depolarizing step are rapidly shut off by the closing of the activation gates.

The principal effect of pyrethroids is to cause a marked prolongation of the Na current associated with membrane depolarization (van den Bercken and Vijverberg, 1980b; Vijverberg et al., 1982b, 1983; Vijverberg and de Weille, 1985). After termination of the depolarizing pulse, when in the control situation all Na channels are closed, a large, slowly decaying Na tail current remains in pyrethroid treated nerve fibres (Fig. 5B). Low concentrations of pyrethroid do not affect the K current through the membrane. All insecticidally active pyrethroids induce similar

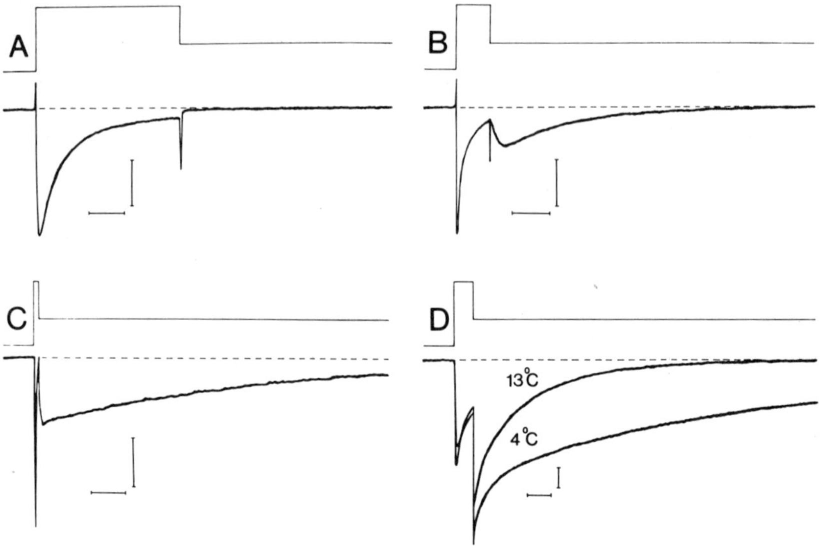

Fig. 5. Effects of pyrethroids on Na currents in myelinated nerve fibres of Xenopus. K currents are eliminated by applying tetraethylammonium chloride (TEA) and by replacing K with Cs. Na currents are elicited by a step depolarization to -5 mV from a hyperpolarized level of -125 mV (upper traces). Dashed lines indicate holding current level.
A. Control Na current. B. Na current followed by a large Na tail current after treatment with permethrin. C. Na current and a long-lasting Na tail current after fenvalerate. D. Na current and Na tail current after cismethrin at the temperatures indicated.
Calibrations: vertical 10 nA (A,B), 2 nA (C), 3 nA (D); horizontal 2 ms (A), 10 ms (B,D), 100 ms (C).

Na tail currents after depolarization, but the rate of Na tail current decay varies markedly for the different compounds. In particular the cyano pyrethroids induce long-lasting Na tail currents (Fig. 5C).

The decaying phase of the Na tail current induced by the various pyrethroids is always exponential and can be characterized by a single time constant. After cyano pyrethroids the decay is at least one order of magnitude slower than after non-cyano pyrethroids (see Table 2). The stereochemistry of the various pyrethroids tested is also depicted in Table 2. The Na tail current induced by the cis- or trans-isomer of permethrin have a different time constant. Both (R)-α-cyano isomers of fenvalerate, which are virtually devoid of insecticidal activity, fail to induce a detectable Na tail current. Hence, it appears that the interaction of pyrethroids with Na channel gating is a highly stereospecific process.

Comparison of Table 2 with Table 1 shows that there is a clear correlation between the time constant of Na tail current decay and the duration of the pyrethroid-induced nerve impulse trains in the lateral-line sense organ.

The amplitude of the Na tail current induced by the various pyrethroids is always proportional to the amplitude of the Na current during depolarization, or in other words, to the number of Na channels that have opened during depolarization. This indicates that pyrethroids preferentially interact with Na channels that are in the open configuration (Vijverberg et al., 1982b). Further, the shape of the initial part of the Na tail current strongly depends on amplitude and duration of depolarization. After short depolarizing pulses the decay of the Na tail current is always monotonic. With increasing amplitude and also with increasing duration of depolarization the Na tail current often shows a marked initial rise before it starts to decay (Fig. 6). These results are most readily explained by postulating that pyrethroids selectively delay the closing of the activation gate of a number of Na channels that open during depolarization (Vijverberg et al., 1982b, 1983).

The principal action of pyrethroids on nerve membrane Na channels is depicted in Fig. 7 which shows a simplified schematic of Na channel gating according to the classical Hodgkin-Huxley model (Hodgkin and Huxley, 1952), along with its modification by pyrethroids (Vijverberg and van den Bercken, 1982).

Table 2. Time constants of decay of Na tail current induced by various pyrethroids at 15 °C.

Compound	Stereochemistry	τ_{tail} (ms)
allethrin	1RS 3RS αRS	9.8
cismethrin	1R 3S	20.7
permethrin	1RS 3RS	17.4
cis-permethrin	1R 3S	28.5
trans-permethrin	1R 3R	6.4
cypermethrin	1R 3R αS	1020
deltamethrin	1R 3S αS	1453
S/S-fenvalerate	2S αS	602
RS/S-fenvalerate	2RS αS	545
R/R-fenvalerate	2R αR	-
RS/R-fenvalerate	2RS αR	-

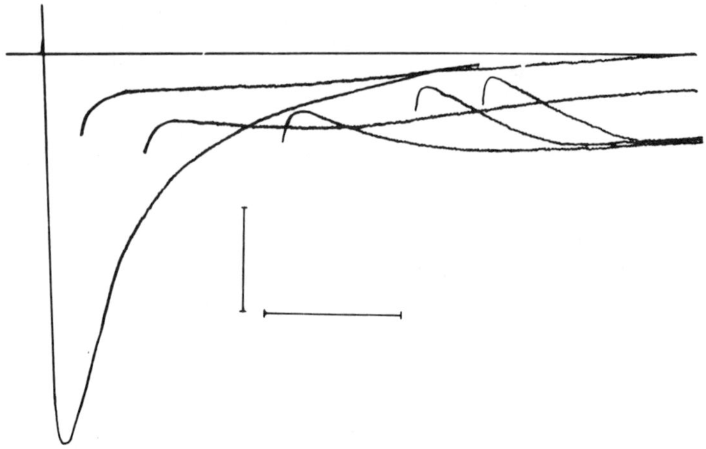

Fig. 6. Influence of duration of depolarization on the initial shape of the Na tail current in a myelinated nerve fibre treated with allethrin. Five superimposed traces of Na currents elicited by depolarizing pulses with increasing duration are shown, together with baseline level. Calibration: vertical 0.5 nA; horizontal 2 ms.

At the resting potential (-75 mV) the activation gate or m-gate is closed, while the inactivation gate or h-gate is in the open position. On depolarization, for instance to a membrane potential of -5 mV, the m-gate opens quickly and Na ions can pass through the channel. At the same time, however, the h-gate starts closing, although at a somewhat lower rate. This accounts for the gradual decline of the Na current during depolarization. On repolarization the m-gate closes quickly shutting off all Na channels which are still open at the end of the depolarizing pulse. Thereafter the h-gate returns to the open position and the resting state is restored.

The right hand panel depicts Na channel gating as modified by pyrethroids. The pyrethroid is symbolized by the arrowhead. The opening of the m-gate on depolarization is not affected by the pyrethroid. However, once the m-gate has opened it is stabilized in its open position by the pyrethroid. On repolarization, the h-gate reopens, while the m-gate remains open causing the Na channel to become conductant again, until the m-gate eventually closes.

According to this interpretation the slow decay of the Na tail current can be regarded as the relaxation of the m-gate in pyrethroid-affected Na channels (Vijverberg et al.,1982b, 1983).

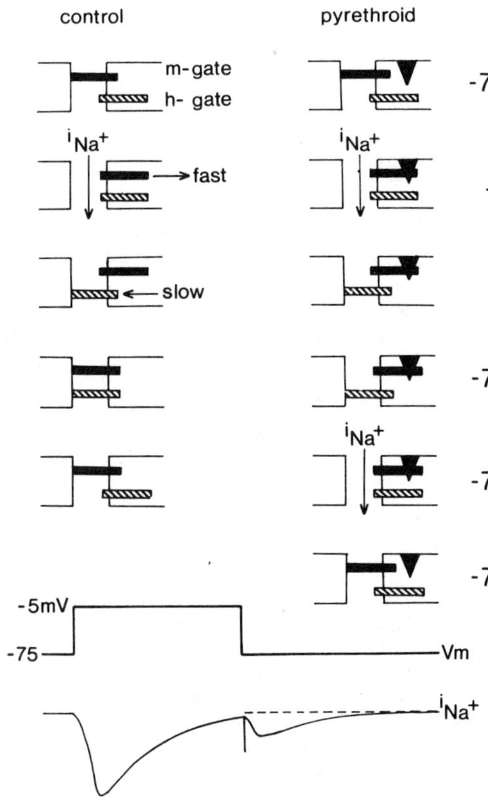

Fig. 7. Simplified schematic of Na channel gating before and after treatment with pyrethroid. The pyrethroid is symbolized by an arrowhead. Right hand figures denote membrane potential. At the bottom the membrane depolarization together with the Na current and Na tail current are also depicted. For details see text.

Since the decay of the Na tail current always follows a single exponential time course with a time constant that is independent of Na tail current amplitude, the relaxation of the m-gate in the modified Na channels is governed by an apparent first order, unimolecular process. The rate of decay of the pyrethroid-induced Na tail current is gradually and reversibly slowed when the temperature is lowered, as illustrated for cismethrin in Fig. 5D. This shows that the relaxation process is positively correlated with temperature. Between 0 ^{o}C and 25 ^{o}C the relation between the rate of Na tail current decay and temperature for the various pyrethroids is in accordance with the Arrhenius equation, i.e., the reciprocal value of the time constant of decay is linearly related to 1/T. This indicates that a single energy barrier limits the rate of relaxation of the m-gate in pyrethroid-affected Na channels. By applying the transition state theory (Eyring et al., 1980) it is possible to calculate the Gibb's free energy of activation of the relaxation process. After cyano pyrethroids the free energy of activation is 9.6 kJ/mol higher than after non-cyano pyrethroids. Apparently, the large difference in Na tail current decay between cyano and non-cyano pyrethroids is associated with a relatively small difference in the height of the energy barrier that has to be crossed for the relaxation of the activation gate in the modified Na channels.

CONCLUDING REMARKS

Our results demonstrate that all pyrethroids thus far studied have essentially the same basic mode of action. Cyano as well as non-cyano pyrethroids specifically interfere with Na channel gating in frog myelinated nerve fibres and selectively delay the closing of Na channels that open during depolarization of the membrane. This results in a marked prolongation of the Na current associated with nerve membrane excitation, which is directly responsible for the pyrethroid-induced repetitive activity. The dramatic increase of repetitive activity by cooling, as observed in the lateral-line sense organ, can be accounted for by a further prolongation of the Na tail current at lower temperatures.

In recent experiments we have found that in cultured mouse neuroblastoma cells pyrethroids also induce a marked prolongation of the Na current evoked by depolarization (Ruigt, 1984). In addition, various pyrethroids interfere with Na channel gating and induce a large, slowly declining Na tail current in nerve membrane of crayfish (Lund and Narahashi, 1981a), squid (Lund and Narahashi, 1981b; 1982) and cockroach (Laufer et al., 1984). Thus it appears that the mechanism of action of the pyrethroid insecticides is qualitatively the same throughout the animal kingdom.

There is now sound evidence that the mechanism of action of pyrethroids on nerve membrane Na channels as described here is similar to that of the classical insecticide DDT and its analogs (van den Bercken et al., 1973; 1979; Vijverberg et al., 1982b; van den Bercken and Vijverberg, 1983; Narahashi, 1983). The structural basis for this similarity is still far from understood. Holan et al. (1978; 1984), however, have succeeded in synthesizing insecticidally active compounds with a chemical structure intermediate between the pyrethroids and DDT. These new compounds also cause repetitive firing in blowfly chemoreceptor hairs.

Recently it has been reported that cypermethrin and other cyano pyrethroids, in contrast to non-cyano compounds, cause a partial, stereospecific inhibition of radioligand binding to the GABA receptor-ionophore complex in rat brain synaptic membranes (Lawrence and Casida 1983; Casida et al. 1983). Whether this effect contributes significantly to the poisoning syndrome has yet to be established.

Finally, because of the strong excitatory action of pyrethroids, especially the cyano pyrethroids, it can be expected that poisoning by these insecticides will seriously disturb the generation and processing of all nervous activity in the central as well as in the peripheral nervous system.

Acknowledgement

This work was supported by the Foundation for Medical Research FUNGO-ZWO and by Shell Internationale Research Maatschappij B.V.

REFERENCES

Akkermans L.M.A., van den Bercken J. and Versluijs-Helder M., 1975, Comparative effects of DDT, allethrin, dieldrin and aldrin-transdiol on sense organs of Xenopus laevis, Pestic. Biochem. Physiol., 5: 451.

van den Bercken J., 1977, The action of allethrin on the peripheral nervous sytem of the frog, Pestic. Sci., 8: 692.

van den Bercken J., Akkermans L.M.A. and van der Zalm J.M., 1973, DDT-like action of allethrin in the sensory nervous system of Xenopus laevis, European J. Pharmacol., 21: 95.

van den Bercken J., Kroese A.B.A. and Akkermans L.M.A., 1979, Effects of insecticides on the sensory nervous system, in: "Neurotoxicology of insecticides and pheromones," T. Narahashi ed., Plenum Press, New York, p. 183.

van den Bercken J. and Vijverberg H.P.M., 1980a, Effects of insecticides on the sensory nervous sytem of Xenopus, in: "Insect neurobiology and pestide action," Society of Chemical Industry, London, p. 391.

van den Bercken J. and Vijverberg H.P.M., 1980b, Voltage clamp studies on the effects of allethrin and DDT on the sodium channels in frog myelinated nerve membrane, in: "Insect neurobiology and pesticide action," Society of Chemical Industry, London, p. 79.

van den Bercken J. and Vijverberg H.P.M., 1983, Interaction of pyrethroids and DDT-like compounds with the sodium channels in the nerve membrane, in: "IUPAC Pesiticide chemistry: Human welfare and the environment," J. Miyamoto et al. eds., Pergamon Press, Oxford, p. 115.

Casida J.E., 1980, Pyrethrum flowers and pyrethroid insecticides, Environm. Health Persp., 34: 189.

Casida J.E., Gammon D.W., Glickman A.H. and Lawrence L.J., 1983, Mechanism of selective action of pyrethroid insecticides, Ann. Rev. Pharmac. Toxic., 23: 413.

Elliott M., 1977, "Synthetic pyrethroids," ACS symposium series, Vol. 12, American Chemical Society, Washington DC.

Elliott M. and Janes N.F., 1978, Synthetic pyrethroids - A new class of insecticide, Chem. Soc. Rev., 7: 473.

Elliott M., Janes N.F. and Potter C., 1978, The future of pyrethroids in insect control, Ann. Rev. Entomol. 23: 443.

Evans M.H., 1976, End-plate potentials in frog muscle exposed to a synthetic pyrethroid, Pestic. Biochem. Physiol., 6: 547.

Eyring H., Lin S.H. and Lin S.M., 1980, "Basic chemical kinetics," John Wiley and Sons, New York.

Harris C.R. and Kinoshita G.B., 1977, Influence of posttreatment temperature on the toxicity of pyrethroid insecticides, J. Econ. Entomol., 70: 215.

Hirano M., 1979, Influence of posttreatment temperature on the toxicity of fenvalerate, Appl. Entomol. Zool., 14: 404.

Hodgkin A.L. and Huxley A.F., 1952, A quantitative description of membrane current and its application to conduction and excitation in nerve, J. Physiol., 117: 500.

Holan G., O'Keefe D.F., Virgona C. and Walser S., 1978, Structural and biological link between pyrethroids and DDT in new insecticides, Nature, 272: 734.

Holan G., Johnson W.M.P., Rihs K. and Virgona C.T., 1984, Insecticidal isosteres of DDT-pyrethroid structures, Pestic. Sci., 15: 361.

Laufer J., Roche M., Pelhate M., Elliott M., Janes N.F. and Satelle D.B., 1984, Pyrethroid insecticides: Actions of deltamethrin and related compounds on insect axonal sodium channels, J. Insect Physiol., 30: 341.

Lawrence L.J. and Casida J.E., 1984, Stereospecific action of pyrethroid insecticides on the γ-aminobutyric acid receptor-ionophore complex, Science, 221: 1399.

Lund A.E. and Narahashi T., 1981a, Modification of sodium channel kinetics by the insecticide tetramethrin in crayfish giant axons, Neurotoxicol., 2: 213.

Lund A.E. and Narahashi T., 1981b, Kinetics of sodium channel modification by the insecticide tetramethrin in squid axon membranes, J. Pharmacol. Exp. Ther., 219: 464.

Lund A.E. and Narahashi T., 1982, Dose dependent interaction of the pyrethroid isomers with sodium channels in squid axon membranes, Neurotoxicol., 3: 11.

Mauck W.L., Olson L.E., and Marking L.L., 1976, Toxicity of natural pyrethrins and five pyrethroids to fish, *Arch. Environm. Contam. Toxicol.*, 4: 18.

Narahashi T., 1976, Nerve membrane as a target for pyrethroids, *Pestic. Sci.*, 7: 267.

Narahashi T., 1983, Nerve membrane sodium channels as the major target site of pyrethroids and DDT, *in*: "IUPAC Pesticide Chemistry: Human welfare and the environment," J. Miyamoto et al. eds., Pergamon Press, Oxford, p. 109.

Naumann K., 1981, Chemie der synthetischen Pyrethroid-Insektizide, *in*: "Chemie der Pflanzenschutz- und Schädlingsbekämpfungsmittel," Band 7, R. Wegler ed., Springer Verlag, Berlin.

Ruigt G.S.F., 1984, "An electrophysiological investigation into the mode of action of pyrethroid insecticides," Thesis, University of Utrecht.

Ruigt G.S.F., 1985, Pyrethroids, *in*: "Comprehensive insect physiology, biochemistry and pharmacology," Vol. 12, G.A. Kerkut and L.I. Gilbert eds., Pergamon Press, Oxford, in press.

Ruigt G.S.F. and van den Bercken J., 1985, Action of pyrethroids on a nerve-muscle preparation of the clawed frog *Xenopus laevis*, *Pestic. Biochem. Physiol.*, accepted.

Vijverberg H.P.M. and van den Bercken J., 1979, Frequency-dependent effects of the pyrethroid insecticide decamethrin in frog myelinated nerve fibres, *European J. Pharmacol.*, 58: 501.

Vijverberg H.P.M. and van den Bercken J., 1982, Action of pyrethroid insecticides on the vertebrate nervous system, *Neuropathol. Appl. Neurobiol.*, 8: 421.

Vijverberg H.P.M., Ruigt G.S.F. and van den Bercken J., 1982a, Structure-related effects of pyrethroid insecticides on the lateral-line sense organ and on peripheral nerves of the clawed frog, *Xenopus laevis*, *Pestic. Biochem. Physiol.*, 8: 315.

Vijverberg H.P.M. and de Weille J.R., 1985, The interaction of pyrethroids with voltage-dependent Na channels, *Neurotoxicol.*, in press.

Vijverberg H.P.M., van der Zalm J.M. and van den Bercken J., 1982b, Similar mode of action of pyrethroids and DDT on sodium channel gating in myelinated nerves, *Nature*, 295: 601.

Vijverberg H.P.M., van der Zalm J.M., van Kleef R.G.D.M. and van den Bercken J., 1983, Temperature- and structure-dependent interaction of pyrethroids with the sodium channels in frog node of Ranvier, *Biochim. Biophys. Acta*, 728: 73.

Wouters W., van den Bercken J., 1978, Review: Action of pyrethroids, *Gen. Pharmacol.*, 9: 387.

Wouters W., van den Bercken J. and van Ginneken A., 1977, Presynaptic action of the pyrethroid insecticide allethrin in the frog motor endplate, *European J. Pharmacol.*, 43: 163.

EXCITOTOXINS AND ANIMAL "MODELS" OF HUMAN DISEASE

Edith G. McGeer and Patrick L. McGeer

Kinsmen Laboratory of Neurological Research

University of British Columbia, Vancouver, Canada

INTRODUCTION

Glutamate, aspartate and a number of structurally related amino acids possess the capacity not only to excite neurons in the CNS, but also to bring about their destruction if administered at a sufficiently high concentration. The neurotoxic effects are diverse and not yet well understood. Nevertheless, they are being exploited by neuroscientists as a means of providing much new information about the operation of neuronal systems. This review will be concerned with a brief description of some of the excitatory and neurotoxic amino acids that have been investigated to date, their diverse modes of action and their use to produce some animal models of human disease.

STRUCTURES AND SUPPOSED MECHANISMS OF ACTION

The excitotoxic amino acids of particular interest are shown in Figure 1. They all have two acidic groups separated by 2-4 atoms, with 1 acidic group being part of an α-amino acid structure or its equivalent. They can be viewed as analogs of L-glutamate and L-aspartate, which are the most abundant amino acids in the CNS and are thought to be the neurotransmitters for many excitatory neuronal pathways[1]. A number of other amino acids of this general type have also been reported to be excitotoxic but the ones shown in Figure 1 are sufficient to illustrate the diverse actions of these compounds.

These compounds are found in a variety of plants or animals. Ibotenic acid is obtained from a mushroom, while KA comes from a

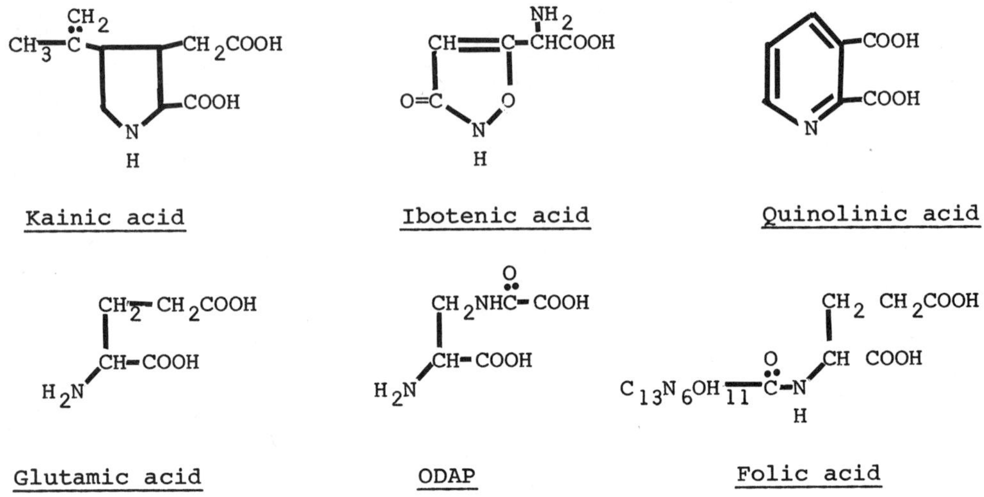

Fig. 1 Structures of some excitatory and neurotoxic amino acids.

Japanese seaweed. β-n-Oxalyl-L-α, β-diaminopropionic acid (ODAP) is found in chickling pea and may be the toxin responsible for the crippling neurodenerative illness neurolathyrism[2]. Quinolinic and folic acids are both widely found in animals as well as plants since quinolinic acid is a metabolite of the essential amino acid tryptophan and folic acid is a required vitamin. Kainic acid is the most active of these derivatives and has been by far the most widely studied. But differences in the mechanisms of action and effects achieved by the other amino acids suggests that they will also come into wide-spread use.

The excitotoxic hypothesis was first articulated by Olney and his colleagues in 1974[3]. It proposes that a depolarization mechanism underlies the neurotoxic effects. The process is initiated by activation of excitatory receptors on the dendrites and soma of cells. It is presumed that the excitotoxin, when present in high concentrations in the vicinity of suitable receptors, produces a state of pathological depolarization in which the neuronal plasma membrane permeability is increased for extended periods of time. This causes energy-dependent homeostatic mechanisms to draw heavily on the cell's energy stores in an effort to restore the ionic balance. If these energy sources become irreversibly depleted, or if the ionic exchange reaches a state where cell membrane pumps can no longer function, then cell death can be expected to occur[4]. The excitatory receptors exist at much lower concentrations, if at all, on axons and nerve endings. Excitotoxic lesions therefore spare these processes unless the cell bodies and dendrites are also within the injected area. This selective action is critical to the value of these excitotoxins as neurobiological tools.

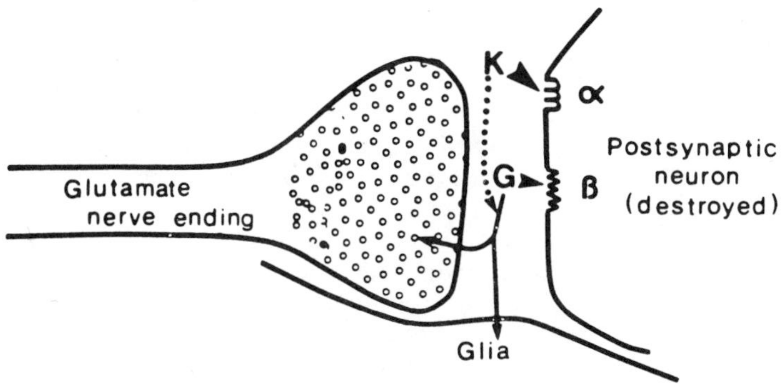

Fig. 2 Hypothesized mechanism of action of KA acid at an extrajunctional receptor (α) which sensitizes the postsynaptic neuron to the action of synaptically released glutamate (at site β). Inhibition by KA of the reuptake of glutamate (dotted line) may contribute to the effect by prolonging the action of glutamate in the synaptic cleft[5]. KA may also act presynaptically to potentiate the release of glutamate from the nerve ending[6-9].

The toxic action is very rapid[3]. Following intracerebral injection of KA or one of the other neurotoxic amino acids, evidence of damage to the dendrites and to the soma appears within a few minutes, with phagocytosis of the necrotic neuronal cell body beginning as early as 3 hours after administration of the neurotoxin. At these early stages, there are large changes in high energy phosphates and glucose metabolism which are consistent with a profound activation of affected neurons[10].

Further work has made it evident that a number of different mechanisms are involved[11-12]. At least 3, and probably more, distinct receptors exist for excitatory amino acids[1]. Kainic acid seems to act on a receptor which is distinct from, but modulatory on, the glutamate postsynaptic receptor[13], and its local neurotoxicity depends upon a cooperative reaction with neurotransmitter glutamate and thus on an intact glutamatergic afferent to the injected area (Figure 2). For example, injections of 5-10 nmoles of KA into rat neostriatum will normally cause degeneration of most neuronal cell bodies in a large portion of that nucleus. However, when the glutamatergic corticostriatal pathway has been sectioned, the neurotoxicity of KA is reduced by at least two orders of magnitude[11]. The neurotoxicity of KA is restored if glutamate is injected along with the KA[14]. Kainic acid, however, also often causes damage in areas remote from the injection site and such remote damage seems to depend upon the severe epileptiform activity which KA often induces, depending upon the conditions of injection[12,15].

Ibotenic and quinolinic acids produce local neuronal lesions with the same type of selectivity as found with KA but have little or no tendency to produce epileptiform activity and remote damage [16-19]. They clearly differ from KA also in the mechanism of local toxicity. Different cell groups in brain show markedly different sensitivities to KA and ibotenate[20]. Moreover, the α-amino-ω-phosphonocarboxylate antagonists, such as 2-amino-7-phosphonoheptanoate, block ibotenate but not KA neurotoxicity in rat hippocampus[21]. Ibotenate is far more toxic than KA in developing rat striatum or hippocampus and even dopaminergic nerve endings are markedly affected in the developing striatum[22]. Unlike KA, ibotenic acid seems to exert its local neurotoxicity by direct action on postsynaptic glutamate receptors and the effect persists even after lesioning of glutamatergic afferents.

Quinolinic acid probably acts at the subclass of excitatory receptors which are more sensitive to N-methyl-D-aspartic acid (NMDA) than to either glutamate or KA. Quinolinic acid seems to have more selective excitatory actions than glutamate or KA and pronounced regional differences have been reported for both its excitatory[23] and neurotoxic effects. Thus, quinolinic acid is effective in killing neurons of rat striatum or hippocampus, but not of several other brain regions, on local infusion[19,24,25].

Folic acid is still different in that it seems to cause little local damage but does elicit convulsions and causes remote damage[26-27]. The kind of receptor involved in the action of folic acid is not yet established.

The distant effects of KA and folic acid are largely blocked by pretreatment of the animal with large doses of an anticonvulsant such as valium[26] which does not affect the local neurotoxicity of KA, ibotenic or quinolinic acids. The distant damage presumably depends upon overexcitation of excitatory pathways but these do not appear to be necessarily neuronal tracts served by excitatory amino acid neurotransmitters. There is some evidence, for example, that overstimulation of the cholinergic neurons of the substantia innominata or pontine reticular formation by either folic acid or KA can cause extensive damage in projection areas[26,28].

MODELS OF HUMAN DISEASE

Movement Disorders

Much of the interest in excitotoxins was first stirred almost a decade ago by reports from two separate laboratories that intrastriatal injections of KA reproduced in rats the histological and chemical pathology then established for Huntington's disease (HD)[29-30].

Huntington's disease is an hereditary condition, transmitted as an autosomal dominant disease. It is world-wide in distribution having first been recognized in Scandinavia, but later described in more detail by a New York physician after whom the disease is named. It has an incidence of about 5/100,000 population in North America which makes it a relatively rare disorder. Typically, it manifests itself in the late 30's or early 40's which is just beyond the normal child bearing age. The time of onset accounts for its genetic preservation despite its devastating physical and social characteristics.

The disease is characterized by jerky, uncontrolled movements and by severe mental deterioration which progress relentlessly. Death usually occurs within 15 years of the onset of symptoms. There is no known preventive measure, nor any effective treatment. Curiously, the mental symptoms can mimic schizophrenia in the early stages, although in the later phases the severe dementia is unmistakable.

The most striking pathological changes in HD occur in the basal ganglia, particularly the caudate, where there is marked atrophy and severe loss of neurons. The putamen is also heavily involved and damage to the globus pallidus is usually prominent. Negligible histological changes are observed in the substantia nigra, although severe biochemical losses are noted. Loss of cells in the cerebral cortex, particularly the frontal cortex, is also characteristic. The histological changes seen in animals following intrastriatal injections of KA have been repeatedly found to resemble those seen in HD[31], particularly in chronic preparations [32-34]. If care is taken with the striatal injections of KA, there is little or no remote damage in the acute phase[15] but there is some scattered neuronal loss in areas such as the cortex and thalamus in chronic preparations[32-33].

A summary of the biochemical changes reported in HD and in rats given intrastriatal injections of KA is shown in Table 1. As can be seen from the table, there are marked decreases in the neostriatum in the levels of neuronal markers for acetylcholine, GABA, enkephalin, substance P and angiotensin converting enzyme. These indices are all associated with neurons originating in the basal ganglia. On the other hand, indices of dopamine, noradrenaline and serotonin, where the cell bodies exist in the substantia nigra, locus coeruleus and raphe, respectively, are unchanged or elevated. This is consistent with the lack of excitatory receptors on axons and nerve endings, and therefore the relative sparing of these neuronal processes when contacted by KA. Many different types of receptors are lost in the striatum since these presumably are located on the neurons that degenerate. In both conditions, the myelinated axons of the internal capsule are preserved.

Table 1 Biochemical Similarities Between Huntington's Disease (HD) and the Kainic Acid "Model"

Biochemical Changes	HD	KA "Model"	Refs.
In Neostriatum:			
Presynaptic GABA indices**	markedly decreased		*
γ-Hydroxybutyrate levels	increased		35,36
GABA transaminase activity	normal	decreased	*
Presynaptic ACh indices**	markedly decreased		*
Presynaptic DA indices##	normal or elevated		*
Presynaptic 5HT indices**	normal or elevated		*,37,38
Presynaptic NA indices**	normal or elevated --		*
Angiotensin converting enzyme	-- decreased --		*
Enkephalin levels	-- decreased --		*,34
TRH levels	increased	decreased	39,40
SRIF levels	increased	decreased	41
CCK levels	normal	decreased	42
Ganglioside levels	-- decreased --		43
DNA levels	-- increased --		43
Aspartate transaminase	-- decreased --		44
Ornithine δ-transaminase	-- decreased --		44,45
Binding sites ("receptors") for:			
Serotonin	-- decreased --		*,46
Dopamine	-- decreased --		*,47
Acetylcholine (muscarinic)	-- decreased --		47,48
Benzodiazepines	-- decreased --***		49.50
Kainic acid	-- decreased --		51-54
GABA	-- decreased --***		*,55
Noradrenaline (β-adrenergic)	-- normal --		56,57
CCK	-- decreased --		42
In Substantia Nigra:			
Presynaptic GABA indices**	-- decreased --		*
Substance P levels	-- decreased --		*
Presynaptic dopamine indices**	-- normal --		*
GABA binding sites	-- increased --		58,59
CCK levels	-- decreased --		42

* References in Coyle et al.[31]

**Including levels, release, turnover, activity of synthetic enzymes, and/or uptake of transmitter or (in the case of cholinergic systems) the precursor.

***At >1 month following KA injections; no decrease in acute preparations. Peripheral-type benzodiazepine binding sites are increased in both KA-lesioned striatum and HD putamen[60].

In the substantia nigra, there is a loss of neuronal markers for GABA and substance P neurons while dopamine and acetylcholine markers are normal or increased. The losses result from destruction of GABA and substance P neuronal cell bodies in the striatum that give rise to projections to the substantia nigra. In keeping with such a picture is the fact that stimulation of KA-lesioned caudates in rats causes a response in only about 58% of nigral neurons as compared to 92% in intact animals; a pure inhibitory response was decreased from 59% to about 30%[61].

Quantitative data differ somewhat from laboratory to laboratory, both in the levels seen in HD and in the KA lesions. Qualitatively, however, there would appear to be marked biochemical similarities between HD and the KA model. It must be pointed out, however, that some chemical differences between the human disease and the KA "model" appear in studies of the striatal levels of three peptide neurotransmitters: thyrotropin releasing hormone (TRH), somatostatin (SRIF) and cholecystokinin (CCK). All of these have been found decreased in the KA "model" and increased or normal in HD; the KA "model" is, of course, generally examined in an "acute" phase shortly after the injections of KA while HD is a chronic condition. The few studies on the chronic model suggest secondary changes may occur[32-34].

Pharmacological and behavioral studies have also indicated marked similarities. Following a bilateral injection of KA into the striatum, rats do not display the bizarre choreiform movements seen with HD patients. However, they do show enhanced activity at night but not during the day[62], abnormal locomotion[63], learning problems[64-65], and body weight changes[66] reminiscent of those seen in HD. Although some rats given such striatal injections of KA may also show hippocampal damage, others do not, and the behavioral impairments thought comparable to HD are attributable to the loss of striatal neurons[67].

Such rats also show a markedly enhanced response to amphetamine, scopolamine and pilocarpine but an attenuated cataleptic response to haloperidol[62,68], sedative effects with apomorphine[69] and some decrease in stereopathy with haloperidol or physostigmine[70]. These findings have all been interpreted as possibly akin to the movement and mentation disorders, as well as the pharmacological responses, seen in HD. Thus, there is a similarity in pathology, behavioral disorder and pharmacology, although the time course of neurotoxicity is different and the genetic factor is lacking.

The model is potentially useful for the pre-clinical testing of potential therapeutic agents[70-71] and has also been used to examine the viability of intracerebral grafts designed to replace destroyed neurons. Cell suspensions from fetal or neonatal rats have been injected into the KA-lesioned striata of adult hosts.

Cells survive for at least two months and form neuronal masses easily distinguished from the surrounding gliotic tissue. Clear evidence of a significant recovery of cholinergic and GABAergic indices has been reported[72], as well as histochemical and autoradiographic evidence for new vascularization, near normal glucose metabolism and possible innervation by dopaminergic afferents[73-74].

It has been proposed[12,30,75] that the mechanism of cell death in HD might be an excitotoxic one. This hypothesis does not require the formation in HD of a unique KA-like neurotoxin, and indeed there is evidence against such a possibility[76]. Rather the hypothesis suggests either excessive production of an endogenous neurotoxic amino acid or some abnormality in the postsynaptic membrane which would render the neurons more sensitive.

Candidates for excessive production are quinolinic acid[19] or glutamate itself which causes striatal cell loss in rats on chronic infusion[77]. Pyroglutamic acid has also been proposed as the endogenous neurotoxin[78] but others have had some difficulty demonstrating neurotoxic effects on intrastriatal injections[79].

If sensitivity changes in the postsynaptic membrane occur in HD, the action of glutamate from the corticostriatal glutamate pathway might be excitotoxic in HD. If such a mechanism of cell death is valid, then an obvious protective treatment might be a drug that inhibits glutamate release or blocks its postsynaptic action. It is on the basis of this hypothesis that clinical trials are presently underway with baclofen (p-chlorophenylGABA) which is reported to inhibit glutamate release[80-81] and to have a very minor protective action against KA-induced damage[82-83]. In a short-term trial of baclofen in HD, no positive results were obtained[84] but, on the postulated mechanism, an agent which inhibited glutamate release could at best slow progression of the disease and could not be expected to affect established symptomatology. Similar reasoning might suggest chronic treatment with naloxone[85-86], hypotaurine or taurine[87] which have all been found to inhibit slightly the neurotoxicity of KA. In the future, better inhibitors of glutamate release or of its postsynaptic action might be found and these would deserve evaluation as inhibitors of the progressive deterioration in HD. The great hope in HD now, however, is that the defective gene and its translation product will soon be identified[88]; it would not be surprising if this gene had something to do with the excitatory amino acid neuronal systems.

A limited number of reports on excitotoxic "models" of other movement disorders have appeared. Hemiballismus and spasmodic torticollis (head tilt), resembling those seen in the human conditions, have been produced in monkeys by KA injections into, respectively, the subthalamus[89] and the interstitial nucleus of Cajal[90]. In each of these cases, the movement disorder was attributed to the local neurotoxic damage elicited by the KA. On the

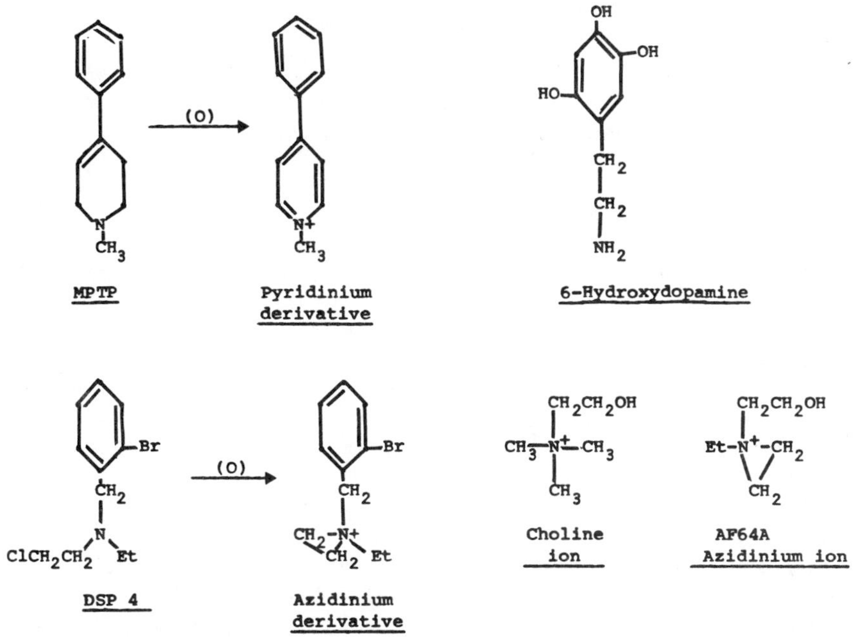

Fig. 3. Structures of some neurotoxins whose selectivity is determined by selective uptake into neurons rather than, as in the case of excitotoxins, selective action at postsynaptic receptors.

other hand, a possible model of Parkinson's disease has been suggested involving the distant effects of KA or folic acid. Injection of either into the pedunculopontine formation of the brain stem resulted in distant damage to the dopaminergic neurons of the substantia nigra[28,91]; loss of these dopaminergic neurons is the hallmark of Parkinson's disease. Interest in this "model" is small, however, compared with the intense interest generated by discovery that peripheral administration of a very small amount of N-methyl-4-phenyl-1,2,3,6-tetrahydropyridine (MPTP) leads to a very selective and drastic loss of these dopamine neurons with production of a severe form of Parkinson's disease[92]. The exact nature and mechanism of action of the active neurotoxic derivative of MPTP is not known but it is probably taken up by the dopamine neurons because of its structural similarity and oxidized to a pyridinium derivative which is toxic to the neurons. Related azidinium derivatives (Figure 3) have been reported to be selectively toxic to noradrenaline and cholinergic neurons; their mode of action is unknown but they are not excitotoxins. Their toxic selectivity, like that of the well known 6-hydroxydopamine, is dependent on neuronal uptake mmechanisms rather than on the types of receptors on the neuron.

Senile Dementia of the Alzheimer Type (SDAT)

SDAT is now recognized as the most common cause of mental deterioration in the elderly. It involves a progressive deterioration of cognitive functions and can occur as early as the third decade, but the incidence increases markedly with age. It is now well established that SDAT cases consistently show marked losses of indices of cholinergic neuronal activity in the hippocampus and some cortical areas[93]. This seems to be due largely, if not entirely, to a loss of the cholinergic neurons of the substantia innominata/diagonal band complex which provides most of the cholinergic innervation to these forebrain regions[94-95]. The cholinergic loss has been connected with the memory deficits characteristic of SDAT[93]. No treatment is presently available for SDAT, and establishment of an animal model would be a major step in facilitating drug screening. Injections of KA after valium pretreatment[26] or of ibotenate into the substantia innominata (nucleus basalis of Meynert) cause local destruction of cholinergic neurons and large drops of indices of cholinergic activity in forebrain regions. Sowewhat surprisingly, ibotenate-lesioned animals seem to show recovery of cortical cholinergic activity with time[96]. Lesioned rats do show significantly impaired retention of shock avoidance performance[97].

A major problem, however, is that the injections are also toxic to non-cholinergic neurons in the area which are not lost in SDAT; these include, for example, local GABAergic neurons[26]. For this reason, more attention is presently being given to the azidinium choline derivatives, such as AF64A (Figure 3), which have been reported to cause loss of cortical and hippocampal cholinergic indices after intracerebroventricular injection[98-99]. Unfortunately, these studies did not include measurement of indices of other neurotransmitter systems so that selectivity was not established. After direct injections into the striatum, AF64A causes large decreases in local cholinergic indices with much less or no change in GABAergic, catecholaminergic and serotonergic indices[100]; the cholinergic cells do not, however, appear to be destroyed[101]. Some selectivity vis-a-vis noradrenaline and serotonin systems has also been reported after intrahippocampal injections[102]. In our hands, injections into the substantia innominata are not a satisfactory way to destroy selectively cholinergic innervation of the cortex; there is extensive histological damage at the injection site and local GABAergic neurons are almost as much affected as the cholinergic system. Levy et al.[103] also report extensive local histological damage and depletion of dopamine after injections into the substantia nigra.

The problem of producing a "model" for SDAT is further complicated by the indications that some other neuronal systems are also affected in the human disease - notably cortical somatostatin neurons and noradrenergic neurons of the locus coeruleus. Studies of animals in which the noradrenergic system has been selectively destroyed by 6-hydroxydopamine or DSP-4 (Figure 3) suggest that such destruction does not affect either memory (as measured by retention of a passive avoidance task) or the enhancement of such memory produced by the cholinomimetic oxotremorine[104]. The effects on memory of selective losses of somatostatin activity, which might be temporarily produced by treatment with cysteamine [105-106] have not been assessed.

Epilepsy

Excitotoxic agents in many circumstances induce various types of epileptic phenomena. This is seen both after systemic and intracerebral injections. It is logical therefore that they should be considered as a means for producing animal models of epilepsy, particularly status epilepticus. Status epilepticus describes a situation where a continuous seizure, or a series of intermittent seizures, extends for over a period of at least an hour without restoration of normal brain function. Both EEG and pathological studies indicate that limbic structures, notably the hippocampus and amygdala, occupy a central position in human temporal lobe epilepsy. At autopsy, humans with such epilepsy show nerve cell loss and gliosis, primarily in specific sites of the limbic system such as the hippocampal formation. Systemic injections of KA in adult rats reproduce this condition with an amazingly broad range of electrographic, clinical, metabolic and histopathologic correlates (for review see 107). Ben-Ari et al.[108-109] found that KA, at a dose of 0.4-1.6 μg injected directly into the amygdaloid nucleus unilaterally, will produce the same effect. With either systemic or intracerebral injection, the EEG epileptoform activity starts in limbic structures. There are behavioral seizures characterized by chewing, "wet dog" shakes, rearing, fore limb clonus and generalized clonic and tonic seizures. These behaviors are dose-dependent and can progress over time (within 3 hrs) to status epilepticus. Termination of the episode, and thus prevention of death, can be brought about by intraperitoneal doses of 20 mg/kg of valium (diazepam). After intra-amygdaloid injections, neuronal lesions occur, as expected, in the amygdala but they also extend to the hippocampus, particularly to the highly vulnerable CA_3 field. This secondary brain hippocampal damage is highly similar to that observed following systemic administration of KA to rats[110-111] or status epilepticus in man[112]. Similar seizure activity and pathological consequences are also seen in baboons given amygdala or temporal pole injections[113]. Pretreatment with valium before intracerebral KA injections into the amygdala in rats reduces the hippocampal and other distant damage, as well as the seizure phenomena, without reducing the toxic effects of the agent at the site of injection[109].

Intrahippocampal injections in both cats[114] and rats[115] result in the long-term in spontaneous recurrent seizures, a finding which further strengthens the clinical relevance of the model, since spontaneity is a characteristic of human epilepsy. This long-term effect seems to depend upon amygdala involvement since prior lesioning of the amygdala increases markedly the acute effects of intrahippocampal injections of KA but delays the recurrent seizures[116]. The importance of the amygdala in the KA epileptic phenomena is further indicated by the finding that very young rats do not show seizures in response to systemic KA[117] and that the appearance of the seizure syndrome correlates with the appearance of KA binding sites in the amygdala but not in the hippocampus[118].

The neuronal circuitry involved in the production of these limbic seizures has not been completely worked out. Many neurotransmitters may be involved. Markedly increased turnover of noradrenaline, dopamine and serotonin seems to occur after seizure-inducing injections of KA[119] and there may well be similarly increased activity of many other, so far unstudied, neurotransmitter systems. Metabolic studies, using the 2-deoxyglucose technique, have demonstrated an increased glucose utilization in the hippocampus, subiculum, pyriform and entorhinal cortices, septum and amygdala associated with KA-induced limbic convulsions[120-121]. These are the areas which are sensitive to distant toxic effects, supporting the hypothesis that the distant damage involves trans-synaptic effects secondary to the hyperactivation of excitatory systems[122].

It may be relevant that these areas are all associated with the substantia innominata/diagonal band forebrain cholinergic system. A role for this cholinergic system in the mechanism of epileptic spread was suggested by Kimura et al.[123]. They reported that amygdaloid kindling, a form of epilepsy induced by frequent, pathological electrical stimulation of the amygdala, is enhanced by the acetylcholinesterase inhibitor, DFP, and reduced by atropine (an acetylcholine blocker). This implies that the spontaneous seizure activity induced by kindling is mediated, at least in part, by a cholinergic system. Animals with lesions of the nucleus of the diagonal band of Broca, the medial septal area, the interpeduncular nucleus and the habenula all could be successfully kindled. However, animals with lesions to the substantia innominata could not be kindled. The substantia innominata contains the largest collection of cholinergic cell bodies in the brain and is the main source of afferents to the neocortex, as well as to the amygdala[94]. There is evidence of reciprocal, though non-cholinergic, connections from the amygdala to the substantia innominata and these may be involved in amygdaloid kindling.

Injections of either KA or folic acid into the substantia

innominata also cause convulsions in rats and distant damage to neurons in the pyriform and other cortices, amygdala and thalamus; some of the neurons destroyed are GABA neurons. Unlike KA, folic acid causes little local damage in the injected substantia innominata. The distant damage can be blocked almost completely by prior administration of valium. Distant damage in all areas except the thalamus is markedly reduced by prior administration of scopolamine, a cholinergic antagonist, which is consistent with the hypothesis that excitation of the cholinergic system is largely responsible for the effects noted. Injections of folic acid into the substantia innominata cause more convulsive activity and far more distant damage than similar injections into either the amygdala or striatum, again emphasizing the probable importance of this widespread cholinergic system in convulsive phenomena[26]. The distant damage again conforms to that observed in the autopsied brains of human epileptics.

These results have led to a reconsideration of older literature in which folic acid was described as having epileptogenic activity in rats[124], enhancing kindling[125] and being elevated in brain during maximum seizure susceptibility following barbiturate withdrawal[126]. The possible relationship of folic acid to human epilepsy was first raised when it was realized that prolonged treatment with diphenylhydantoin lowered serum folate levels[127-128]. While epileptic activity was not exacerbated in most patients by replacement therapy[128-130], in some patients it clearly had such an effect[131-133]. Brennan et al.[134] found CSF folate levels significantly raised (by 3-fold) following grand mal seizures in untreated patients and suggested that folates released from nerve endings might interact with receptors to play a role in the spread of seizures. The suggestion has also been put forward on the basis of experiments in rats that, if the blood-brain barrier is breached in epilepsy, then folic acid could concentrate in the epileptic focus itself.[135] Tremblay et al.[136], however, found that on intra-amygdaloid injection folic acid was much less able than KA to induce limbic seizures or hippocampal damage.

There is continued, intense interest in the study of these neurotoxin-induced "models" as a means of identifying the mechanism and improving the pharmacology of human epilepsy, particularly temporal lobe epilepsy.

Interstitial Myocardial Necrosis

Rats injected bilaterally with 2-3 nmol of KA into the thalamus almost invariably show hematuria, elevated blood fibrinogen levels, and acute myocardial necrosis. The type of cardiac damage differs markedly from that observed after myocardial infarction where there is necrosis of all tissues beyond the thrombosed vessels. Instead, the changes are those of focal myocardial cell injury where the integrity of large vessels is unaffected and where the damage does not follow the perfusion bed of any particular vessel. Cells are often damaged even though they are close to vessels whose integrity is intact. This type of focal myocardial necrosis is seen in humans and animals following strokes, subarachnoid hemorrhage or traumatic brain damage. It has also been noted following extremely stressful conditions[137]. It is not readily detected clinically, but is often detected at autopsy and may be a far more important contributing factor to cardiac failure, and even to the long term consequences of a classical myocardial infarction, than is commonly recognized. Such cardiac damage has been produced erratically after repetitive electrical stimulation of certain brain regions, but KA has the advantage of being rapid and highly reproducible. Thus, it forms a model for investigation of this interesting phenomenon which may have important clinical implications. The hematuria appears to come from tissue destruction in the bladder. Although cases showing gross hematuria all display myocardial damage, the reverse is not true. In contrast to thalamic injections of KA, focal myocardial necrosis is not detected following electrolytic lesions of the thalamus or injections of KA into the cerebellum, cortex or periphery, even when the doses are 10 mg/kg subcutaneously or 5 mg/kg intraperitoneally.

It cannot be said with certainty whether the myocardial damage is humoral, neurogenic or both. However, the most likely hypothesis on the basis of current evidence is that circulating catecholamines play an important part. Urinary levels of catecholamines increase 2-10 fold following thalamic injections and the cardiac effects are partially blocked by pretreatment with reserpine or 6-hydroxydopamine[137]; no treatment was found which entirely blocks the effect.

Chelly et al.[138] found that L-glutamate (10^{-5}-10^{-7} mol/kg) or KA (10^{-8}-10^{-10} mol/kg), injected into the cisterna magna of dogs, produced a dose-dependent increase in blood pressure and slowing of the heart rate. Intravenous injections of larger doses were ineffective. This again suggests the possibility that excitation of CNS structures can produce effects in the cardiovascular system.

Hypothalamic-Pituitary Disturbances

In infant animals the arcuate nucleus seems particularly sensitive to the neurotoxic effects of systemically administered excitotoxins. Animals treated in this fashion may be extremely useful in studying possible mechanisms underlying various hypothalamic-pituitary disturbances in man[139]. For example, in mice treated in infancy with either single or multiple subcutaneous injections of glutamate, Olney[140] described an obesity syndrome in which treated animals, initially lower in body weight, surpassed the weight of littermate controls at about 45 days of age and thereafter continued to amass considerable carcass fat at a slow but steady pace through adulthood. Despite this, the treated animals were slightly hypophagic compared to controls. All workers who have attempted to measure food intake in glutamate-treated obese animals have reported them to be either hypophagic or normophagic but never hyperphagic. Thus, the glutamate-obese mouse may be a promising model for studying human obesity.

Cameron and his colleagues[141] have employed the glutamate-obese mouse as a model for studying mechanisms of carbohydrate disturbance in diabetes. Such mice are insulin-sensitive, hyperinsulinemic and mildly hypoglycemic on fasting. In KK mice, an inbred strain with a high genetic susceptibility to diabetes, the disease was unmasked by a glutamate challenge in infancy. Such mice became markedly obese and developed hyperglycemia accompanied by gross hyperinsulinemia, implying a state of insulin resistance. Food restriction restored glucose levels to normal. Cameron et al. considered the hyperglycemia and hyperinsulinemia to be a direct result of the hypothalamic abnormality in this diabetes-prone strain and suggested that further study of this model might shed light on the role of the hypothalamus in obesity and diabetes

SUMMARY

The use of excitotoxic amino acids has already produced interesting animal "models" which may be useful in exploring diseases as diverse as Huntington's, Parkinsonism, torticollis, senile dementia, epilepsy, myocardial necrosis and hypothalamic-pituitary disturbances. Many other possibilities exist. As the range of excitotoxic amino acids with different properties is extended, their application to producing modes of human disease states should also expand.

REFERENCES

1. P.L. McGeer and E.G. McGeer, Amino acid neurotransmitters, in: "Basic Neurochemistry", G.J. Siegel, A.W. Albers, B.W. Agranoff and R. Katzman, eds., Little Brown & Co., Boston, pp. 233-254, 1981.
2. J.W. Olney, C.K. Misra and V. Rhee, Brain and retinal damage from lathyrus excitotoxin, β-N-oxalyl-L-α,β-diaminopropionic acid, Nature 264:659 (1976).
3. J.W. Olney, Neurotoxicity of excitatory amino acids, in: "Kainic Acid as a Tool in Neurobiology", E.G. McGeer, J.W. Olney and P.L. McGeer, eds., Raven Press, New York, pp. 95-122, 1978.
4. I.R. Duce, P.L. Donaldson and P.N.R. Usherwood, Investigations into the mechanism of excitant amino acid cytotoxicity using a well-characterized glutamatergic system, Brain Res. 263:77 (1983).

5. P.L. McGeer, E.G. McGeer and T. Hattori, Kainic acid as a tool in neurobiology, in: "Kainic Acid as a Tool in Neurobiology", E.G. McGeer, J.W. Olney and P.L. McGeer, eds., Raven Press, New York, pp. 123-138, 1978.
6. G.G.S. Collins, J. Anson and L. Surtees, Presynaptic kainate and N-methyl-D-aspartate receptors regulate excitatory amino acid release in the olfactory cortex, Brain Res. 265:157 (1983).
7. J.W. Ferkany and J.T. Coyle, Kainic acid selectively stimulates the release of endogenous excitatory acidic amino acids, J. Pharmacol. Exp. Ther. 225:399 (1983).
8. J.W. Ferkany, R. Zaczek and J.T. Coyle, The mechanism of kainic acid neurotoxicity, Nature 308:561 (1984).
9. S.J. Potashner and D. Gerard, Kainate-enhanced release of D-[3H]aspartate from cerebral cortex and striatum: reversal by baclofen and pentobarbital, J. Neurochem. 40:1548 (1983)).
10. K.C. Retz and J.T. Coyle, Kainic acid lesion of mouse striatum: effects on energy metabolites, Life Sci. 27:2495 (1982
11. E.G. McGeer, P.L. McGeer and K. Singh, Kainic acid-induced degeneration of neostriatal neurons: dependency upon corticostriatal tract, Brain Res. 139:381 (1978).
12. P.L. McGeer and E.G. McGeer, Kainate as a selective lesioning agent, in: "Glutamate: Transmitter in the Central Nervous System", P.J. Roberts, J. Storm-Mathisen and G.A.R. Johnston, eds., John Wiley & Sons Ltd., London, pp. 55-75 (1981).
13. K. Fuxe, L.F. Agnati and F. Celani, Evidence for interactions between [3H]glutamate and [3H]kainic acid binding sites in rat striatal membranes. Possible relevance for kainic acid neurotoxicity, Neurosci. Lett. 35:233 (1983).
14. K. Biziere and J.T. Coyle, Influence of cortico-striatal afferents on striatal kainic acid neurotoxicity, Neurosci. Lett. 8:303 (1981).
15. E.G. McGeer and P.L. McGeer, Some factors influencing the neurotoxicity of intrastriatal injections of kainic acid, Neurochem. Res. 3:501 (1978).
16. W.O. Guldin and H.J. Markowitsch, No detectable remote lesions following massive intrastriatal injections of ibotenic acid, Brain Res. 225:446 (1981).
17. R. Schwarcz, T. Hokfelt, K. Fuxe, G. Jonsson, M. Goldstein and L. Terenius, Ibotenic acid-induced neuronal degeneration: A morphological and neurochemical study, Exp. Brain Res. 37:199 (1979).
18. R. Schwarcz, C. Kohler, K. Fuxe, T. Hokfelt and M. Goldstein, On the mechanism of selective neuronal degeneration in the rat brain: studies with ibotenic acid, in: "Advances in Neurology", Vol. 23, T.N. Chase, N.S. Wexler and A. Barbeau, eds., Raven Press, New York, pp. 655-668, 1979.
19. R.C. Schwarcz, W.O. Whetsell Jr and R.M. Mangano, Quinolinic acid: an endogenous metabolite that produces axon-sparing

lesions in rat brain, Science 219:316 (1983).
20. C. Kohler and R. Schwarcz, Comparison of ibotenate and kainate neurotoxicity in rat brain: a histological study, Neuroscience 8:819 (1983).
21. R. Schwarcz, J.F. Collins and D.A. Parks, α-Amino-ω-phosphono carboxylates block ibotenate but not kainate neurotoxicity in rat hippocampus, Neurosci. Lett. 33:85 (1982).
22. H.X. Steiner, G.J. McBean, C. Kohler, P.J. Roberts and R. Schwarcz, Ibotenate-induced neuronal degeneration in immature rat brain, Brain Res. 307:117 (1984).
23. M.N. Perkins and T.W. Stone, Quinolinic acid: regional variations in neuronal sensitivity, Brain Res. 259:172 (1983).
24. R. Schwarcz and C. Kohler, Differential vulnerability of central neurons of the rat to quinolinic acid, Neurosci. Lett. 38: 85 (1983).
25. R. Schwarcz, G.S. Brush, A.C. Foster and E.D. French, Seizure activity and lesions after iontrahippocampal quinolinic acid injection, Exp. Neurol. 84:1 (1984).
26. P.L. McGeer, E.G. McGeer and T. Nagai, GABAergic and cholinergic indices in various regions of rat brain after intracerebral injections of folic acid, Brain Res. 260:107 (1983).
27. J.W. Olney, T.A. Fuller, T. de Gubareff and J. Labruyere, Intrastriatal folic acid mimics the distant but not the local brain damage properties of kainic acid, Neurosci. Lett. 25:185 (1981).
28. E.G. McGeer and P.L. McGeer, Substantia nigra cell death from kainic acid or folic acid injections into the pontine tegmentum, Brain Res. 298:339 (1984).
29. J.T. Coyle and R. Schwarcz, Lesion of striatal neurons with kainic acid provides a model for Huntington's Chorea, Nature 263:244 (1976).
30. E.G. McGeer and P.L. McGeer, Duplication of biochemical changes of Huntington's chorea by intrastriatal injections of glutamic and kainic acids, Nature 263:517 (1976).
31. J.T. Coyle, E.G. McGeer, P.L. McGeer and R. Schwarcz, Neostriatal injections: a model for Huntington's chorea, in: "Kainic Acid as a Tool in Neurobiology", E.G. McGeer, J.W. Olney and P.L. McGeer, eds., Raven Press, New York, pp. 139-160, 1978.
32. E. Krammer, Anterograde and transynaptic degeneration 'en cascade' in basal ganglia induced by intrastriatal injection of kainic acid: an animal analogue of Huntington's disease, Brain Res. 196:209 (1980).
33. E.G. McGeer, P.L. McGeer, T. Hattori and S.R. Vincent, Kainic acid neurotoxicity and Huntington's disease, Adv. Neurol. 23:577 (1979).
34. R. Schwarcz, K. Fuxe, T. Hokfelt, L. Terenius and M. Goldstein, Effects of chronic striatal kainate lesions on some dopaminergic parameter and enkephalin immunoreactive neurons in the basal ganglia, J. Neurochem. 34:772 (1979).

35. N. Ando, B.I. Gold, E.D. Bird and R.H. Roth, Regional brain levels of γ-hydroxybutyrate in Huntington's disease, J Neurochem. 32: 617 (1979).
36. N. Ando, J.R. Simon and R.H. Roth, Inverse relationship between GABA and γ-hydroxybutyrate levels in striatum of rats injected with kainic acid, J. Neurochem. 32:623 (1979).
37. L.M. Neckers, N.H. Neff and R.J. Wyatt, Increased serotonin turnover in corpus striatum following an injection of kainic acid: evidence for neuronal feedback regulation of synthesis, Naunyn-Schmied. Arch. Pharmacol. 306:173 (1979).
38. G. Sperk, M. Berger, H. Hortnagl and O. Hornykiewicz, Kainic acid-induced changes of serotonin and dopamine metabolism in the striatum and substantia nigra of the rat, Eur. J. Pharmacol. 74:279 (1981).
39. E.R. Spindel, R.J. Wurtman and E.D. Bird, Increased TRH content of the basal ganglia in Huntington's disease, N. Engl. J. Med. 303:1235 (1980).
40. E.R. Spindel, D.J. Pettibone and R.J. Wurtman, Thyrotropin-releasing hormone (TRH) content of rat striatum: modification by drugs and lesions, Brain Res. 216:323 (1981).
41. G.D. Burd, P.E. Marshall, M.F. Beal, D.M.D. Landis and J.B. Martin, Effects of kainic and ibotenic acid on the neostriatal somatostatin system of the rat. Neurosci. Absts. 12:140 (1982).
42. D.C. Emson, J.F. Rehfeld, H. Langvin and M. Rossor, Reduction in cholecystokinin-like immunoreactivity in the basal ganglia in Huntington's disease, Brain Res. 198:497 (1980).
43. M.R. Higatsberger, G. Sperk, H. Bernheimer, K.S. Shannak and O. Hornykiewicz, Striatal ganglioside levels in the rat following kainic acid lesions comparison with Huntington'd disease, Exp. Brain Res. 44:93 (1981).
44. P.-T. Wong, E.G. McGeer and P.L. McGeer, Effects of kainic acid injection and cortical lesion on ornithine and aspartate transaminases in rat striatum, J. Neurosci. Res. 8: 643 (1982).
45. P.-T. Wong, P.L. McGeer, M. Rossor and E.G. McGeer, Ornithine aminotransferase in Huntington's disease, Brain Res. 231: 466 (1982).
46. G. Fillion, D. Beaudoin, J.C. Rousselle, J.M. Deniau, M.P. Fillion, F. Dray and J. Jacob, Decrease of [^{3}H]-5-HT high affinity binding and 5-HT adenylate cyclase activation after kainic acid lesion in rat brain striatum, J. Neurochem. 33:567 (1979).
47. J.Z. Fields, T.D. Reisine and H.I. Yamamura, Loss of striatal dopaminergic receptors after intrastriatal kainic acid, Life Sci. 23:569 (1978).
48. R.S. Briggs, P. Redgrave and S.R. Nahorski, Effect of kainic acid lesions on muscarinic agonist receptor subtypes in rat striatum, Brain Res. 206:451 (1981).
49. H. Mohler and T. Okada, The benzodiazepine receptor in normal

and pathological human brain, Br. J. Psychiatr. 133:261 (1978).
50. G. Sperk and E. Schlogl, Reduction of number of benzodiazepine binding sites in the caudate nucleus of the rat after kainic acid injections, Brain Res. 170:563 (1979).
51. K. Beaumont, Y. Maurin, T.D. Reisine, J.Z. Fields, E. Spokes, E.D. Bird and H.I. Yamamura, Huntington's disease and its animal model. Alterations in kainic acid binding, Life Sci. 24: 809 (1979).
52. H. Henke, Kainic acid binding in human caudate nucleus; effect of Huntington's disease, Neurosci. Lett. 14:47 (1979).
53. E.D. London, H.I. Yamamura, E.D. Bird and J.T. Coyle, Decreased receptor-binding sites for kainic acid in brains of patients with Huntington's disease, Biol. Psychiatry 16: 155 (1981).
54. S.R. Vincent and E.G. McGeer, Kainic acid binding to membranes of striatal neurons, Life Sci. 24:265 (1979).
55. R. Zaczek, R. Schwarcz and J.T. Coyle, Long-term sequelea of striatal kainate lesion, Brain Res. 152:626 (1978).
56. S.J. Enna, E.D. Bird, J.P. Bennett, D.B. Bylund, H.I. Yamamura, L.L. Iversen and S. Snyder, Huntington's chorea: changes in neurotransmitter receptors in the brain, N. Engl. J. Med. 294:1305 (1976).
57. N.R. Zahniser, K.P. Minneman and P.B. Molinoff, Persistence of β- adrenergic receptors in rat striatum following kainic acid administration, Brain Res. 178:589 (1979).
58. A.J. Cross and J.L. Waddington, Substantia nigra γ-aminobutyric acid receptors in Huntington's disease, J. Neurochem. 37:321 (1981).
59. J.L. Waddington and A.J. Cross, The striatonigral GABA pathway: functional and neurochemical characteristics in rats with unilateral striatal kainic acid lesions, Eur. J. Pharmacol. 67:27 (1980).
60. H. Schoemaker, M. Morelli, P. Deshmukh and H.I. Yamamura, [3H]Ro5-4864 benzodiazepine binding in the kainate lesioned striatum and Huntington's diseased basal ganglia, Brain Res. 248:396 (1982).
61. S. Nakamura, K. Iwatsubo, C.T. Tsai and K. Iwama, Neuronal activity of the substantia nigra (pars compacta) after injection of kainic acid int the caudate nucleus, Exp. Neurol. 66:682 (1979).
62. H.C. Fibiger, Kainic acid lesions of the striatum: a pharmacological and behavioral model of Huntington's disease, in "Kainic Acid as a Tool In Neurobiology", E.G. McGeer, J.W. Olney and P.L. McGeer, eds., Raven Press, New York, pp. 161-176 (1978).
63. R.E. Hruska and E.K. Silbergeld, Abnormal locomotion in rats after bilateral intrastriatal injection of kainic acid, Life Sci. 25:181 (1979).
64. I. Divac, H.J. Markowitsch and M. Pritzel, Behavioral and

anatomical consequences of small intrastriatal injections of kainic acid in the rat, Brain Res. 151:523 (1978).
65. P.R. Sanberg, J. Lehmann and H.C. Fibiger, Impaired learning and memory after kainic acid lesions of the striatum: a behavioral model of Huntington's disease, Brain Res. 149: 546 (1978).
66. P. Sanberg and H.C. Fibiger, Body weight, feeding and drinking behaviors in rats with kainic acid-induced lesions of striatal neurons - with a note on body weight symptomatology in Huntington's disease, Exp. Neurol. 66:444 (1979).
67. M. Pisa, P.R. Sanberg and H.C. Fibiger, Locomotor activity, exploration and spatial alternations learning in rats with striatal injections of kainic acid, Physiol. Behav. 24:11 (1980).
68. P.R. Sanberg, M. Pisa and H.C. Fibiger, Kainic acid injections in the striatum alter the cataleptic and locomotor effects of drugs influencing dopaminergic and cholinergic systems. Eur. J. Pharmacol. 74:347 (1981).
69. P.R. Sanberg, J. Lehmann and H.C. Fibiger, Sedative effects of apomorphine in an animal model of Huntington's disease, Arch. Neurol. 36:349 (1979).
70. R.L. Borison and B.I. Diamond, Kainic acid model predicts therapeutic agents in Huntington's disease, Trans. Am. Neurol. Assoc., 104:67 (1979).
71. R.T. Owen, Intrastriatal kainic acid - a possible model for antidyskinetic/antichoreic agents? Methods Exp. Clin. Pharmacol. 2:133 (1980).
72. R.H. Schmidt, A. Bjorklund and U. Steveni, Intracerebral grafting of dissociated CNS tissue suspensions: a new approach for neuronal transplantation to deep brain sites, Brain Res. 218:347 (1981).
73. H. Kimura, P.L. McGeer, Y. Noda and E.G. McGeer, Brain transplants in an animal "model" of Huntington's disease, Neurosci. Abstrs. 6:235 (1980).
74. P.L. McGeer, H. Kimura and E.G. McGeer, Transplantation of newborn brain tissue into adult kainic acid lesioned neostriatum, in: "Neural Transplants", J.R. Sladek Jr. and D.M. Gash, eds., Plenum Press, N.Y., pp. 361-371, 1984.
75. J.W. Olney and T. de Gubareff, Glutamate neurotoxicity and Huntington's disease, Nature 271: 557 (1978).
76. B.A. Beutler, A.B.C. Noronha, M.M. Poon and B.G.W. Arnason, The absence of unique kainic acid-like molecules in urine, serum, and CSF from Huntington's disease patients, J. Neurol. Sci. 5:355 (1981).
77. G.J. McBean and P.J. Roberts, Chronic infusion of L-glutamate causes neurotoxicity in rat striatum, Brain Res. 290:372 (1984).
78. G.K. Rieke, A.D. Scarfe and J.F. Hunter, L-Pyroglutamic acid: A neurotoxic imino acid that produces a drug induced model of Huntington's disease and with a potential role in the

etiology of Huntington's disease, Neurosci. Abs. 9:269 (1983).

79. E.G. McGeer and E. Singh, Neurotoxic effects of endogenous materials: quinolinic acid, L-pyroglutamic acid and thyroid releasing hormone (TRH), Exp. Neurol. in press.

80. S. Fox, K. Krnjevic, M.E. Morris, E. Puil and R. Werman, Action of baclofen on mammalian synaptic transmission, Neuroscience 3:495 (1978).

81. S.J. Potashner, Baclofen effects on amino acid release and metabolism in slices of guinea pig cerebral cortex, J. Neurochem. 32:103 (1979).

82. J.M. Liebman, G. Pastor, P.S. Bernard and J.K. Saelens, Antagonism of intrastriatal and intravenous kainic acid by various anticonvulsants and GABAmimetics, Life Sci. 27:1991 (1980).

83. E.G. McGeer, A. Jakubovic and E.A. Singh, Ethanol, baclofen and kainic acid neurotoxicity, Exp. Neurol. 69:359 (1980).

84. A. Barbeau, GABA and Huntington's chorea. Lancet 2:1499 (1979).

85. T.A. Fuller and J.W. Olney, Effects of morphine or naloxone on kainic acid neurotoxicity, Life Sci. 24:1793 (1979).

86. E.G. McGeer, P.L. McGeer and S.R. Vincent, Morphine, naloxone and kainic acid neurotoxicity, Res. Commun. Chem. Path. Pharmac. 25:411 (1979).

87. P.R. Sanberg, W. Staines and E.G. McGeer, Chronic taurine effects on various neurochemical indices in control and kainic acid-lesioned neostriatum, Brain Res. 161:367 (1979).

88. J.F. Gusella, N.S. Wexler, P.M. Conneally, S.L. Naylor, M.A. Anderson, R.E. Tanzi, P.C. Watkins, K. Ottina, M.R. Wallace and A.Y. Sayaguchi, A polymorphic DNA marker genetically linked to Huntington's disease, Nature 306:234 (1983).

89. C. Hammond, J. Feger, B. Bioulac and J.P. Souteyrand, Experimental hemiballism in the monkey produced by unilateral kainic acid lesion in corpus Luysii, Brain Res. 171:577 (1979).

90. F. Malouin and P.J. Bedard, Frontal torticollis (head tilt) induced by electrolytic lesion and kainic acid injection in monkeys and cats, Exp. Neurol. 78:551 (1982).

91. G. Ricciardi, C. Forchetti, A. Gasbarri, E. Scarnati and C. Pacitti, Neuroexcitatory properties of kainic acid. II) Neuronal damages following intracerebral microinjections in behavioral rats, Boll. Soc. Ital. Biol. Sper. 57:919 (1981).

92. R. Lewin, Trail of ironies to Parkinson's disease, Science 224:1083 (1984).

93. J.T. Coyle, D.L. Priceand M.R. DeLong, Alzheimer's disease: a disorder of cortical cholinergic innervation, Science 219:1184 (1983).

94. P.L. McGeer, E.G. McGeer and J.H. Peng, Choline acetyltransferase: purification and immunohistochemical localization, Life Sci. 34:2319 (1984).

95. P.L. McGeer, E.G. McGeer, J. Suzuki, C.E. Dolman and T. Nagai,

Aging, Alzheimer's disease, and the cholinergic system of the basal forebrain, Neurology 34:741 (1984).
96. G.L. Wenk and D.S. Olton, Recovery of neocortical choline acetyltransferase activity following ibotenic acid injection into the nucleus basalis of Meynert in rats, Brain Res. 293:184 (1984).
97. H.J. Altman, R.D. Crosland, D.J. Jenden and R.F. Berman, Impairment of memory following destruction of the major cholinergic projection to the neocortex, Brain Res., in press.
98. A. Fisher and I. Hanin, Choline analogs as potential tools in developing selective animal models of central cholinergic hypofunction, Life Sci. 27:1615 (1980).
99. C.R. Mantioni, A. Fisher and I. Hanin, The AF64A-treated mouse: possible model for central cholinergic hypofunction. Science 213:579 (1981).
100. I. Hanin, W.C. DeGroat, C.R. Mantione, J.T. Coyle and A. Fisher, Chemically-induced cholinotoxicity in vivo: studies utilizing ethylcholine aziridinium ion (AF64A), in: "Banbury Report 15: Biological Aspects of Alzheimer's Disease", Cold Spring Harbor Laboratory, 1983.
101. K. Sandberg, I. Hanin, A. Fisher and J.T. Coyle, Selective cholinergic neurotoxin: AF64A's effects in rat striatum, Brain Res. 293:49 (1984).
102. C.R. Mantioni, M.J. Zigmond, A. Fisher and I. Hanin, Selective presynaptic cholinergic neurotoxicity following intrahippocampal AF64A injection in rats, J. Neurochem. 41:251 (1983).
103. A. Levy, G.J. Kant, J.L. Meyerhoff and L.E. Jarrard, Non-cholinergic neurotoxic effects of AF64A in the substantia nigra, Brain Res.: 305:169 (1984).
104. I.B. Introini, C.M. Baratti and P. Huygens, Selective brain noradrenaline depletion induced by the neurotoxin N-(2-chloroethyl)-N-ethyl-2-bromo- benzylamine (DSP 4) does not prevent the memory facilitation induced by a muscarinic agonist in mice, Psychopharmacology (Berlin) 82:107 (1984).
105. M. Palkovits, M.J. Brownstein, L.E. Eiden, M.C. Beinfeld, J. Russell, A. Arimura and S. Szabo, Selective depletion of somatostatin in rat brain by cysteamine, Brain Res. 240:178 (1982).
106. S.M. Sagar, D. Landry, W.J. Millard, T.M. Badger, M.A. Arnold and J.A. Martin, Depletion of somatostatin-like immunoreactivity in the rat central nervous system by cysteamine, J. Neurosci. 2:225 (1982).
107. J.V. Nadler, Kainic acid as a tool for the study of temporal lobe epilepsy, Life Sci. 29:2031 (1981).
108. Y. Ben-Ari, J. Lagowska, E. Tremblay and G. Le Gal La Salle, A new model of focal status epilepticus: intra-amygdaloid application of kainic acid elicits repetitive secondarily generalized convulsive seizures, Brain Res. 163:176 (1979).

109. Y. Ben-Ari, E. Tremblay, O.P. Ottersen and R. Naquet, Evidence suggesting secondary epileptogenic lesions after kainic acid: pretreatment with diazepam reduces distant but not local brain damage, Brain Res. 165:362 (1979).
110. D.B. Clifford, E.W. Lothman, W.E. Dodson and J.A. Ferendelli, Effect of anticonvulsant drugs on kainic acid-induced epileptiform activity, Exp. Neurol. 76: 156 (1982).
111. E.W. Lothman, R.C. Collins and J.A. Ferrendell, Kainic acid-induced limbic seizures: electrophysiological studies, Neurology 31:806 (1981).
112. W. Blackwood and J.A.N. Corsellis eds., "Greenfield's Neuropathology", Arnold, London, 1976.
113. C. Menini, B.S. Meldrum, D. Riche, C. Silva-Comte and J.M. Stutzmann, Sustained limbic seizures induced by intraamygdaloid kainic acid in the baboon: Symptomatology and neuropathological consequences, Ann. Neurol. 8:501 (1980).
114. T. Tanaka, M. Kaijima, G. Daita, S. Ohgami, Y. Yonemasu and D. Riche, Electroclinical features of kainic acid-induced status epilepticus in freely moving cats. Microinjection into the dorsal hippocampus, EEG Clin. Neurophysiol. 54: 288 (1982).
115. E.A. Cavalheiro, D.A. Riche and G. Le Gal La Salle, Long-term effects of intrahippocampal kainic acid injection in rats: a method for inducing spontaneous recurrent seizures, EEG Clin Neurophysiol. 53:581 (1982).
116. E.A. Cavalheiro, L.S. Calderasso Filho, D. Riche, S. Feldblum and G. Le Gal La Salle, Amygdaloid lesion increases the toxicity of intrahippocampal kainic acid injection and reduces the late occurrence of spontaneous recurrent seizures in rats, Brain Res. 262:201 (1982).
117. E. Cherubini, M.R. De Feo, O. Mecarelli and G.F. Ricci, Behavioral and electrographic patterns induced by systemic administration of kainic acid in developing rats, Dev. Brain Res. 9:69 (1983).
118. Y. Ben-Ari, E. Tremblay, M. Berger and L. Nitecka, Kainic acid seizure syndrome and binding sites in developing rats, Dev. Brain Res. 14:284 (1984).
119. G. Sperk, H. Lassman, H. Baran, S.J. Kish, F. Seitelberger and O. Hornykiewicz, Kainic acid induced seizures: neurochemical and histopathological changes, Neuroscience 10: 1301 (1983).
120. Y. Ben-Ari, E. Tremblay, D. Riche, G. Ghilini and R. Naquet, Electrographic, clinical and pathological alterations following systemic administration of kainic acid, bicuculline or pentetrazole: metabolic mapping using the deoxyglucose method with special reference to the pathology of epilepsy, Neuroscience 7:1361 (1981).
121. E.W. Lothman and R.C. Collins, Kainic acid induced limbic seizures: metabolic, behavioral, electrographic and neuropathologic correlates, Brain Res. 218:299 (1981).

122. E.C. Tremblay, O.P. Ottersen, C. Rovira and Y. Ben-Ari, Intra-amygdaloid injections of kainic acid: regional metabolic changes and their relation to the pathological alterations, Neuroscience 8:299 (1983).

123. H. Kimura, A. Kaneko and J.A. Wada, Catecholamine and cholinergic systems and amygdaloid kindling, in: "Kindling", vol. 2, J.A. Wada, ed., Raven Press, New York, pp. 265-287, 1981.

124. O.R. Hommes and E.A.M.T. Obbens, The epileptogenic action of sodium folate in the rat, J. Neurol. Sci. 16:271 (1972).

125. D. Goff, A.A. Miller and R.A. Webster, Anticonvulsant drugs and folic acid on the development of epileptic kindling in rats. Brit. J. Pharmacol. 64:406P (1978).

126. S. Cooke and J. Crossland, Effect of short- and long-term administration of some anticonvulsant drugs on the folate content of rat brain, Brit. J. Pharmacol. 64:407P (1978).

127. R.L. Blakely, "The Biochemistry of Folic Acid and Related Pteridines", (Frontiers of Biology, Vol. 13), Amsterdam, North-Holland Publishing Co, 1969.

128. P.F.M. Houben, O.R. Hommes and P.J.H. Knaven, Anti-convulsant drug an folic acid in young mentally retarded epileptic patients. A study of serum folate, fit frequency and I.Q., Epilepsia (Amst.) 12:235 (1971).

129. O.N. Jensen and O.V. Olesen, Folic acid and anti-convulsive drugs, Arch. Neurol. Psychiat. (Chic.) 21:208 (1969).

130. A.J. Ralston, R.P. Snaith and J.B. Hinley, Effects of folic acid on fit frequency and behaviour in epileptics on anti-convulsants, Lancet 1970i:867.

131. E.M. Baylis, J.M. Crowley, J.M. Preece, P.E. Sylvester and V. Marks, Influence of folic acid on blood-phenytoin levels, Lancet 1:62 (1971).

132. I. Chanarin, J. Laidlaw, L.W. Loughridge and D.L. Mollin, Megaloblastic anaemia due to phenobarbitone. The convulsant action to therapeutic doses of folic acid, Brit. med. J. 1:1099 (1960).

133. E.H. Reynolds, I. Chanarin and D.M. Matthews, Neuropsychiatric aspect of anticonvulsant megaloblastic anemia, Lancet 1968i:394.

134. M.J.W. Brennan, J. Costa, P. Ruff and P. Sutej, Elevation of CSF folate levels following grand mal seizures in untreated patients. Neurosci. Absts. 12:139 (1982).

135. A. Mayersdorf, R.R. Streiff, B.J. Wilder and R.H. Hammer, Folic acid and vitamin B_{12} alterations in primary and secondary epileptic foci induced by metallic cobalt powder, Neurology 21:418 (1971).

136. E.C. Tremblay, E. Cavalheiro and Y. Ben-Ari, Are convulsant and toxic properties of folates of the kainate type? Eur. J. Pharmacol. 93:283 (1983).

137. W.J. Boyko, C.K. Galabru, E.G. McGeer and P.L. McGeer, Thalamic injections of kainic acid produce myocardial

necrosis, Life Sci. 25:87 (1979).

138. J. Chelly, J.C. Kouyoumdjian, P. Mouille, A.M, Huchet and H. Schmitt, Effects of L-glutamic acid and kainic acid on central α-cardiovascular control, Eur. J. Pharmacol. 60:91 (1979).

139. J.W. Olney and M.T. Price, Excitotoxic amino acids as neuroendocrine probes, in: "Kainic Acid as a Tool in Neurobiology", E.G. McGeer, J.W. Olney and P.L. McGeer, eds., Raven Press, New York, pp. 239-264, 1978.

140. J.W Olney, Brain lesions, obesity and other disturbances in mice treated with monosodium glutamate, Science 164:719 (1969).

141. D.P. Cameron, T.K.-Y. Poon and G.C. Smith, Effects of monosodium glutamate administration in the neonatal period on the diabetic syndrome in KK mice, Diabetologia 12:621 (1976).

RETINOTOXIC AGENTS AND ITS PATHOGENESIS

W. Meier-Ruge

Department of Neuropathology
Institut of Pathology, University of Basle
CH-4056 - Basle, Switzerland

The pathogenesis of toxic lesions of the retina

Toxic agents display a remarkable predilection for the retina. This becomes particularly evident when the retina is compared with the brain or the other chief metabolic organs, which normally do not display concomitant toxic changes. This peculiar vulnerability of the retina is explicable on considering its special anatomy and physiology (93, 95).

The most important parts of the retina are:

the visual cells,
the pigmented epithelium and
the choriocapillaris.

The retina is supplied by two vascular systems:

1. The inner layers of the retina receive blood from the central retinal artery. This part of the retina, the cerebral part, is characterized by capillaries presenting a blood-retina barrier.

2. The visual cells and the pigmented epithelium receive oxygen and nutrients from the choroidal vessels, via the choriocapillaris. The occurrence of localized drug-induced injuries in the pigmented epithelium and/or the visual cells is explained by the fact that more than 80% of the total retinal blood flow passes through the melanin-bearing choroid (41, 42, 52) in which

drugs may be accumulated on the melanin (68, 76, 83, 89, 94, 109, 111). Furthermore, the choroidal capillaries, like those in the anterior lobe of the pituitary gland, do not possess a blood-tissue barrier.

It was shown by Potts[109] in 1962 that many compounds are accumulated in the uvea, but only few are toxic to the retina. From later work (39, 69, 83, 90, 94) we know that the preconditions for toxic damage confined to the retina are:

a) the accumulation (adsorption) of the drug on the melanin of the uvea

b) the melanin content of the choroid

c) the toxic properties of the drug, together with

d) the dosage and duration of drug administration.

The general clinical picture

A toxic retinopathy is characterized by:

- a maculopathy of symmetrical pattern (92) pigmentary changes in the fundus (27, 89, 93) or patchy exudative foci, and

- facultative temporary progression (66, 81).

Symmetry of the retinal lesions is a distinctive funduscopic finding. This symmetry results from the pathogenetic process giving rise to the toxic retinal lesion (93, 95). Toxic retinopathy occurs when the toxic compound has been presented for a sufficient time at a sufficiently high level in the blood of the choroidal capillaries. The concentration of the compound will always be higher in the choroidal capillaries than in the systemic circulation. This difference is due to the steady state of melanin adsorption of the toxic compound (e.g. chloroquine, phenothiazine, etc.). Since the melanin content of the choroid is the same in both eyes, the toxic levels attained and the subsequent deterioration in the metabolism of the pigmented epithelium and/or visual cells will therefore always be the same in both eyes. Conversely, the blood level of the drug in the vessels of the central retinal artery, which supplies the cerebral part of the retina (inner retinal layers), will be low, because it is the same as in the rest of the brain.

Retinal pigmentation may develop by the following mechanisms (27, 90, 91):

1. A primary lesion of the pigmented epithelium with narrowing of the visual field (e.g. chloroquine retinopathy) (86, 87, 152).

2. Increased shedding or disruption of peripheral segments of rods, and overloading of the capacity of the pigmented epithelium to break down sudanophilic, light-absorbing material which thus accumulates in the pigmented epithelium (27, 77, 90, 93). In the acute phase of retinopathy the fundus may also be pigmented by disintegrated light-absorbing rod material which has not yet been phagocytosed by the pigmented epithelium (77, 90).

3. Diffuse pigmentation of the macula results from a lipofuscinosis of the optic nerve cells, which have their highest density in the macula, equalling that of the cones (125). Macular pigmentation as a symptom of a general lipofuscinosis (e.g. in psychiatric patients receiving long-term phenothiazine treatment) does not affect visual acuity (17, 93).

When the known retinotoxic compounds are reviewed and evaluated, only chloroquine is seen to be of importance. All other compounds which are potentially retinotoxic (after an acute intoxication or a long-term treatment at high dosage) are of minor importance. Such compounds, known to have a direct or indirect retinotoxic effect, are: quinine, cytotoxic drugs, steroid hormones, indomethacin, ethambutol, digitalis and phenothiazines.

Chloroquine retinopathy

On reviewing the known retinotoxic compounds, chloroquine is found to be most important. The literature contains many case reports (81, 82, 104, 108), critical reviews (19, 34, 80, 136) and recommendations concerning the diagnosis of chloroquine retinopathy (10, 21, 26, 40, 49, 120, 132, 136). Clinically, chloroquine retinopathy comprises maculopathy with a central scotoma, disturbance of colour vision and a reduction in the b- and c-wave amplitude of the ERG (120, 122) which may eventually result in disappearance of the c-wave (4, 30).

In 1965, we achieved the first convincing experimental induction of chloroquine retinopathy in the rabbit and the cat (9, 86, 87, 113). Funduscopic examinations showed a finely punctate pigmentation of the retina (Fig. 1). The retinal changes progressed even after withdrawal of chloroquine. The morphological picture accorded with that in human cases observed at necropsy (15, 99, 145): the pigmented epithelium was markedly thickened. At the same time there was a marked increase in acid phosphatase activity and in levels of PAS-positive substances (Fig. 2). Today we know that the material stored in the pigmented epithelium is an acidic phospholipid (64). In the melanin-containing pigmented epithelial cells a loss of melanin was observable. As a rule, the changes in the pigmented epithelium were patchy, but in later stages they were diffuse. In the later stages atrophic change was observed, leading to a decline in the number of visual cells (Fig. 3). Similar find-

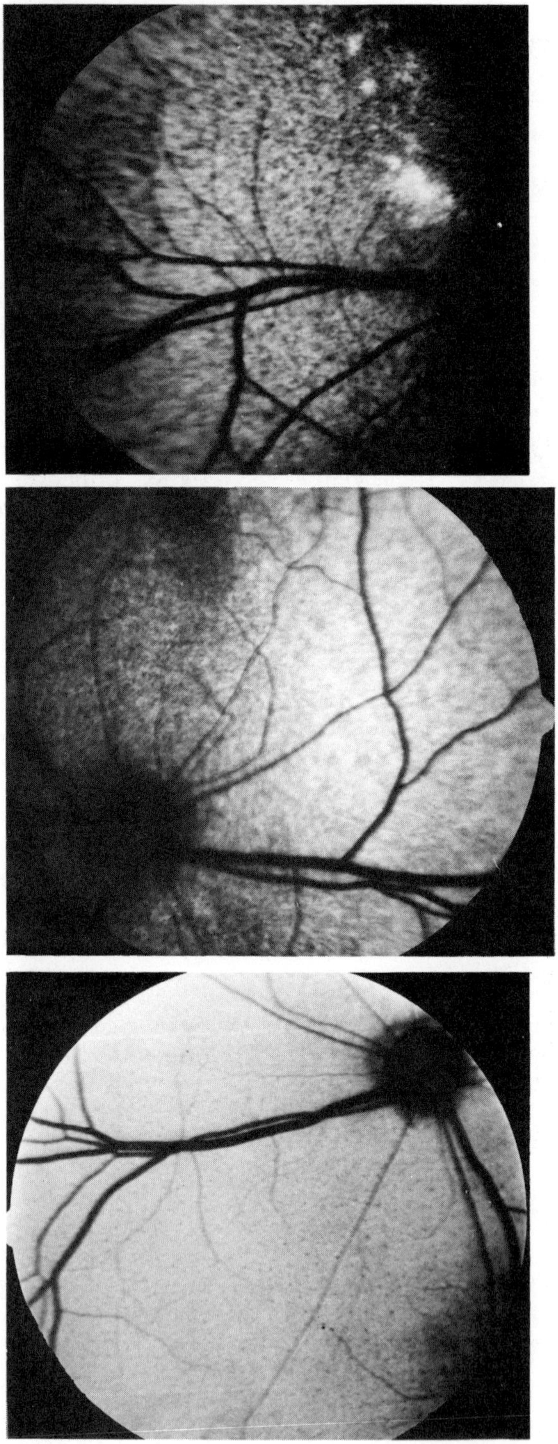

Fig. 1

(top)
Normal fundus of the cat retina.

(middle)
Chloroquine retinopathy. Finely punctate fundus after 16 weeks oral chloroquine application with increasing doses up to 9 mg/kg/day.

(bottom)
Advanced state of chloroquine retinopathy. Spotts with increased light reflection in the (left) lower segment (27 weeks oral chloroquine dosage, 1.5 to 9 mg/kg/day).

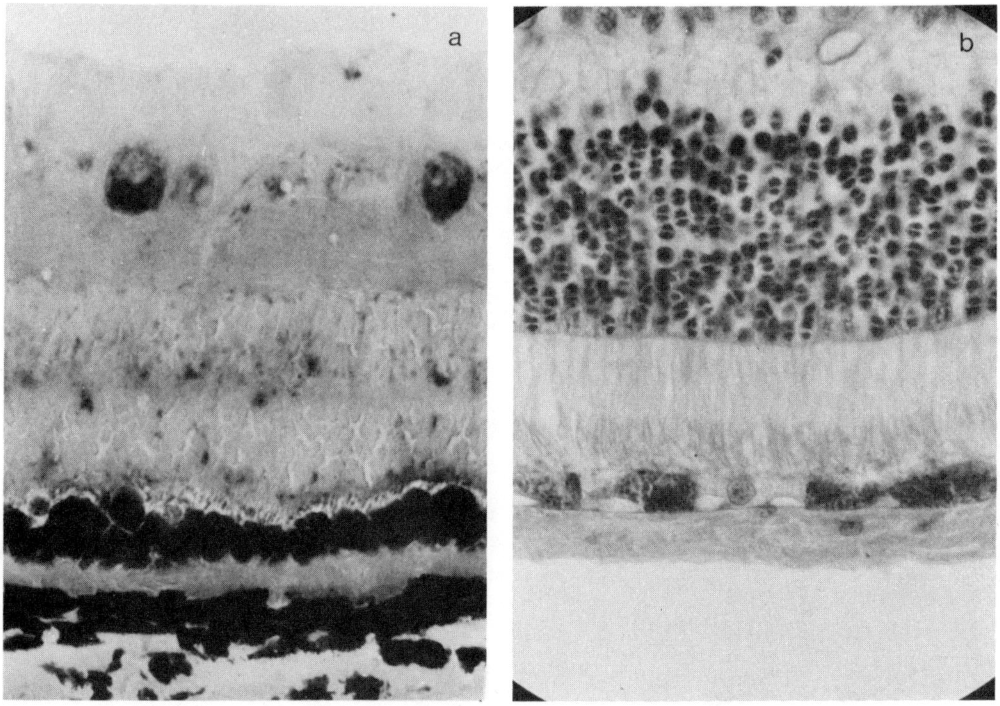

Fig. 2

a) Chloroquine retinopathy. Thickening of the pigmented epithelium with marked increase of PAS-positive material (native cryostat slice, PAS reaction, magnific. 290 x).

b) Chloroquine retinopathy. The thickening of the pigmented epithelium is less obvious if the tissue is dehydrated and embedded in paraffin. The PAS-positive material in the pigment epithelium appears granulated (magnific. 580 x).

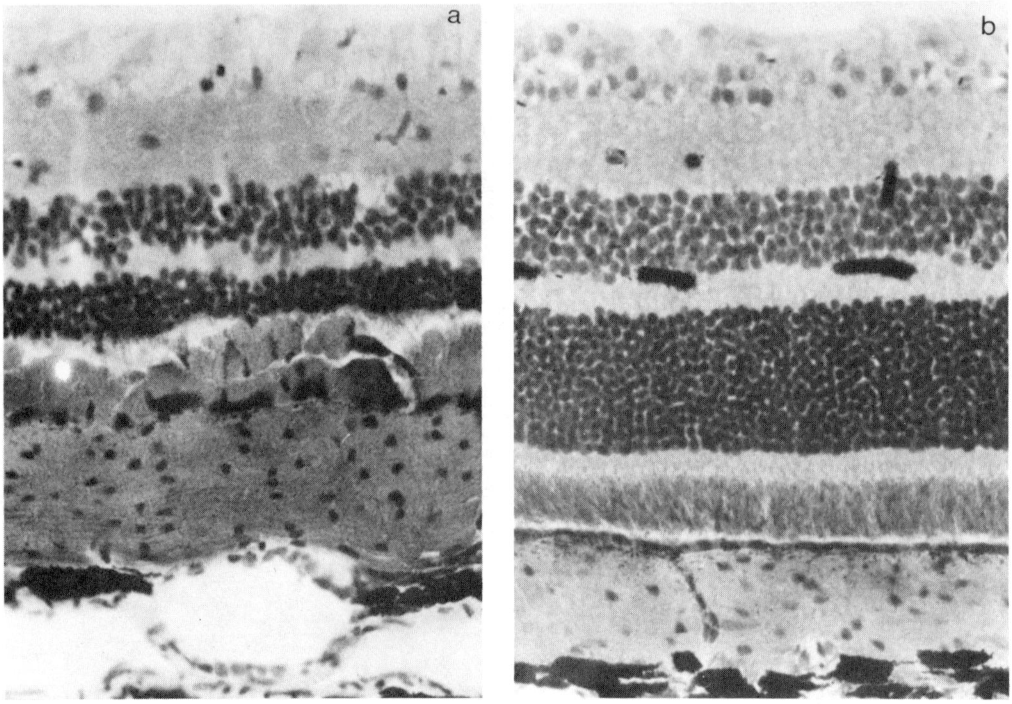

Fig. 3

a) Chloroquine retinopathy. Numerical atrophy of the visual cell layer after a two years treatment with 9 mg chloroquine/kg/day. The pigmented epithelium is swollen and shows nuclear pyknosis. (Alkaline phosphatase reaction with hemalum counterstaining, magnific. 290 x).

b) Normal retina of a control animal (alkaline phosphatase reaction with hemalum counterstaining, magnific. 290 x).

ings have been described in monkeys by Rosenthal et al. (1978)[115]. Chloroquine retinopathy has also been induced in rats (131), monkeys (115) and pigs (65).

With regard to the loss of melanin from melanin-containing cells of the pigmented epithelium, we know from studies by Rubin an Slonicki (1966)[117] that chloroquine interferes with the enzymatic activity of the melanocytes (118) by inhibiting protein metabolism (72), resulting in the synthesis of melanin with a low protein content. Similarly the defects of colour vision observed in chloroquine-induced retinal damage may also be regarded as the consequence of disturbed protein metabolism (10, 49, 102). A reversible pigmentation of the hair observed during treatment with chloroquine is another manifestation of the inhibition of protein metabolism (31, 147, 151). Destruction of tapetal cells has been observed in cats (67, 69). In the latter study only minor effects were seen in the melanin-containing pigmented epithelium.

The disappearance of the c-wave in the ERG (4, 30, 56) and the decrease of the b-wave amplitude are evidence in favour of primary chloroquine damage to the pigmented epithelium.

Marked changes induced by chloroquine in the pigmented epithelium have been described in experimental studies in rabbits (9, 87, 113), cats (86, 88), rats (107), pigs (65) and monkeys (115). Electron microscopic investigations by Babel and Englert (1969)[9] have demonstrated a reduction in melanin content and the appearance of lamellar granules in the pigmented epithelium and in the retinal ganglion cells. Narrowing of the field of vision obviously results from derangement of normal protein metabolism in the pigmented epithelium. An intact protein metabolism is necessary for normal synthesis of rhodopsin (88, 93, 149).

The neurotoxic action of chloroquine was shown in the preceding section to result from disturbance of protein metabolism (46, 99) and ganglioside metabolism (64, 65). Lamellar inclusion bodies, similar to those seen in cerebral neurons, were found in the retinal ganglion cells, in addition to changes in the lysosomes and the coarse endoplasmic reticulum (45, 46, 48, 64, 112, 114). The observation of similar changes in the retinal ganglion cells of albino rats (1, 2, 54, 70) has led to the hypothesis that abnormalities in the retinal ganglion cells are responsible for chloroquine retinopathy. In particular, ERG findings in albino rats which have received sublethal doses of chloroquine also suggested primary damage to the neuronal layer of the retina (73). Lesions of this type affecting peripheral nerves, the brain and the retina were observed in experimental studies in pigs by Gleiser et al (45, 46). They therefore regarded these lesions as systemic tissue damage and not as specific retinal changes, as also did Ramsey and Fine (1972)[112]. Finally, Klinghardt et al. (1981)[65] demonstrated that chloroquine causes extensive accumulation of gangliosides in brain and retina (the most abundant substances were G_{M2} and three fucogangliosides); the equivalent submicroscopical observation is the presence of lamellar inclusion bodies and membranous lysosomal residual bodies(64).

The identification of a predisposition to the development of chloroquine retinopathy has become a matter of major interest for the avoidance of toxic side effects in the retina. The following facts must be borne in mind whenever chronic treatment with chloroquine is started:

1. The safe single dose of chloroquine is considered to be 100 to 120 mg (58, 103).

   A daily dosage over 250 mg may lead to retinal damage, depending on the duration of treatment (25, 30, 80, 110).

2. 100 g chloroquine per year is regarded as the critical total dose (26, 140, 141).

   With a cumulative dose of 300 g chloroquine administered over a period of 3 years the probability of a toxic retinopathy developing is believed to be as high as 80% (103).

3. The incidence of chloroquine retinopathy is three times greater in patients with lupus erythematosus than in other patients (102, 103, 140).

4. The risk of developing chloroquine retinopathy increases with age (and is greatest after the age of 60 years). The risk in adults under 50 years of age seems to be negligible (34).

The development of a chloroquine maculopathy in man is known as bull's-eye formation; its cause is at present obscure. Light may be the most important additional factor in the development of chloroquine maculopathy (24, 78, 79, 92, 117). Up to now animal experiments have yielded no convincing evidence that light is instrumental in the development of a toxic maculopathy. The maculopathy is rather to be regarded as a manifestation of a systemic retinopathy.

Chloroquine retinopathy was unknown while chloroquine was used only as an antimalarial drug. The increased dosage required when chloroquine was used to treat rheumatoid arthritis resulted in a greater toxic effect, leading to the first observations of chloroquine retinopathy (3, 104). Although retinotoxic side effects are unlikely to occur at antimalarial dose levels of chloroquine (105) there have been a number of reports over recent years from two groups of authors (13, 28, 97, 98, 138). If in these few cases it is confirmed that retinopathy was linked to an antimalarial treatment with chloroquine, as suggested by these authors, light must be taken into consideration as an enhancing secondary factor (78, 79, 117).

Mackenzie (1970)[78], in particular, believes that light energy is an essential factor in the induction of a chloroquine retinopathy, and that the eye should be well protected against light if ocular lesions due to chloroquine are to be avoided. In fact, if a fluorescent substance such as chloroquine accumulates in the pigmented epithelium or in the retinal ganglion cells, short wavelength irradiation could cause sufficient bioelectric response to induce irreversible damage (24).

Retinotoxic effects of hydroxychloroquine and 4-aminoquinoline

Hydroxychloroquine is stated to be half as toxic as chloroquine (30, 78, 132). A maximal daily dosage of 400 mg is regarded as safe (119, 132). Its retinotoxic activity, however, is identical with that of chloroquine.

4-aminoquinolines are similar to hydroxychloroquine. Experiments in dogs have revealed morphological changes closely resembling chloroquine retinopathy with typical alterations of the pigmented epithelium and ERG changes (116). Like chloroquine, 4-aminoquinoline may induce retinal lesions, particularly in non-malarial indications, if given in excessive dosage for a long period (71). A few cases of retinal lesions have also been described in patients receiving 4-aminoquinoline for malaria prophylaxis for periods of 12 to 20 years (139).

Hydroxyquinolines

Hydroxyquinolines are regarded as potentially retinotoxic, since a few patients with acrodermatitis enteropathica who were treated with 1200 to 3600 mg hydroxyquinoline developed atrophy of the optic nerve (14, 35, 128, 134). Hydroxyquinoline would appear to possess neurotoxic properties if given at a daily dosage exceeding 1.5 g, but is not retinotoxic (60, 61).

Toxic retinal lesions induced by quinine

Toxic ocular side effects of quinine were described as early as 1913 in a monograph by Lewin and Guillery[75] on retinal side effects of drugs.

Case reports of quinine amblyopia mainly relate to quinine taken in overdosage with suicidal intent (20, 135, 152).

The ERG of patients with quinine intoxication exhibits a decrease in the amplitude of the b-wave, indicating a neurotoxic process (56, 152). Low doses affect the c-wave, and this is regarded as a direct retinotoxic action (55, 59).

Cytotoxic drugs

Cytotoxic drugs must be regarded as potentially retinotoxic because of their inhibitory action on protein metabolism. In recent years the number of reports of toxic retinopathies following cytotoxic treatment has increased remarkably.

A change in the pigmented epithelium resembling that induced by chloroquine was observed after administration of the antimetabolite sparsomycin which inhibits nucleic acid metabolism (84). Similar lesions were described with tilorone (144). Tilorone is an experimental cytotoxic drug which, like chloroquine, affects free radical scavenging mechanisms in the pigmented epithelium.

A lesion of the pigmented epithelium and a cystoid maculopathy were observed as retinotoxic side effects of treatment with tamoxifen (85). Submicroscopic investigations of retinal tissue obtained at autopsy revealed axonal degeneration in the nerve fibre layer and inner plexiform layer (62).

Retinotoxic side effects were reported in patients with malignant intracerebral tumours treated by intracarotid infusion of cis-diammineplatinum (II) dichloride. These lesions, characterized by a decrease of visual acuity (and auditory acuity) seem to be linked to the neurotoxicity of this cytotoxic compound (126).

Experimental studies of methylnitrosourea derivatives have been reported by several authors (6, 53, 101, 124). Lesions were demonstrated morphologically in the pigmented epithelium and in the rods and cones of the visual cells.

Oncologists would be wise to give careful attention in future to the possibility of retinotoxic side effects with cancer chemotherapy.

Retinal lesions due to oral contraceptives and steroid hormones

Following the introduction of oral contraceptives, numerous papers have been published since 1965 on retinal complications occurring during long-term treatment (for a review see Wood, 1977)[150].

The retinal changes occurring during administration of oral contraceptives cannot be regarded as primary toxic effects. These changes, like vascular thrombosis (5, 127, 137), haemorrhage (121, 137) and localized retinal oedema (47, 57) are, in fact, all changes resulting from vascular lesions (8, 121, 150) and abnormal blood coagulation profiles (5).

With reference to the incidence of retinal lesions during chronic contraceptive treatment, Ambrus et al., (1975)[5] have screened 5877 women taking oral contraceptives over a 10-year period. In this population they found 4 women with vascular complications, while 348 (6%) had abnormal blood coagulation profiles.

Corticosteroids appear to produce the same ophthalmic complications as do oral contraceptives. The case reports also mention retinal oedema, vascular complications and macular exudates (33, 44, 146).

Indomethacin

There are only isolated case reports of retinal side effects of indomethacin. No thorough experimental toxicity studies are available. The case reports describe macular pigmentation, decline of dark adaptation and ERG changes (22, 51). All changes were reversible after withdrawing the drug.

Ethambutol

In the treatment of tuberculosis, ethambutol given long term at high dosage causes amblyopia. Dose-dependent side effects in the retina can be detected fairly early by ERG examination (11, 12, 129). The critical total dose of ethambutol at which changes in retinal function may be expected is 150 g (74). Symptoms of an ethambutol lesion of the retina are disturbance of colour vision and a decline in the ERG amplitudes (12). These retinotoxic side effects are reversible on stopping ethambutol. With regard to pathogenesis, chelation of metal ions has been proposed as the chief explanation for the retinal side effects of ethambutol (23, 36).

Digitalis

Retinotoxic effects of digitalis deserve mention more for historical reasons than because of their actual importance. The reversible amblyopia and disturbance of colour vision induced by digitalis, described as xanthopsia, was described by Withering as early as 1785[148].

Literature reports on the disturbance of colour vision by digitoxin intoxication are rather sporadic. ERG studies have shown that red and green sensitivity decline and blue sensitivity increases (29, 43, 133).

The red-green scotoma may result from protein binding of digitoxin in the visual cells, particularly the cones, which are important for colour vision (142), or the outer plexiform layer.

Phenothiazine retinopathy

The importance of phenothiazine retinopathy has rapidly declined since a knowledge of the aetiology and pathogenesis (27, 48, 89, 91, 93) has made it possible to avoid iatrogenic hazard. However, it is appropriate to present here an account of phenothiazine retinopathy, because there have been many misinterpretations of retinal changes observed in patients on psychotropic drugs.

The pathogenesis of phenothiazine retinopathy was studied in cats treated with the experimental drug piperidylchlorophenothiazine (NP 207) (18, 27, 89, 93). NP 207 lesion of the retina begins with a finely punctate and circumscribed pigmentation of the fundus (Fig. 4). The pigmentation is due to the accumulation of light-

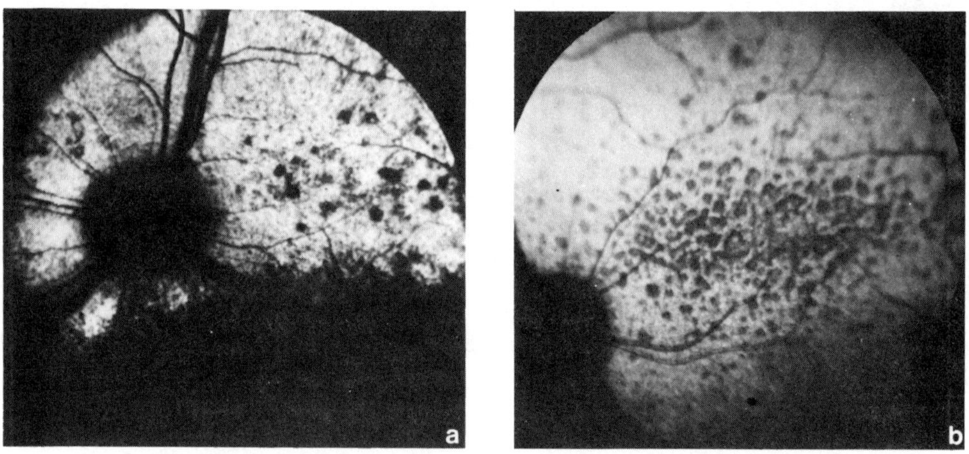

Fig. 4 Phenothiazine retinopathy.

a) Coarsely punctate pigmentation of the cat fundus after 7 weeks oral application of piperidylchlorophenothiazine (NP 207).

b) After 16 weeks further application of NP 207. The intensity of pigmentation has disappeared and swollen areas of pigmented epithelium can be observed.

absorbing distal segments of disrupted rods. In a few areas disrupted still unabsorbed rod material can be found in the vicinity of the pigmented epithelium (Fig. 5). In later stages atrophy of visual cells and nummular areas of the tapetum having increased reflectivity can be observed in the fundus (Fig. 6).

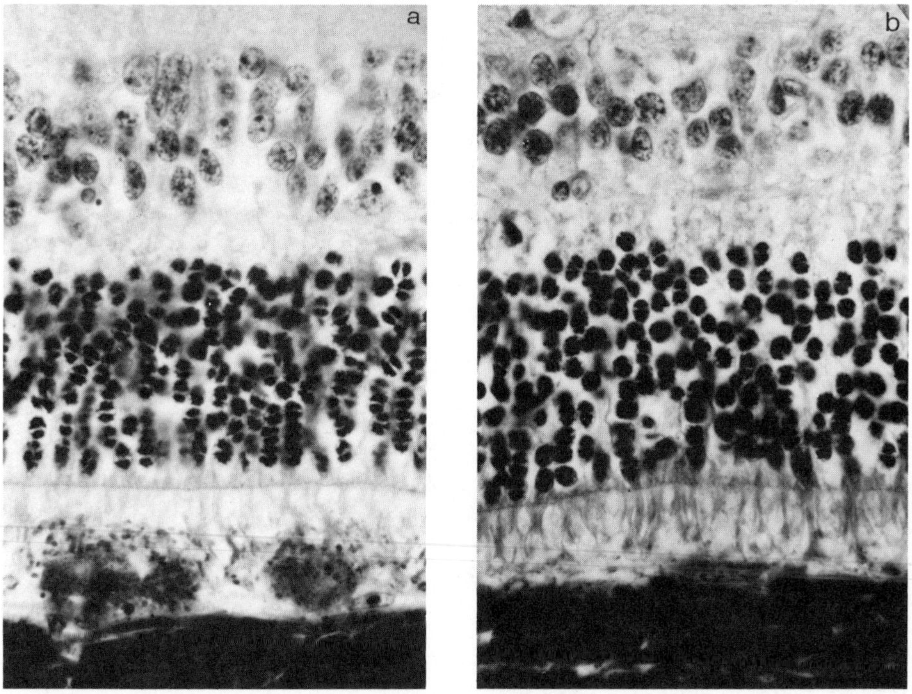

Fig. 5 Phenothiazine retinopathy

a) Associates of disrupted unabsorbed rod material in the vicinity of the pigmented epithelium. (Heidenhain hematoxylin staining, magnif. 580 x).

b) Phenothiazine retinopathy with total loss of distal rod segments (Heidenhain hematoxylin, magnific. 580 x).

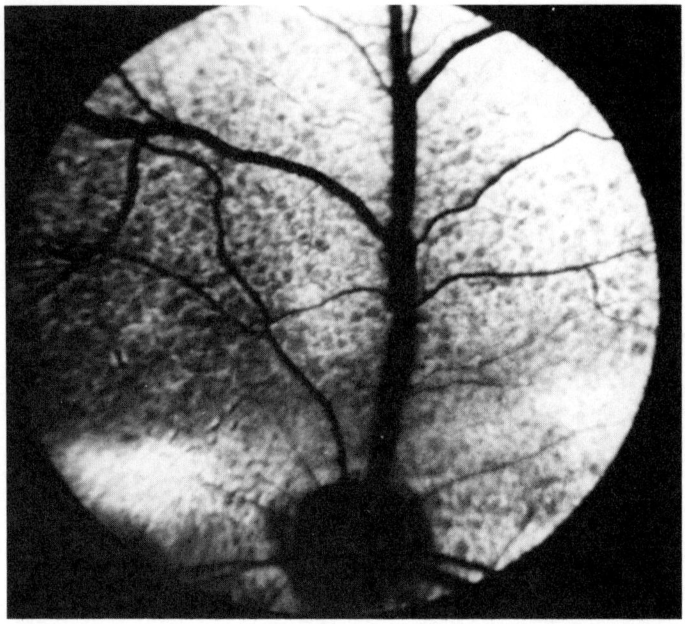

Fig. 6 Phenothiazine retinopathy.

After 52 weeks if MNP 207 dosing zones of retinal degeneration with increased reflectivity in the fundus.

Enzyme histochemical studies (27, 89, 93) have shown that piperidylchlorophenothiazine (NP 207) retinopathy is a primary lesion of the visual cells. There is a massive fall in the activity of the enzymes involved of energy metabolism in the ellipsoids of the rods (Fig. 7), to which changes producing accumulation of lipophilic material in the pigmented epithelium are secondary. It is accepted today that disturbance in the function of rods and cones attenuates the a- and c-waves of the ERG (106). Bornschein et al. (1974)[18] showed that in cats receiving chronic treatment with piperidylchlorophenothiazine this retinopathy is characterized by a dose-dependent decrease in the amplitude of the ERG c-wave.

In the light of present knowledge of the pathogenesis and pathophysiology of phenothiazine retinopathy it should be possible to determine the retinotoxic potency of any psychotropic drug in toxicological trials.

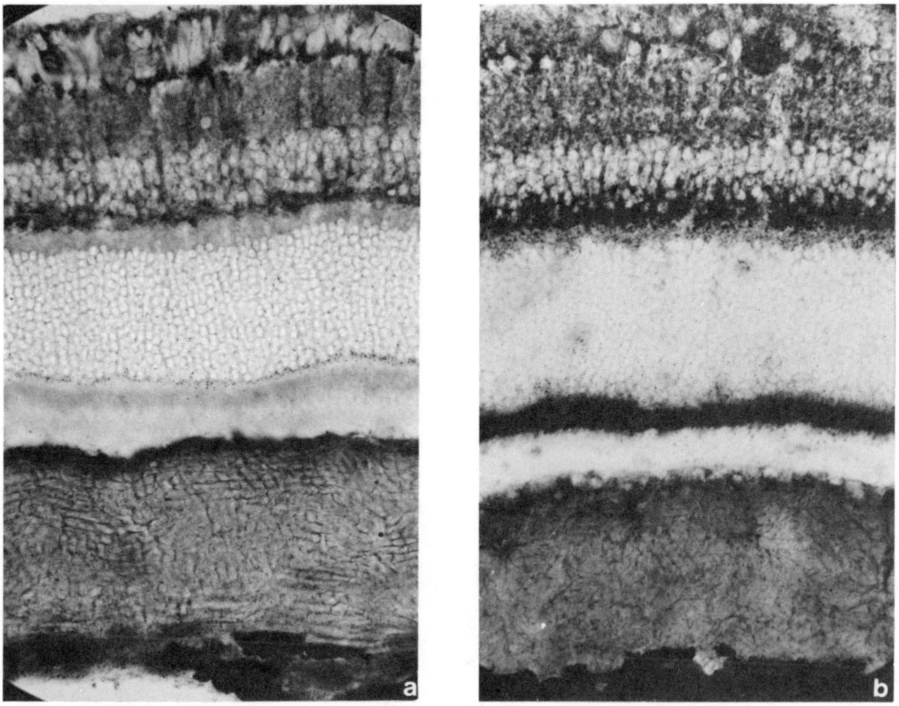

Fig. 7 Phenothiazine retinopathy.

a) Inhibition of isocitric dehydrogenase in the ellipsoids of the rods and cones, and in the outer plexiform layer.

b) Normal retina (magnif. 290 x).

Thioridazine can also cause a phenothiazine retinopathy if given for a long time in doses above the maximum tolerated dosage (32, 37, 96, 130, 143).

The safe upper limit for thioridazine is now accepted as 800 mg per day. No evidence has been obtained that thioridazine causes retinal damage in doses of less than 600 mg per day (7, 38, 50). The recommended dose at the present time is 100 to 600 mg/day (as originally recommended by Potts, 1968)[110].

The pathogenesis and morphological changes in thioridazine retinopathy are similar to those in piperidylchlorophenothiazine retinopathy (114). Moster (1972)[100] has shown that thioridazine inhibits functionally important enzymes in the visual cells; this effect resembles those produced by piperidylchlorophenothiazine (NP 207). Electrophysiological studies in a patient with thioridazine retinopathy showed that early receptor potentials in response to a light flash had a lower than normal initial amplitude. These studies further confirmed that thioridazine retinopathy involves predominantly the rods (130).

Two reports show that a fully developed thioridazine retinopathy, following daily doses of 1600 to 1800 mg for 1 to 6 months, may induce persistent progressive pigmented retinopathy (32, 96). Since the observance of an upper limit of thioridazine dosage in psychiatric treatment there have been extremely few reports of such cases in the literature.

The so-called "phenothiazine maculopathy", described by Kirk et al., (1970)[63] is not a toxic retinopathy in the narrower sense. The ophthalmologist observes a diffuse pigmentation of the macula without any effect on visual acuity. Boet (1969, 1970)[16, 17] investigated this phenomenon extensively. This special form of macula pigmentation, in which a macula lutea becomes a macula fusca, is simply the result of an accumulation of lipofuscin in the layer of optic nerve cells - as already outlined in the introductory section - without any disturbance of retinal function (92, 93). With advancing age there is likewise a gradually increasing deposition of lipofuscin in the optic nerve cells, giving the macula a more or less brown coloration. Pigmentation of this type - often misdiagnosed as retinopathy - is a harmless side effect not related to toxic retinal degeneration and not impairing visual acuity.

SUMMARY

In a brief introduction the aetiology and pathogenesis of toxic retinal lesions are outlined.

The production of side effects in the retina is dependent first of all on the metabolic toxicity of the drug. The vulnerability of the retina to toxic drug effects results from the adsorption of polycyclic aromatic compounds on the melanin of the choroid, a process which is regulated by an adsorption isotherm. In this way an increased blood level of the drug is attained in the choroidal capillaries which - having no blood-retina barrier - supply the pigmented epithelium and the visual cells. A critical high blood level of the drug is reached at which the binding capacity of melanin for an adsorbed drug is exhausted. This means that duration of therapy and dosage level are important determinants in the development of a retinopathy due to a retinotoxic drug. Therefore three conditions are essential do the causation of a toxic retinopathy:

1. adsorption of the active compound on to the melanin of the choroid

2. metabolic toxicity of the compound

3. high doses and long duration of the treatment

The following compounds are reviewed, which are important in drug therapy and have various levels of retinal toxicity: chloroquine, hydroxychloroquine, 4-aminoquinoline, hydroxyquinolines, quinine, cytotoxic drugs, oral contraceptives, steroid hormones, indomethacin, ethambutol, digitoxin, piperidylchlorophenothiazine (NP 207) and thioridazine.

A tentative critical evaluation is presented of the degree of retinotoxicity possessed by the various compounds. At the present time only chloroquinine and its derivatives, which are still important drugs in the treatment of rheumatic diseases, carry any risk of inducing toxic retinopathy.

REFERENCES

1. Abraham,R. and Handy,R.J., 1970, Irreversible lysosomal damage induced by chloroquine in the retinae of pigmented and albino rats, Exp.Molec.Path., 12:185
2. Abraham,R. and Handy,R.J., 1970, Retinal lysosomal changes in pigmented and albino rats treated with chloroquine, Toxicol.Appl.Pharmacol., 17:298
3. Adams,S.T., 1963, Retina and optic nerve, Arch.Ophthal., 69:642
4. Adlakha,D., Crews,S.J., Shearer,A.C.I., 1968, Electrodiagnosis in drug-induced disorders of the eye, Trans. Ophthal.Soc., 87:267
5. Ambrus,J.L., Mink,.B., Courey,N.G., Niswabder,K., Moore, R.H., Ambrus,C.M., Lillie,M.A., 1975, Thromboembolic complications of oral contraceptive therapy, Res.Comm. Chem.Path.Pharmacol., 10:197
6. Amemiya,T., 1972, Electron microscopic study of the retina of rats repeatedly treated with urethane, Acta Soc. Ophthal.Jap., 72:293
7. Appelbaum,A., 1963, An ophthalmoscopic study of patients under treatment with thioridazine, Arch.Ophthal., 69:578

8. Ardouin,M., Urvoy,M., Lavenant,F., 1978, Accidents neuro-ophthalmologiques de la contraception hormonale, Bull. Mem.Soc.Fr.Ophthalmol., 90:261
9. Babel,J. et Englert,U., 1969, Etude experimentale de la retinopathie par chloroquine, Bull.Mem.Soc.Fr.Ophthalmol., 82:491
10. Babel,J. et Meyer,E., 1965, Fréquence et prévention des lésions rétiniennes dues à la chloroquine, Schweiz.Med. Wschr., 95:1125
11. Barron,G.J., Trepper,L., Iovine,G., 1974, Ocular toxicity from ethambutol, Amer.J.Ophthal., 77:256
12. Bourgin,C. et Korol,S., 1974, Toxicité oculaire du myoambutol, Schweiz.Med.Rundschau (Praxis), 63:1382
13. Bec,P., Arne,J.L., Barrioulet,Y., Poitevin,B., Pene, P., 1975, L'électrorétinographie en fluorescence (A.E. R.G.) dans le dépistage précoce de la maculopathie par antipaludéens de synthèse, Bull.Soc.Ophthalmol.France, 75:353
14. Berggren,L. and Hansson,L., 1968, Absorption of intestinal antiseptics derived from 8-hydroxyquinolines, Clin. Pharmacol.Ther., 9:67
15. Bernstein,H.N. and Ginsberg,J., 1964, The pathology of chloroquine retinopathy, Arch.Ophthal., 71:238
16. Boet,D.J., 1969, Phenothiazine retinopathy, Ophthalmologica (Basel) Suppl., 158:574
17. Boet,D.J., 1970, Toxic effects of phenothiazines on the eye, Uitgeverij Dr. W. Junk N.V.
18. Bornschein,H., Hoyer,J., Heilig,P., Lützow,A., Heiss, W.D., Thaler,A., Wündsch,L., Hommer,K., 1974, Tierexperimentelle Untersuchungen mit einer das visuelle System schädigenden Substanz (NP 207), Albrecht v. Graefes Arch.Klin.Exp.Ophthal., 190:13
19. Brinkley,J.F. Jr., Dubois,E.L., Ryan,S.J., 1979, Long-term course of chloroquine retinopathy after cessation of medication, Am.J.Ophthalmol., 88:1
20. Brinton,G.S., Norton,E.W., Zahn,J.R., Knighton,R.W., 1980, Ocular quinine toxicity, Am.J.Ophthalmol., 90:403
21. Brückner,R., 1969, Frühdiagnose medikamentöser Schäden von Netzhaut und Sehnerv, Ophthalmologica (Basel), 158:245
22. Bruns,C.A., 1966, Ocular effects of indomethacin. Slit lamp and electroretinographic (ERG) study, Invest. Ophthal., 5:325

23. Campbell,I.A. and Elmes,P.C., 1975, Ethambutol and the eye; zinc and copper, Lancet, 2:711
24. Capri,R., Cordella,M., Franchi,A.,Neri,F., 1980, L'elettro-retinografia in fluorescenza come metodo di controllo della terapia con antimalarici di sintesi, Ateneo Parmense (Acta Biomed.), 51:445
25. Carr,R.E., Chloroquine and organic chenges in the eye, 1968, Dis.Nerv.Syst., 29, Supp. 3:36
26. Carr,R.E., Gouras,P., Gunkel,R.D., 1966, Chloroquine retinopathy. Early detection by retinal threshold test, Arch.Ophthal., 75:171
27. Cerletti,A. and Meier-Ruge,W., 1967, Toxicological studies on phenothiazine induced retinopathy, Proc.Europ.Soc. Drug Tox., Excerpt. Med.Intl.Congr.Ser. 145, 9:170
28. Chovet,M., Vedy,J., Fauxpoint,B., Vingtain,P., 1979, Un cas de rétinopathie par la chloroquine au cours de la prophylaxie du paludisme chez l'adulte, Rev.Int. Trach.Pathol.Ocul.Trop.Subtrop., 56:91
29. Cozijnsen,M., Pinckers,A.J.L.G., 1969, OOgheelkundige aspecten van digoticine-intoxicatie, Ned.Tijdschr.Geneesk., 113:1735
30. Crews,S.J., 1969, Some aspects of retinal drug toxicity, Ophthalmologica (Basel), 158:232
31. Dall,J.L.C. and Keane,J.A., 1959, Disturbances of pigmentation with chloroquine, Brit.Med.J., 1:1378
32. Davidorf,F.H., 1973, Thioridazine pigmentary retinopathy, Arch.Ophthalmol., 90:251
33. Ellis,Ph.P., 1968, Visual loss following tonsillectomy, Arch.Otolaryng., 87:128
34. Elman,A.,Gulberg,R.,Nilsson,E., Rendahl,I., Wachtmeister, L.,1976, Chloroquine retinopathy in patients with rheumatoid arthritis, Scand.J.Rheumatol., 5:161
35. Etheridge,J.E. and Stewart,G.T., 1966, Treating acrodermatitis enteropathica, Lancet, i:261
36. Figueroa,R., Weiss,H., Smith,J.C., 1971, Effect of ethambutol on the ocular zinc concentration in dogs, Am. Rev.Resp.Dis., 104:592
37. Finn,R., 1964, Pigmentary retinopathy associated with thioridazine: a report of a case with a maximum daily dose of 1400 mgm, Am.J.Psychiat., 120:913
38. Forrest,F.M. and Snow,H.L., 1968, Prognosis of eye complications caused by phenothiazines, Dis.Nerv.Syst., 29 (Suppl.3):26

39. Francois,J., 1979, Rétinopathies toxiques, Arch.Ophthalmol. (Paris), 2:639
40. Friedmann,A.I., 1969, The early detection of chloroquine retinopathy with the Friedmann visual field analyser, Ophthalmologica (Basel), Suppl. 158:583
41. Friedman,E., Smith,T.R., Kuwabara,T., 1964, Retinal microcirculation in vivo, Inv.Ophthal., 3:217
42. Friedman,E., Kopald,H.H., Smith,T., Mimura,S., 1964, Retinal and choroidal blood flow determined with krypton-85 in anesthetized animals, Inv.Ophthal., 3:539
43. Gibson,H.C., Smith,D.M., Alpern,M., 1965, Specificity in digitoxin toxicity, Arch.Ophthal., 74:154
44. Giovannini,A. and Consolani,A., 1979, Contraceptive-induced unilateral retinopathy, Ophthalmologica, 179:302
45. Gleiser,C.A., Bay,W.W., Dukes,T.W., Brown,R.S., Read, W.K., Pierce,K.R., 1968, Study of chloroquine toxicity and a drug-induced cerebrospinal lipodystrophy in swine, Am.J.Pathol., 53:27
46. Gleiser,C.A., Dukes,T.W., Lawwill,T., Read,W.K., Bay, W.W., Brown,R.S., 1969, Ocular changes in swine associated with chloroquine toxicity, Am.J.Ophthal., 67:399
47. Goren,S.B., 1967, Retinal edema secondary to oral contraceptives, Am.J.Ophthal., Ser.3, 64:447
48. Gregory,M.H., Rutty,D.A., Wood,R.D., 1970, Differences in the retinotoxic action of chloroquine and phenothiazine derivatives, J.Path., 102:139
49. Grützner,P., 1969, Acquired color vision defects secondary to retinal drug toxicity, Ophthalmologica (Basel), Suppl. 158:592
50. Hagopian,V., Stratton,D.B., Busiek,R.D., 1966, Five cases of pigmentary retinopathy associated with thioridazine administration, Am.J.Psychiat., 123:97
51. Henkes,H.E. and van Lith,G.H.M., 1971, Indocid-retinopathie, Ned.Tijdschr.Geneesk, 115:820
52. Henkind,P., 1966, The retinal vascular system of the domestic cat, Exp.Eye Res., 5:10
53. Herrold,K.M., 1967, Pigmentary degeneration of the retina induced by N-methyl-N-nitrosourea. An experimental study in syrian hamsters, Arch.Ophthal., 78:650
54. Hodgkinson,B.J. and Kolb,H., 1970, A preliminary study of the effect of chloroquine on the rat retina, Arch. Ophthal., 84:509

55. Hommer,K., 1968, Ueber die Chininvergiftung der Netzhaut. Mit einer Bemerkung zur experimentellen Chlorochinvergiftung, Klin.Mbl.Augenheilk., 152:785
56. Hommer,K., Ulrich,W.D., Wündsch,L., 1968, Direkte und indirekte Beeinflussung des ERG durch Antimalariamittel, Albrecht v. Graefes Arch.Klin.Exp.Ophthal., 175:121
57. Huismans,H., 1977, Weitere Mitteilung einer Komplikation unter einer Langzeittherapie oraler hormonaler Kontrazeptiv Klin.Monatsbl.Augenheilk., 171:781
58. Jeremy,R., 1968, A critical appraisal of therapy in rheumatoid arthritis, Med.J.Austr., 1:818
59. Jünemann,G., Schulze,J., 1968, Elektroretinographische Untersuchungen zur Entstehung der Chinin- bzw. Resochin-Retinopathie, Klin.Monatsbl.Augenheilk., 152:562
60. Kaeser,H.E., Scollo-Lavizzari,G., 1970, Akute zerebrale Störungen nach hohen Dosen eines Oxychinolinderivates, Dtsch.Med.Wschr., 95:394
61. Kaeser,H.E., Wüthrich,R., 1970, Zur Frage der Neurotoxizität der Oxychinoline, Dtsch.Med.Wschr., 95:1685
62. Kaiser-Kupfer,M.I., Kupfer,C., Rodrigues,M.M., 1981, Tamoxifen retinopathy. A clinicopathologic report, Ophthalmology (Rochester), 88:89
63. Kirk,L., Rasmussen,K.B., Faurbye,A., 1970, Retinopathy following thioridazine treatment, Acta Psychiat.Scand., 46, Suppl. 217:56
64. Klinghardt,G.W., 1981, Pathology of the neuron,preferences and differences in the participation of neuronal system in experimental storage dystrophy due to chloroquine, Acta Histochem. (Suppl.), 24:41
65. Klinghardt,G.W., Fredman,P., Svennerholm,L., 1981, Chloroquine intoxication induces ganglioside storage in nervous tissue: A chemical and histopathological study of brain, spinal cord, dorsal root ganglia and retina in the miniature-pig, J.Neurochem., 37:897
66. Kolb,H., 1965, Electro-oculogram findings in patients with antimalarial drugs, Brit.J.Ophthal., 49:573
67. Kuhn,H., Keller,P., Kovacs,E., Steiger,A., 1981, Lack of correlation between melanin affinity and retinopathy in mice and cats treated with chloroquine or flunitrazepam, Albrecht v. Graefes Arch.Klin.Exp.Ophthal., 216:177
68. Kuhn,H., 1980, Autoradiographic evidence for binding for ^{3}H-flunitrazepam (Rohypnol) to melanin granules in the cat eye, Experientia, 36:863

69. Kuhn,H., Steiger,A., 1981, Structural alterations of tapetal cells in the retina of cats induced by prolonged treatment with chloroquine, Cell Tissue Res., 215:263

70. Kurtz,M.S., Kaump,D.H., Schardein,J.F., Roll,D.E., Reutner, T.F., Fisken,R.A., 1967, The effect of long-term administration of amopyroquine, a 4-amino quinoline compound, on the retina of pigmented and non-pigmented laboratory animals, Inv.Ophthal., 6:420

71. Labat,P., Fauxpoint,B., Carrica,A., Rivaud,C., Vedy, J., 1979, La rétinopathie par les antipaludéens de synthèse du groupe des amino-4-quinoléines, Med.Trop. (Marseille), 39:307

72. Lefler,C.F., Filja,H.S., Holbrook,D.J., 1973, Inhibition of aminoacylation and polypeptide synthesis by chloroquine and primaquine in rat liver in vitro, Biochem.Pharmacol., 22:715

73. Legros,J. and Rosner,I., 1971, Electroretinographic modificationsin albino rats after chronic administration of toxic doses of hydroxychloroquine and desethylhydroxychloroquine, Arch.Ophthal.(Paris), 31:165

74. Leibold,J.E., 1966, The ocular toxicity of ethambutol and its relation to dose, Ann.N.Y. Acad.Sci., 135:904

75. Lewin,L.,Guillery,H., 1913, "Die Wirkung von Arzneimitteln und Giften auf das Auge", August Hirschwald, Berlin 1913

76. Lindquist,N.G., Sjöstrand,S.E., Ullberg,S., 1970, Accumulation of chorio retinotoxic drugs in the foetal eye, Acta Pharmacol.Toxicol., 28, Suppl. 1:64

77. Lüllmann-Rauch,R., 1976, Retinal lipidosis in albino rats treated with chlorphentermine and with tricyclic antidepressants, Acta Neuropath., 35:55

78. Mackenzie,A.H., 1970, An appraisal chloroquine,Arthritis Rheum., 13:280

79. Mackenzie,A.H., Szilagy,P.J., 1968, Light may provide energy for retinal damage during chloroquine treatment, Arthritis Rheum., 11:496

80. Marks,J.S., 1982, Chloroquine retinopathy: is there a safe daily dose ?, Ann.Rheum.Dis., 41:52

81. Marks,J.S., Power,B.J., 1979, Is chloroquine obsolete in treatment of rheumatic disease ?, Lancet, i:371

82. Martin,L.J., Bergen,R.L., Dobrow,H.R., 1978, Delayed onset chloroquine retinopathy: case report, Ann.Opthal., 10:723

83. Mason,C.G., 1977, Ocular accumulation and toxicity of certain systemically administered drugs, J.Toxicol.Environ. Health, 2:977
84. McFarlane,J.F., Yanoff,M., Scheie,H., 1966, Toxic retinopathy following sparsomycin therapy, Arch.Ophthal., 76:532
85. McKeown,C.A., Swartz,M., Blom,J., Maggiano,J.M., 1981, Tamoxifen retinopathy, Brit.J.Ophthalmol., 65:177
86. Meier-Ruge,W., 1965, Experimental investigation of the morphogenesis of chloroquine retinopathy, Arch.Ophthal., 73:540
87. Meier-Ruge,W., 1965, Die Morphologie der experimentellen Chlorochinretinopathie des Kaninchens, Ophthalmologica, 150:127
88. Meier-Ruge,W., 1968, The functional significance of Müller cells in the retina, in "Biochemistry of the Eye", U. Dardenne & J. Nordmann eds., pp.526-531, Karger, Basel/New York
89. Meier-Ruge,W., 1967, "Die medikamentöse Retinopathie", G. Thieme, Stuttgart
90. Meier-Ruge,W., 1968, The pathophysiological morphology of the pigmented epithelium and its importance for retinal structures and functions, Mod.Probl.Ophthal., 8:32
91. Meier-Ruge,W., 1970, The toxicology of neuroleptics on the eye, Acta Psychiat.Belg., 70:688
92. Meier-Ruge,W., 1973, Toxische Maculaschäden, Dtsch. Ophthalmol.Ges., 73:536
93. Meier-Ruge,W., 1981, Drug-induced retinopathy:I.Causal and clinical aspects (Lectures in Toxicology,No.6),II. Pathogenesis and Experimental Pathology (Lectures in Toxicology,No.7), in "Lectures in Toxicology", G. Zbinden ed., Pergamon Press, Oxford,New York,Paris,Frankfurt, Toronto,Sydney
94. Meier-Ruge,W., Cerletti,A., 1966, Zur experimentellen Pathologie der Phenothiazin-Retinopathie,Ophthalmologica, 151:512
95. Meier-Ruge,W., Cerletti,A., 1968, The significance of the melanin-bearing choroid in the retina, in "Biochemistry of the Eye", U. Dardenne ed.,pp.521-525, Karger, Basel/ New York
96. Meredith,T.A., Aaberg,T.M., Willerson,W.D., 1978, Progressiv chorioretinopathy after receiving thioridazine, Arch. Ophthal., 96:1172

97. Metge,P., Rodor,F., 1980, Rétinopathie à la chloroquine lors de la prophylaxie du paludisme à posologie correcte, Therapie, 35:439

98. Metge,P., Rodor,F., Chovet,M., Montabone,M., Llavador, M., 1979, A propos de 6 cas de rétinopathie chloroquinique consécutive à une prophylaxie antipalustre, Bull.Soc. Ophthalmol.France, 29:347

99. Monahan,R.H., Horns,R.C., 1964, The pathology of chloroquine in the eye, Trans.Am.Acad.Ophthal.Otolaryng., 68:40

100. Moster,M.F., 1972, The mechanism of the effect of phenothiazines on the eye, Scr.Med., 45:505

101. Murthy,A.S.K., Vawter,G.F., Kopito,L., Rossen,E., 1972, Retinal atrophy and cataract in rats following administration of N-methyl-N-nitrourea, Proc.Soc.Exper.Biol. Med., 139:84

102. Nylander,U., 1966, Ocular damage in chloroquine therapy, Acta Ophthal.(Kbn.), 44:335

103. Nylander,U., 1967, Ocular damage in chloroquine therapy, Acta Ophthal.(Kbn.), Suppl. 92:1

104. Okun,E., Gouras,P., Bernstein,H., Sallmann,L., 1963, Chloroquine retinopathy. A report of eight cases with ERG and dark-adaptation findings, Arch.Ophthal., 69:59

105. Olansky,A.J., 1982, Antimalarials and ophthalmologic safety, J.Am.Acad.Dermatol., 6:19

106. Penn,R.D., Hagins,W.A., 1969, Signal transmission along retinal rods and the origin of the electroretinographic a-wave, Nature, 223:201

107. Perääsalo,R., Rechardt,L., Palkama,A., 1973, Chloroquine-induced ultrastructural changes in the pigment epithelium of the albino rat, Acta Ophthalmol., :94

108. Percival,S.P.B., Meanock,I., 1968, Chloroquine: Ophthalmological safety and clinical assessment in rheumatoid arthritis, Brit.Med.J., III:579

109. Potts,A.M., 1962, Uveal pigment and phenothiazine compounds, Trans.Am.Ophthal.Soc., 60:517

110. Potts,A.M., 1968, Agents which cause pigmentary retinopathy, Dis.Nerv.Syst., 29, Suppl. 3:16

111. Potts,A.M., 1974, Drug toxicity as related to ocular melanin, Psychopharmacol.Bull., 10:40

112. Ramsey,M.S., Fine,B.S., 1972, Chloroquine toxicity in the human eye. Histopathologic observations by electron microscopy, Am.J.Ophthalmol., 73:229

113.Ramsey,M.S., Bloodworth,J.M.B., Engerman,R.L., 1970, Chloroquine retinopathy in the rabbit, Canad.J.Opthal., 5:264

114.Reinert,H., Rutty,D.A., 1969, Mechanisms of chloroquine and phenothiazine retinopathies, Toxicol.Appl.Pharmacol., 14:635

115.Rosenthal,A.R., Kolb,H., Bergsma,D., Huxsoll,D., Hopkins, J.L., 1978, Chloroquine retinopathy in the rhesus monkey, Inv.Ophthalmol.Vis.Sci., 17:1158

116.Rosner,I., Legros,J., 1970, Etude expérimentale des effets oculaire de deux 7-chloro-4-amino quinoléines chez le chien, Arch.Ophthal.(Paris), 30:865

117.Rubin,M., Slonicki,A., 1966, A mechanism for the toxicity of chloroquine, Arthritis Rheum., 9:537

118.Rubin,M.L., Zvaifler,N., Bernstein,H., Mansour,A., 1965, Chloroquine toxicity, in "Drugs and Enzymes", B.B. Brodie & J.R. Gillette eds., p.467, Pergamon Press,Oxford

119.Rynes,R.I., Krohel,G., Falbo,A., Reineck,R.D., Wolfe, B., Bartholomew,L.E., 1979, Ophthalmologic safety of long-term hydroxychloroquine treatment, Arthritis Rheum., 22:832

120.Sassman,F.W., Cassidy,J.T., Alpern,M.,Maaseidvaag,F., 1970, Electroretinography in patients with connective tissue diseases treated with hydroxychloroquine, Am. J.Ophthalmol., 70:515

121.Svarc,E.D., Werner,D., 1977, Isolated retinal hemorrhages associated with oral contraceptives, Am.J.Ophthalmol., 84:50

122.Sverak,J., Erbenova,Z., Peregrin,J., Salavec,M., 1970, Die ERG- und EOG-Potentiale nach einer langfristigen Resochin-Therapie, Klin.Monatsbl.Augenheilkd., 157:389

123.Schaller,J.P., Wyman,M., Weisbrode,S.E., Olsen,R.G.,1981, Induction of retinal degeneration in cats by methylnitroso-urea and ketamine hydrochloride, Vet.Pathol., 18:239

124.Steinberg,R.H., Reid,M., Lacy,P.L., 1973, The distribution of rods and cones in the retina of the cat, J.Comp.Neur., 148:229

125.Stewart,D.J., Wallace,S., Feun,L., Leavens,M., Young,S.E., Handel,S., Mavligit,G., Benjamin,R.S., 1982, A phase I study of intracarotid artery infusion of cisdiaminedi-chloroplatinum (II) in patients with recurrent malignant intracerebral tumors, Cancer Res., 42:2059

126.Stowe,C.G., Zakov,Z.N., Albert,D.M., 1978, Central retinal vascular occlusion associated with oral contraceptives, Am.J.Ophthalmol., 86:798

127.Strandvik,B., Zetterstrom,R., 1968, Amaurosis after broxyquinoline, Lancet, i:922

128.Tamai,A., 1972, Studies on the early receptor potential in human eye.II. ERP in a case of ethambutol intoxication, Yonago Acta Med., 16:97

129.Tamai,A., Holland,M.G., 1975, Electrophysiological studies on a case of thioridazine pigmentary retinopathy, Yonago Acta Med., 19:188

130.Thompson,S.W., 1975, Chloroquine retinopathy in the rat, Vet.Pathol., 12:71

131.Tobin,D.R., Krohel,G., Rynes,R.I., 1982, Hydroxychloroquine. Seven years experience, Arch.Ophthalmol., 100:81

132.Towbin,E.J., Pickens,W.S., Doherty,J.E., 1967, The effects of digoxin upon color vision and the electroretinogram, Clin.Res., 15:60

133.Van Balen,A.T.M., 1970, Toxische Beschadiging van de nervus opticus door joodchloorhydroxychinoline, Ned. Tijdschr.Geneek., 114:489

134.Vancea,P., Tacorian,D., 1969, La valeur ERG dans l'interprétation et la prognose de l'intoxication quininique, Ophthalmologica(Basel), Suppl., 158:653

135.van Lith,G.H., Mak,G.T., Wijnands,H., 1976, Clinical importance of the electro-oculogram with special reference to the chloroquine retinopathy, Bibl.Ophthalmol., :2

136.Varga,M., 1976, Recent experiences on the ophthalmologic complications of oral contraceptives, Ann.Ophthalmol., 8:925

137.Vedy,J., Fauxpoint,B., Labat,P., Carrica,J., Rivaut,C., 1978, Un nouveau cas de rétinopathie à la chloroquine au cours de la prophylaxie du paludisme chez l'adulte, Bull.Soc.Ophthalmol.France, 78:415

138.Vedy,J., Graveline,J., Carrica,J., Rivaud,C., Chanut, G., 1979, La rétinopathie par les amino-4-quinoléines dans la prophylaxie du paludisme, Bull.Soc.Pathol.Exot. Filiales, 72:353

139.Voipio,H., 1966, Incidence of chloroquine retinopathy, Acta Ophthalmol., 44:349

140.Voipio,H., 1967, Aminoquinolines and visual field, Acta Neurol.Scand., 43, Suppl. 31:149

141.Wald,G., 1966, Defective color vision and its inheritance, Proc.US Natl.Acad.Sci., 55:1347

142.Weekley,R.D., Potts,A.M., Reboton,J., May,R.H., 1960, Pigmentary retinopathy in patients receiving high doses of a new phenothiazine,A.M.A., Arch.Ophthalmol., 64:65

143.Weiss,J.N., Ochs,A.L., Abedi,S., Selhorst,J.B., 1980, Retinopathy after tilorone hydrochloride, Am.J.Ophthalmol., 90:846

144.Wetterholm,D., Winter,F.C., 1964, Histopathology of chloroquine retinal toxicity, Arch.Ophthalmol., 71:82

145.Williamson,J., 1970, A new look at the ocular side-effects of long-term systemic corticosteroid and adrenocorticotrophic therapy, Proc.Roy.Soc.Med., 63:791

146.Wilson,W., 1961, Retinopathy during chloroquine therapy, Brit.J.Ophthal., 45:756

147.Withering,W., 1785, "An Account of the Foxglove". Printed by M. Swinney G.G.J. and J. Robinson, Paaternoster Row, London. An account of the foxglove.

148.Wong,V.G., Lietman,P.S., Seegmiller,J.E., 1967, Alterations of pigment epithelium in cystinosis, Arch.Ophthal., 77:361

149.Wood,J.R., 1977, Ocular complications of oral contraceptives, Ophthalmic Semin., 2:371

150.Wroblowa,W., 1969, Toxic effect of nivaquine, Pol.Tyg. Lek., 24:1387

151.Zahn,J.R., Brinton,G.F., Norton,E., 1981, Ocular quinine toxicity followed by electroretinogram,electro-oculogram, and pattern visually evoked potential, Am.J.Optom.Physiol. Opt., 58:492

152.Zinn,K.M., Greenseid,D.Z., 1975, Toxicology of the retinal pigment epithelium, Intl.Ophthalmol.Clin., 15:147

NEUROTOXIC AGENTS

in the

HUMAN ENVIRONMENT

ANALYSIS OF NEUROTOXIC DISEASE:

THE ACRYLAMIDE EXPERIENCE

Peter S. Spencer and Herbert H. Schaumburg

Institute of Neurotoxicology, Departments of Neuroscience Neurology and Pathology, Albert Einstein College of Medicine Bronx, New York 10461, USA

INTRODUCTION

The neurotoxicologist is commonly consulted when it is suspected that exposure to a chemical substance has led to an outbreak of human neurological disease. Questions emerge for which answers must be sought by experimental investigation: Is the suspect chemical the culpable agent? What type of disorder is produced? Is it reversible, can it be treated, and what is the prognosis? This paper addresses the orderly analysis of neurotoxic disease, based on experience with a number of human neurotoxins, notably the industrial monomer acrylamide.

EVALUATING THE HUMAN DISORDER

Investigation of a human neurotoxic disorder logically follows from a full understanding of the circumstances surrounding the outbreak and the findings from clinical examination of affected individuals.

Clinical History

The history is often the cornerstone of diagnosis in neurotoxicology. In addition to the usual queries regarding past medical records of patient and family, questions should seek to establish the type, route, duration and degree of chemical exposure. Enquiry should be made into the manner in which the disease appeared and subsequently developed. Was the onset abrupt or slowly evolving? Was it featured by double vision, fever, pain, weakness, abnormal sensations, unsteady gait, bizarre behavior, convulsions, altered consciousness etc.? Did the disorder progress steadily or were the symptoms recurrent? The answers to these and other questions provide valuable information concerning the possibilities of intoxication and the nature of the disorder, toxic or otherwise.

Physical Examination

Findings on physical examination often provide important clues in certain types of chemical intoxications. Examples include: hair loss (vincristine, thallium); horizontal white stripes in the fingernails (certain heavy metal intoxications); brown skin (arsenic, bromide); green-colored tongue (clioquinol). Some of these signs subsequently may be reproducible in experimental animals.

Neurological Examination

This is crucial in defining the nature and location of nervous system disease. Examination includes a systematic evaluation of mental status, cranial-nerve function, sensory and motor function, coordination, gait and tendon reflexes. Supplementary tests are used to evaluate autonomic function (De Jong, 1976).

Evaluation of mental status includes assessment of level of consciousness, attention span, orientation to time, place and person, immediate, recent and remote memory, general knowledge, calculating ability, abstract thinking, mood, behavior, and ability to copy designs. Toxic encephalopathies characteristically produce alterations in consciousness (toxic delerium), while chronic encephalopathy may result in cognitive deterioration (dementia).

Cranial nerves are examined sequentially or in groups. Identification and discrimination of odors is used to test the olfactory nerve (I), while the optic nerve (II) is directly inspected with an ophthalmoscope and its function tested by investigation of visual acuity and visual fields. Electroretinography and assessment of visual evoked potentials provide objective assessment of the retina, optic nerves and its radiations. Different parts of the visual system may be affected by toxic chemicals, such as the retina (chloroquine), optic nerves (clioquinol), and visual cortex (methylmercury) (see Spencer and Schaumburg, 1980). Function of the oculomotor (III), trochlear (IV) and abducens (VI) is tested by observing the pupillary reflex to light and eye movements when following a moving object. Motor function of the trigeminal (V) is assessed by the patient's ability to chew or clench the teeth, and sensory function can be evaluated by testing facial sensibility and the corneal reflex. Impure trichloroethylene has a special predilection for the trigeminal nerve, and the corneal reflex is commonly depressed early in carbon disulfide intoxication. The facial nerve (VII) is tested by examining muscles of facial expression in actions of smiling, blowing or whistling, and by testing taste on the anterior two-thirds of the tongue. Both cochlear and vestibular portions of the auditory (VIII) nerve may be tested. Ability to detect low sound (whisper, watch, tuning-fork) crudely demonstrates a functional cochlea, and a normal oculocephalic ("dolls eyes") maneuver and absence of nystgamus is consistent with normal vestibular function. Auditory evoked potentials, abnormal in individuals addicted to toluene, reveal the integrity of the brainstem auditory relay system. More sophisticated tests of vestibular function include caloric testing (responses to stimulation of the semicircular canals by the instillation of cold water into the ear) and electronystagography. The glossopharyngeal nerve (IX) is tested by examining taste over the posterior third of the tongue and the vagus (X) by observing pharyngeal movements and the gag reflex. Function of the spinal accessory nerve (XI), innervating the trapezius and sternomastoid muscles, is demonstrated by shrugging the shoulders and flexing the head against resistance. Finally, hypoglossal (XII) function is examined by testing ability to protrude the tongue and looking for atrophy and/or fasciculations.

The motor system, commonly affected in neurotoxic disorders, is evaluated by assessing muscle power, bulk and tone, looking for involuntary movements and assessing muscle stretch reflexes. Power in extremities is evaluated by attempting to overcome contracted muscles in proximal and distal regions; the latter are commonly weakened in toxic neuropathies. Resistance to passive movement of the limbs at selected joints is used to assess muscle tone, and changes such as flaccidity, spasticity or rigidity must be identified and the distribution of the abnormality established. Muscles are examined for atrophy or fasciculation, and any involuntary movements of limbs or head (chorea, athetosis, dystonia, tremor, tics, or myoclonus) recorded. Electrophysiological assessment of both motor nerve conduction and electromyograms aids in localizing the pathology to nerve or muscle and, on occasion, may provide evidence to determine the nature of the underlying disorder (neuronal, demyelinating, axonal, myopathic).

Assessment of muscle stretch and superficial reflexes is used to assay somatic sensory-motor pathways. Testing of muscle stretch reflexes will reveal evidence of weak or brisk responses, seen respectively in toxic diseases of peripheral nerves and spinal cord. The level of the disorder can be evaluated by eliciting a variety of reflexes: jaw (pons), scapulohumeral (C5-6), triceps (C7-D1), biceps (C5-6), radial (C5,6), patellar (L3,4) and Achilles (S1,S2). Similarly, certain superficial reflexes have localizing value: corneal (pons), pharyngeal and palatal (medulla), epigastric (D7-9), abdominal (D8-12), cremasteric (L1,2), gluteal (L4,5), bulbocavernous (S3,4) and superficial anal (S5 and coccygeal). Pyramidal function is assessed in the legs by observing the response to plantar stimulation: normally the toes flex, but in pyramidal-tract diseases, such as lathyrism, extension of the great toe and fanning of the small toes, collectively known as the Babinski sign, can be demonstrated. Other simple but less reliable tests are available to evaluate pyramidal function in the lower and upper limbs.

Reflex examination is supplemented by tests of cerebellar function, including the finger-to-nose test, rapid alternate pronation and supination of the extended arm, ability to check movements quickly, finger dexterity, foot and hand patting, and ability to stand with eyes closed (Romberg).

Sensory function is examined by determining cutaneous sensibility to touch, pin-prick, vibration, hot and cold objects, digit position (proprioception) and pinching. Discriminative tests include ability to tell the distance between two sharp points, to identify the shape and identity of common objects (stereognosis), numbers traced on the skin (graphesthesia), a spot on the skin touched by the examiner, and differences in the texture and weight of objects. More sophisticated laboratory tests are available to quantify nerve terminal function (eg. vibratory sensation) and the integrity of sensory pathways (nerve conduction, somatosensory function).

The autonomic nervous system is affected in certain neurotoxic disorders (acrylamide). Useful tests of autonomic function include evaluation of cardiovascular reflexes, including the measurement of blood pressure, respiration and pulse rate in response to postural change, deep breathing and hyperventilation, carotid artery massage, acute mental and physical stress, or various pharmacological challenges (Bannister, 1983).

Neurological Assessment

The results of the neurological examination should provide an assessment of the type of disorder and its localization. Sometimes, as with acrylamide poisoning, the neurotoxic disorder may present different clinical features depending on the duration and degree of intoxication (Le Quesne, 1980). Acute acrylamide intoxication has led to encephalopathy with confusion, disorientation, memory disturbances, hallucinations and truncal ataxia, with peripheral neuropathy appearing 2-3 weeks later (Igisu et al., 1975). With less intense exposure, truncal ataxia is prominent, dysarthria and nystagmus may appear, and there is weakness and loss of sensation in the extremities (Fujita et al., 1960). With chronic intoxication, the neurological disorder may be limited to distal-extremity numbness and weakness (Garland and Patterson, 1967). Examination of chronically exposed individuals reveals depressed vibratory sensation, tendon reflexes and weakness distally in the hands and feet. Excessive sweating of limb extremities, with erythematous, peeling skin, are other features (Auld and Bedwell, 1967; Garland and Patterson, 1967). Taken in concert, these signs and symptoms suggest that chronic acrylamide intoxication affects peripheral somatic and autonomic nerves supplying the limbs, with cerebellar and then cerebral dysfunction occurring at progressively higher doses.

Involvement of the peripheral nervous system has been confirmed by electrophysiological examination of selected nerves and histological analysis of sural nerve sampled by biopsy (Fullerton, 1969; Takahashi et al., 1971). These studies demonstrated little change in maximum conduction velocity of motor and sensory fibers, marked dispersion of the muscle action potential, and reduced numbers of large-diameter myelinated fibers. Such results confirmed the involvement of extremity nerves and suggested that the condition was a distal neuropathy. This is consistent with the recovery of sensory and motor function that follows within weeks or months of withdrawal from mild exposure to acrylamide. More heavily exposed individuals may experience residual ataxia, suggesting irreversible changes in the cerebellum, while those with acute encephalopathy from heavy exposure recover rapidly, indicating an absence of structural damage to this region of the nervous system (Le Quesne, 1980). Subsequent experimental animal studies have shown these predictions to be remarkably accurate, thereby demonstrating the power of a detailed neurological examination.

Other features of the human disorder often aid in the subsequent experimental investigation of the disease. These include the clinical laboratory examination of blood, cerebrospinal fluid, and the histological study of brain, spinal cord, peripheral nerves, and muscle at autopsy. This type of pathological examination has been unavailable in human acrylamide intoxication, and the evaluation of tissue fluids has proved unremarkable in this disorder.

NEUROTOXIC DISEASE IN ANIMALS

The panic surrounding a major outbreak of human neurotoxic disease unfortunately often obscures the value of collecting domestic animals that also show signs and symptoms comparable to those seen in humans exposed to the same substance. One outstanding exception was the outbreak of Minamata disease when cats dwelling in the area displayed severe dysfunction with neurological and neuropathological features comparable to those found in man (Chang, 1980). The demonstration that identical changes were reproducible in experimentally intoxicated cats provided conclusive evidence that methyl mercury was responsible for this disorder.

PRODUCING AN ANIMAL MODEL

Experimental animal studies are optimally designed with a full understanding of the human disease under investigation. Part of this understanding concerns the duration of intoxication required to precipitate the neurotoxic disorder. It is often mistakenly assumed that chronic disease in humans can be reproduced more rapidly in animals simply by raising the administered dose, that different doses of a single agent elicit similar experimental disorders, and that the development of <u>any</u> neurological signs in animals provides evidence that the substance caused the neurological disorder in man, a disorder that may be markedly different from the experimental picture! An experienced researcher will persist until a valid animal model mimicking the human disorder is obtained. In some cases, it may be necessary to dose animals for months to reproduce a syndrome that appears in humans after prolonged low-level exposure to a chemical substance.

Experimental animal studies with acrylamide bear out some of these principles. Early investigations utilized large doses administered acutely by various routes to cats. Animals developed postural and ataxic tremors combined with behavioral changes and periodic tonic-clonic convulsions prior to death (Kuperman, 1958), features not reported in humans with acrylamide neurotoxicity. Lower doses of acrylamide administered to animals over a longer period of time resulted in incoordination followed by leg weakness, features typical of the intoxicated human (Fullerton and Barnes, 1966; Hopkins, 1970).

Pathophysiological Studies

After the establishment of a valid animal model, the next logical step is to examine the pathophysiological basis for the disorder. On those occasions when a specific region of the nervous system is likely to be involved, such as the peripheral nerves in acrylamide neuropathy, it is useful to conduct appropriate electrophysiological studies prior to sacrifice or, preferably, serially during the evolution of the disease. The first electrophysiological studies of acrylamide neuropathy in rats demonstrated a progressive reduction in motor conduction velocity in small muscles of the foot during the development of weakness (Fullerton and Barnes, 1966; Sumner and Asbury, 1973). Comparable effects were found in cats, monkeys and baboons (Leswing and Ribelin, 1969; Hopkins and Gilliatt, 1971).

Morphological techniques are then applied to define the nature of any pathological change and to characterize its spatial-temporal evolution. Optimally, a global examination of the nervous system of animals with the fully-developed neurological disease is carried out to allow the investigator to detect all the areas of the nervous system vulnerable to toxic attack. Once this is established, similar examination of animals less severely compromised provides insight into the differential susceptibility of individual structures as well as the spatial-temporal progression of the disorder. Eventually, it is possible to pinpoint the most vulnerable regions if questions of threshold dose are to be addressed.

Morphological studies of experimental acrylamide neurotoxicity have provided an explanation for the clinical and electrophysiological findings in humans and animals repeatedly exposed to this substance. No morphological changes have been identified in the brains of acutely intoxicated animals, consistent with the rapid and complete reversibility of the cerebral dysfunction in comparably intoxicated humans. Animals with hindlimb weakness following subchronic intoxication show a predominantly distal loss of large-diameter nerve fibers in peripheral nerves (Fullerton and Barnes, 1966; Hopkins, 1970). These early studies demonstrated that the lesion occurred within the axon compartment and that the myelin sheath was secondarily involved. In addition, degeneration ascended affected nerve trunks with time suggesting the disorder was a dying-back process (Fullerton and Barnes, 1966; Prineas, 1969). This was confirmed by studies showing comparable distal involvement of long ascending gracile and spinocerebellar tracts in the spinal cord and cerebellum, respectively (Prineas, 1969; Spencer and Schaumburg, 1977). Acrylamide neuropathy therefore fits into a recognized pattern of toxic-metabolic disorders of the nervous system known as central-peripheral distal axonopathies (Spencer and Schaumburg, 1974). Much later it was discovered that in certain animals, acrylamide induced an early loss of Purkinje cells (Cavanagh and Gysbers, 1983).

Once it was established that acrylamide neuropathy was associated with degeneration of distal axons, the next step was to determine whether axons of different functional type displayed different susceptibilities that could explain the clinical observation in humans of decreased vibratory sensation, abnormal proprioception and depressed deep tendon reflexes, coupled with the appearance of distal-extremity weakness. Schaumburg et al. (1974) demonstrated by serial examination of nerve terminals from the hindfeet of cats that Pacinian corpuscles (that respond to touch and vibration) were the first to display axon terminal changes similar to those seen in Wallerian degeneration. The onset of these alterations was followed by degenerative changes occurring in the primary annulospiral endings of adjacent muscle spindles. Somewhat later, similar abnormalities began to appear in nearby secondary terminals of muscle spindles and in adjacent motor nerve terminals. Degenerative changes were also found in axons of joint receptors (Spencer and Schaumburg, 1974). These morphological findings were reinforced by the results of independent electrophysiological studies which demonstrated early functional abnormalities of muscle stretch receptors and Pacinian corpuscles (Sumner and Asbury, 1975; Lowndes et al., 1978; Spencer et al., 1977b). Examination of the membranes of frozen-fractured corpuscles inactivated by acrylamide revealed that the functional loss was unassociated with morphological change (Spencer et al., 1977a). Studies of the hindlimb somatosensory evoked response in primates intoxicated with low levels of acrylamide disclosed an initial reversible decrement in the early component of the complex waveform recorded over the occipital region (Arezzo et al., 1982). These electrophysiological changes correspond to the early degenerative changes in the distal axons of the underlying gracile fasciculus discovered in previous experimental studies of acrylamide intoxication.

Animals with severe acrylamide neuropathy also develop structural and functional changes in the autonomic nervous system (McLeod, 1983). Paralyzed cats showed a progressive impairment of conduction in the splanchnic nerves and loss of myelinated fibers in splanchnic and vagus nerves. This was associated with an impairment of the vasoconstrictor response to splanchnic nerve stimulation (Post and Mcleod, 1977a,b). Baroreceptors and vagal afferents from the aortic arch, cardiothoracic and eosophageal wall were also affected in dogs, leading to abnormalities in postural regulation of blood pressure and megaoesophagus (Satchell and McLeod, 1981, Satchell et al., 1982). Comparable changes have not been looked for in humans with acrylamide neuropathy, although the presence of hyperhydrosis in affected individuals suggests autonomic involvement.

PROGNOSIS AND EARLY DETECTION OF HUMAN NEUROTOXICITY

Once a detailed analysis of a valid experimental model of a human neurotoxic disorder has been accomplished, it is possible to estimate the severity of the condition and prospects for recovery. In the example of acrylamide neuropathy, experimental investigation demonstrated this was predominantly a disorder of somatic and autonomic myelinated axons, elements that could be expected to regenerate and reestablish end-organ connection. Axonal regeneration does follow cessation of intoxication, and recovery from distal sensori-motor dysfunction is usually satisfactory (Fullerton and Barnes, 1966).

Detailed analysis of the spatial-temporal sequence of changes in a neurotoxic disorder may also provide information on vulnerable targets whose function may be monitored in humans exposed to the substance in question. In the case of acrylamide neuropathy, where Pacinian corpuscles develop early changes, quantitative measurement of vibratory sensibility has proved useful. Exceptionally high thresholds were found in certain asymptomatic individuals occupationally exposed to acrylamide. On neurological examination, they showed absent tendon reflexes in the lower extemities and mildly diminished sensation to pinprick. Some of the cases proved to be diabetic, others alcoholic, and one appeared to have subclinical neuropathy from acrylamide exposure (Arezzo et al., 1982). Quantitative sensory testing may therefore be an effective means of screening large populations exposed to axonal neurotoxins.

STUDIES OF PATHOGENESIS

A complete analysis of the pathophysiology of experimental disorders may also reveal important clues on the pathogenesis of the disease and lay the foundation for biochemical enquiry into the mechanism of the neurotoxic damage. From this understanding, a rational treatment of the disorder may emerge. The unfinished enquiry into the pathogenesis of acrylamide neuropathy illustrates these points.

The observation from clinical, electrophysiological and morphological studies of acrylamide neuropathy that nerve-fiber susceptibility to distal axonal degeneration was a function of axon length and fiber diameter led investigators to develop hypotheses about the underlying mechanism of the disease (Spencer and Schaumburg, 1974). An early idea, and one that has not been conclusively disproved, is that acrylamide may disrupt the anabolic activity of neuronal perikarya. As a consequence, the distal axons of long and large neurons would fail to receive their normal metabolic support and undergo degeneration. Another idea was that anterograde axonal transport, the mechanism by which materials are delivered from the perikaryon to the axon, was disrupted by acrylamide. Direct examination of anterograde axon transport showed differing degrees of slowing in animals with hindlimb weakness (Bradley and Williams, 1973; Chretien et al., 1981; Sidenius and Jakobsen, 1983; Wier et al., 1978). Subsequently, changes were found in retrograde axon transport (Sahenk and Mendell, 1981). However, it is unclear from these results whether the defect of transport is a primary event responsible for axonal damage or is secondary to the onset pathological changes (ie. neurofilament accumulation) developing within the axon (Miller and Spencer, in press).

The next logical step was to investigate axonal transport before the appearance of any pathological changes in nerve fibers of treated animals. Initial studies demonstrated that reduced amounts of materials were carried by retrograde transport before the appearance of hindlimb dysfunction (Jakobsen and Sidenius, 1983; Miller et al., 1983). Subsequently, it was shown that a dose-dependent reduction in the rate of retrograde transport occurs within hours of the administration of a single dose of acrylamide (Miller and Spencer, in press), days before structural changes would appear upon repeated intoxication. In addition, retrograde axon transport in sensory neurons seemed more susceptible to acrylamide than in motor neurons, a finding reminiscent of earlier clinical and morphological studies showing involvement of sensory terminals prior to motor terminals.

Since changes in retrograde axonal transport may be involved in the initiation of repair and regenerative processes by the neuronal perikaryon (Bisby and Bulgar, 1977), acrylamide might produce axonal degeneration by blocking retrogradely transported messages signalling the need to repair non-specific axonal lesions. This idea was supported by previous observations that acrylamide impaired terminal axon sprouting and increased the degree of degeneration in the proximal stump of a severed nerve (Cavanagh and Gyspers, 1980; Griffin et al., 1977; Morgan-Hughes et al., 1974). Nerve transection initiates a sequence of neuron perikaryal events preparatory to axon regeneration, changes that may be seen biochemically as an increase in the rate of RNA synthesis and an induction of ornithine decarboxylase, the rate-limiting enzyme in polyamine synthesis (Russell and Snyder, 1968). Single and repeated doses of acrylamide substantially attenuate these changes, possibly by retarding the retrograde transport of signals required to initiate these perikaryal responses (Miller and Spencer, submitted).

MECHANISTIC STUDIES

Biochemical studies of mechanisms underlying neurotoxic disorders naturally follow from earlier investigations defining pathophysiology. Because the nervous system is composed of multiple cellular compartments, the location and character of the disorder under study is required to construct a logical biochemical investigation. In the case of acrylamide neuropathy, it was evident from the study of humans and experimental animals that axons were involved primarily and that morphological changes were preceded by alterations in axonal transport and sensory terminal dysfunction. Since a constant supply of high-energy phosphate is required for maintenance of axonal transport (Ochs, 1982), a logical course of investigation was to determine whether acrylamide interrupted energy transformation. Several investigators demonstrated that acrylamide inhibited the action of key glycolytic enzymes (Sabri and Ochs, 1971; Sabri and Spencer, 1980; Sabri, 1983; Howland et al., 1980a,b), but changes in energy flux have yet to be demonstrated.

PREVENTION OF NEUROTOXICITY

Rational treatment of a human neurotoxic disorder is greatly enhanced by an understanding of the underlying mechanism of disease. Although a full mechanistic explanation of acrylamide neuropathy is unavailable at this time, the possible involvement of energy dysfunction in the development of axonal degeneration led investigators to test agents that might prevent the development of energy dysfunction, namely pyridoxine and pyruvate. Pyridoxine is a cofactor required for many enzymatic reactions, including those that supply substrates to the tricarboxylic acid cycle. Pyruvate was tested because it was hypothesized that blockade of glycolytic enzymes by acrylamide would lead to deficits in pyruvate production. Administration of pyruvate or pyridoxine to animals receiving acrylamide substantially delays, but does not prevent, the onset of neuropathy, thereby a result consistent with the notion that defective energy metabolism may play a role in this disorder (Loeb and Anderson, 1981; Dairman et al., submitted). Whether the administration of these agents would have an effect in delaying or ameliorating human acrylamide neurotoxicity has yet to be tested.

SUMMARY

This paper draws on experience with acrylamide to illustrate the appropriate method to investigate a human neurotoxic disorder. The mandatory first step is to define the human syndrome in detail. Next the experimentalist must develop a valid animal model, one that reproduces as many features of the human disorder as possible. Once this is in hand, the spatial-temporal sequence of pathophysiological events may be established. Identification of the initial pathological change often provides clues to the nature of the disorder, and this is a logical point of departure for biochemical studies designed to address basic mechanisms.

Methods to detect the early stages of the disease in humans may also be designed from this information. Finally, the identification of disease mechanisms will often reveal methods to circumvent the disorder, methods that may prove valuable in the design of drugs to prevent or ameliorate the human disease. In the case of acrylamide neurotoxicity, this entire sequence of investigation, as yet unfinished, has spanned 30 years!

ACKNOWLEDGMENTS

Supported in part by: NS19611, OH00851, OH2065. Gloria Warkenthien kindly typed the manuscript.

REFERENCES

Arezzo, J.C., Schaumburg, H.H., Vaughan, H.G., Jr., Spencer, P.S., and Barna, J., 1982, Hindlimb somatosensory evoked potentials in the monkey: the effects of distal axonopathy. Ann. Neurol. 12: 24.

Auld, R.B., and Bedwell, S.F., 1967, Peripheral neuropathy with sympathetic overactivity from industrial contact with acrylamide. Can. Med. Assoc. J. 96: 652.

Bannister, R., 1983, "Autonomic Failure. A Textbook of Clinical Disorders of the Autonomic Nervous System," Oxford University Press, Oxford.

Bisby, W.G., and Bulgar, V.T., 1977, Reversal of axonal transport at a nerve crush. J. Neurochem. 29: 313-320.

Bradley, W.G., and Williams, M.H., 1973, Axoplasmic flow in axonal neuropathies. Brain 96: 235.

Cavanagh, J.B., and Gysbers, M.F., 1980, "Dying-back" above a nerve ligature produced by acrylamide. Acta Neuropathol. 51: 169.

Cavanagh, J.B., and Gysbers, M.F., 1983, Ultrastructural features of the Purkinje cell damage caused by acrylamide in the rat: a new phenomenon in cellular neuropathology. J. Neurocytol. 12: 413.

Chang, L.W., 1980, Mercury. in: "Experimental and Clinical Neurotoxicology," P.S. Spencer and H.H. Schaumburg, eds., Williams and Wilkins, Baltimore, MD.

Chretien, M., Patey, G., Souyri, F., and Droz, B., 1981, Acrylamide induced neuropathy and impairment of axonal transport of proteins. II. Abnormal accumulations of smooth endoplasmic reticulum at sites of focal retention of fast transported proteins. Electron microscope radioautographic study. Brain Research, 205: 15-28.

De Jong, R.N., 1967, "The Neurological Examination," Harper & Row, New York.

Fujita, A., Shibata, M., Kato, H., Amoni, Y., Itomi, K., Sujuki, K., Nakajawa, T., and Takahashi, T., 1960, Clinical observations on acrylamide poisoning. Nippon Iji Shimpo 1869: 37.

Fullerton, P.M., 1969, Electrophysiological and histological observations on peripheral nerves in acrylamide poisoning in man. J. Neurol. Neurosurg. Psychiat. 32: 186.

Fullerton, P.M., and Barnes, J.M., 1966, Peripheral neuropathy in rats produced by acrylamide. Brit. J. Ind. Med. 23: 210.

Garland, T.O., and Patterson, M.W.H., 1967, Six cases of acrylamide poisoning. Brit. Med. J. 4: 134.

Griffin, J.L., Price, D.L., and Drachman, D.B., 1977, Impaired axonal regeneration in acrylamide intoxication. J. Neurobiol. 8: 355.

Hopkins, A.P., 1970, The effect of acrylamide on the peripheral nervous system of the baboon. J. Neurol. Neurosurg. Psychiat. 33: 805.

Hopkins, A.P., and Gilliatt, R.W., 1971, Motor and sensory nerve conduction velocity in the baboon: normal values and changes during acrylamide neuropathy. J. Neurol. Neurosurg. Psychiat. 35: 163.

Howland, R.D., Vyas, I.L., and Lowndes, H.E., 1980a, The etiology of acrylamide neuropathy: possible involvement of neuron specific enolase. Brain Res. 190: 529.

Howland, R.D., Vyas, I.L., Lowndes, H.E., and Argentieri, T.M., 1980b, The etiology of toxic peripheral neuropathies: In vitro effects of acrylamide and 2,5-hexanedione on brain enolase and other glycolytic enzymes. Brain Res. 202: 131.

Igisu, H., Goto, I., Kawamura, Y., Kato, M., Izumi, K., and Kuroiwa, Y., 1975, Acrylamide encephalopathy due to well water pollution. J. Neurol. Neurosurg. Psychiat. 38: 581.

Jakobsen, J., and Sidenius, P., 1983, Early and dose-dependent decrease of retrograde axonal transport in acrylamide-intoxicated rats. J. Neurochem. 40: 447.

Kuperman, A.S., 1958, Effects of acrylamide on the central nervous system of the cat. J. Pharmacol. Exp. Therapeut. 123: 180.

Le Quesne, P., 1980, Acrylamide. in: "Experimental and Clinical Neurotoxicology", P.S. Spencer and H.H. Schaumburg, eds., Williams and Wilkins, Baltimore, MD.

Leswing, R.J., and Ribelin, W.E., 1969, Physiologic and pathologic changes in acrylamide neuropathy. Arch. Environ. Hlth. 18: 22.

Loeb, A.L., and Anderson, R.J., 1981, Anatagonism of acrylamide neurotoxicity by supplementation with vitamin B6. Neurotoxicology 2: 625.

Lowndes, H.E., Baker, T., Cho, E., and Jortner, B.S., 1978, Position sensitivity of de-afferented muscle spindles in experimental acrylamide neuropathy. J. Pharmacol. 205: 40.

McLeod, J.G., 1983, Distal autonomic neuropathy. in: "Autonomic Failure. A Textbook of Clinical Disorders of the Autonomic Nervous System", R. Bannister, ed., Oxford University Press, Oxford.

Miller, M.S., Miller, M.J., Burks, T.F., and Sipes, I.G., 1983, Altered retrograde axonal transport of nerve growth factor after single and repeated doses of acrylamide in the rat. Toxicol. Appl. Pharmacol. 69: 96.

Miller, M.S., and Spencer, P.S., in press (a), Single doses of acrylamide reduce retrograde transport velocity. J. Neurochem.

Miller, M.S., and Spencer, P.S., in press (b), Mechanisms of acrylamide axonopathy. Ann. Rev. Pharmacol. Therapeut.

Miller, M.S., and Spencer, P.S., in press, Inhibition by acrylamide of increased ornithine decarboxylase activity and RNA synthesis in dorsal root ganglion following sciatic nerve transection. J. Neurochem.

Morgan-Hughes, J.A., Sinclair, S., and Durston, J.H.J., 1974, The pattern of peripheral nerve regeneration induced by crush in rats with severe acrylamide neuropathy. Brain 97: 235.

Ochs, S., 1982, "Axoplasmic Transport and its Relation to Other Nerve Functions", John Wiley & Sons, New York.

Pleasure, D.E., Mischner, K.C., and Engel, W.K., 1969, Axonal transport of proteins in experimental neuropathies. Science 166: 524.

Post, E.J., and McLeod, J.G., 1977a, Acrylamide autonomic neuropathy in the cat. I. Neurophysiological and histological studies. J. Neurol. Sci. 33: 353.

Post, E.J., and McLeod, J.G., 1977b, Acrylamide autonomic neuropathy in the cat. II. Effects on mesenteric vascular control. J. Neurol. Sci. 33: 375.

Prineas, J., 1974, The pathogenesis of dying-back polyneuropathies. II. An ultrastructural study of experimental acrylamide intoxication in the cat. J. Neuropathol. Exp. Neurol. 33: 260.

Russell, D.H., and Snyder, S.H., 1968, Amine synthesis in rapidly growing tissues: Ornithine decarboxylase in rat liver. Endocrinology 86: 1414.

Sabri, M.I., 1983, Mechanism of action of acrylamide on the nervous system. Biol. Mem. 8: 16.

Sabri, M.I., and Ochs, S., 1971, Inhibition of glyceraldehyde-3-phosphate dehydrogenase in mammalian nerve by iodoacetate. J. Neurochem. 13: 1509.

Sabri, M.I., Dairman, W., Juhasz, L., Bischoff, M.C., Spencer, P.S., 1981, Is acrylamide neurotoxicity pyruvate sensitive? Trans. Amer. Soc. Neurochem. 12: 147.

Sabri, M.I., and Spencer, P.S., 1980, Inhibition of glyceraldehyde-3-phosphate and other glycolytic enzymes by acrylamide. Neurosci. Lett. Suppl. 5: 455.

Sahenk, Z., and Mendell, J.R., 1981, Acrylamide and hexanedione neuropathies: abnormal bidirectional transport rate in distal axons. Brain Res. 219: 397.

Satchell, P.M., and McLeod, J.G., 1981, Megaoesophagus due to acrylamide neuropathy. J. Neurol. Neurosurg. Psychiat. 44: 906.

Satchell, P.M., Harper, B., and Goodman, A.H., 1982, Abnormalities in the vagus nerve in acrylamide neuropathy. J. Neurol. Neurosurg. Psychiat. 45: 609.

Schaumburg, H.H., Wisniewski, H.M., and Spencer, P.S., 1974, Ultrastructural studies of the dying-back process. I. Peripheral nerve terminal and axon degeneration in systemic acrylamide intoxication. J. Neuropathol. Exp. Neurol. 33: 260.

Sidenius, P., and Jakobsen, J., 1983, Anterograde axonal transport in rats during intoxication with acrylamide. J. Neurochem. 40: 687.

Spencer, P.S., Hanna, R.B., and Pappas, G.D., 1977a, Acrylamide inactivation of Pacinian corpuscle function: a freeze-fracture study. J. Neuropathol. Exp. Neurol. 36: 631.

Spencer, P.S., Hanna, R.B., Sussman, M., and Pappas, G., 1977b, Inactivation of Pacinian corpuscle mechanosensitivity by acrylamide. J. Gen. Physiol. 70: 17a.

Spencer, P.S., and Schaumburg, H.H., 1974, A review of acrylamide neurotoxicity. II. Experimental animal neurotoxicity and pathologic mechanisms. Canad. J. Neurol. Sci. 1: 152.

Spencer, P.S., and Schaumburg, H.H., 1977, Ultrastructural studies of the dying-back process. IV. Differential vulnerability of PNS and CNS fibers in experimental central-peripheral distal axonopathies. J. Neuropathol. Exp. Neurol. 36: 300.

Spencer, P.S., and Schaumburg, H.H., 1980, "Experimental and Clinical Neurotoxicology". Williams and Wilkins, Baltimore, MD.

Sumner, A.J., and Asbury, A.K., 1975, Physiological studies of the dying-back phenomenon. Muscle stretch afferents in acrylamide neuropathy. Brain 98: 91.

Takahashi, M., Ohara, T., and Hashimoto, K., 1971, Electrophysiological study of nerve injuries in workers handling acrylamide. Int. Arch. Arbeitsmed. 28: 1-11.

Weir, R.L., Glaubiger, G., and Chase, N., 1978, Inhibition of fast axoplasmic transport by acrylamide. Environ. Res. 17: 251.

NEUROTOXIC EFFECTS OF METALS AND THEIR INTERACTIONS

J.B. Cavanagh

Institute of Neurology, Queen Square
London WC1N 3BG, U.K.

Metal intoxications as a pathological grouping command attention only because they are metals. They each have very specific individual pathological effects, so far as we can judge the issues at the present moment, and it is only apparently by chance that two very dissimilar metals, arsenic and thallium, produce clinical and pathological changes that have a great deal in common. This is the product of a purely accidental involvement of the same important metabolic pathway.

The toxic effects of metal on the nervous system have been well studied only in four of those known to be neurotoxic (Table 1). These are arsenic, thallium, mercury and lead. For most of the remainder too little is known about their modes of action to construct even the most tenuous hypotheses.

ARSENIC INTOXICATION

Arsenic, the well known resort of poisoners over the ages, has from its forensic interest as well as from its industrial uses been much studied metabolically and chemically, and although our understanding of biochemical actions *in vitro* and *in vivo* is now very thorough (Webb, 1966), how the pathological changes come about in nervous tissue is still largely conjecture. The absence of a suitably developed animal model allows us only to draw conclusions from human clinical cases of poisoning.

Pentavalent Arsenic

To the nervous system, trivalent arsenic is certainly much more poisonous than pentavalent forms, a fact made much use of in the field of chemotherapy. However, pentavalent forms, unless degraded to the trivalent state (Crecelius, 1977), while being capable of uncoupling oxidative phosphorilation (arsenolysis), do not have neurotoxic effects except by virtue of being part of the organic ring structure. The use of several types of organic arsenical in the treatment of syphilis (arsphenamine; '606'; neoarsphenamine; etc.) and more lately in the treatment of tropical conditions, such as trypanosomiasis, has produced and still continues to produce a small number of cases of haemorrhagic vascular lesions of the eye and the brain ('haemorrhagic leucoencephalopathy') in consequence of this treatment (Globus and Ginsburg, 1933). This type of lesion, with a very unclear relation to dose and to time of injection as well as it's constant relationship to a ring formation in the drug's chemical structure, is very likely to be the result of an anaphylactoid type of immune response. The studies in which lesions of the eye or the brain have been successfully produced in animals have tended to support this conclusion (Longley et al., 1942; Weston Hurst, 1959).

Trivalent Arsenic

Trivalent arsenic is of more importance for our understanding of the direct effects of arsenic, whether absorbed as the oxide or as the gas arsene (AsH_3), involve the gastro-intestinal tract, the skin and its appendages and the nervous system. This last is characteristically a sensory neuropathy that is produced with some degree of motor weakness (Jenkins, 1966). The neuropathy, indeed, is remarkably similar to that caused by chronic vitamin B_1 deficiency (beri-beri). Indeed the similarity is so close that when there was a severe outbreak of arsenic poisoning due to contamination of sugar for making beer in the North of England in 1900, there was much discussion in the literature by those experienced with tropical diseases as to whether this was beri-beri or not (Reynolds, 1901). The skin changes and the finding of arsenic in the urine can often be the only deciding diagnostic factors. Electrophysiological examination of the peripheral nerves will show a marked slowing of the conduction velocity and loss of sensory action potentials, indicating a greater involvement of sensory nerves (Murphy et al., 1981).

Table 1. Metal Intoxications of the Nervous System

Metal	Type of Effects	Probable Mechanism
Aluminium	Dementia (local injection -filaments)	?
Arsenic	'dying back' degeneration of long PNS axons	Inhibition of respiration -lipoate
Cadmium	vascular damage	? Ca^{++} ion interaction
Lead -inorganic	focal vascular damage -encephalopathy -neuropathy.	? Ca^{++} ion interaction
-organic	neuronal degeneration	?
Mercury -inorganic	small cell degener.^{n} in CNS and large sensory cells in PNS	? ribosomal damage
-organic	ditto.	ditto.
Manganese	basal ganglia degener^{n}.	?
Thallium	'dying back' degeneration of long PNS axons	inhibition of respiration-FAD
Tin -trimethyl	neuronal degeneration. c.f. trimethyl-Pb	?
-triethyl	myelin membrane splitting	?

The loss of sensory and motor functions are always distal in distribution and shorter nerves, such as the cranial nerves, have never been reported to be affected. Recovery is slow but usually complete (LeQuesne and McLeod, 1977). It may take many months for regeneration of the axons to be completed due to the lenghts of fibres that have undergone degeneration and thus the distance the regenerating neurites have to travel. There is very little reason to believe that the intoxication itself continues for any great period of time after absorption of arsenic has ceased. The recovery rate will thus be an expression of the severity of the original amount of denervation.

Metabolic background

Trivalent arsenic appears to be readily absorbed from the intestines (Webb, 1966) and it accumulates in the tissues in an organ specific manner, there being no apparent blood-brain barrier (Valkonen et al., 1983). Concentration in the brain, however, is substantially less than in the liver. Excretion is by the kidneys and the faeces and the curves of disappearance from the urine in human cases (Jenkins, 1966; Murphy et al., 1981) show that the 50% level tends to be reached in about 3 weeks after dosing (or diagnosis) and the fall off is probably exponential (Figure 1). Whether agents such as B.A.L. (dimercaptopropanol) and D-penicillamine really have any definite effect in poisoned subjects once poisoned is a matter for debate. As noted above the relative slowness of the return of the conduction properties of the nerves to normal, commented upon LeQuesne and McLeod (1977), is almost certainly due to the length of 'die-back' of the axons and therefore the distances for the regenerating axons to travel at the rate of 1 mm/day. Biopsy studies have shown only the banal changes of wallerian degeneration without any specific features (Ohta, 1970).

Trivalent arsenic binds readily to -SH groups as well as to many other radicles in tissues. Many aspects of cell metabolism are thus modified (Webb, 1966). Pre-eminent, so far as the brain is concerned, is the binding of As^{+++} to the cofactor, lipoate, since pyruvate and α-ketoglutarate decarboxylation are major pathways in nervous tissue for the production of energy. The formation of a fairly stable six-membered ring with lipoate thereby blocks the forward progress of the utilisation of pyruvate. Moreover, since this is the step next after the step requiring thiamine pyrophosphate, it is, perhaps, hardly surprising that there are great similarities in the two syndromes. The success

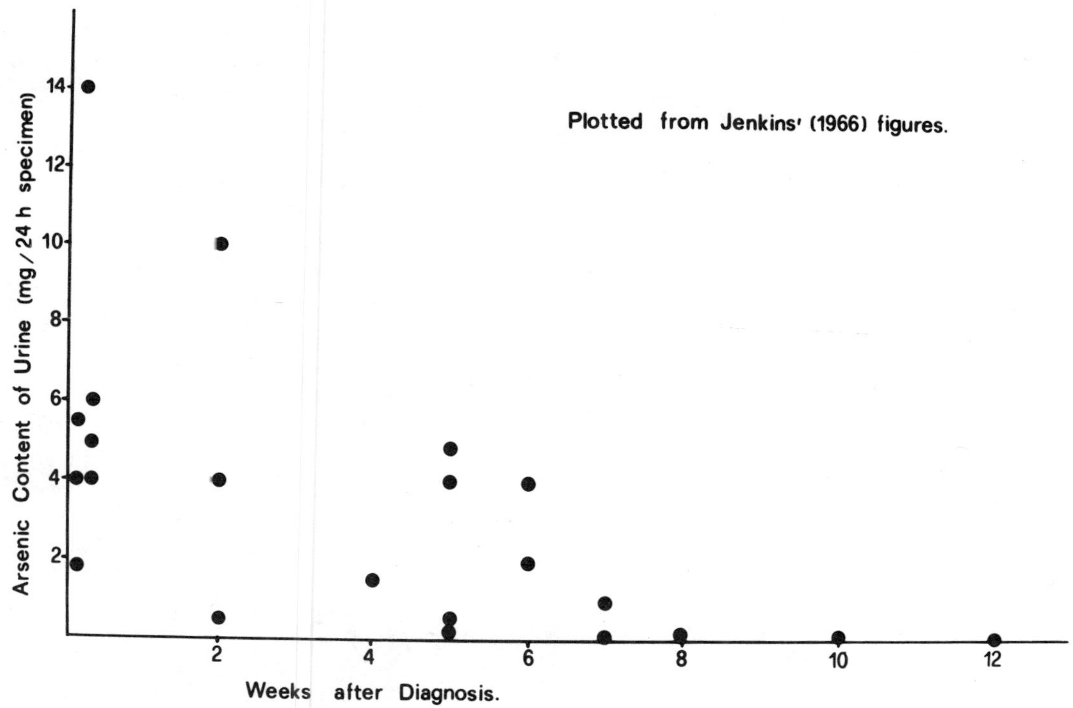

Fig. 1

Arsenic content of 24 hour specimens of urine from patients at various times after diagnosis. Normal is less than 0.1 mg/ 24 hour specimen. Data taken from Jenkins (1966).

of B.A.L. (British Anti-lewisite) in combating the intoxication is due largely to the somewhat greater stability of the five membered ring that it forms with the arsenic as compared with the six-membered ring noted above. Many of the details of the intoxication, particularly the reason for the particular pattern of the nerve fibre degeneration and what is the role of the rate of penetration of the As^{+++} ion into the cell body have yet to be fully worked out. It is certainly probable that one reason for the greater sensitivity of the sensory root ganglion cells, as evidenced by the predominantly sensory symptomatology in the early stages, may well be because they are exposed to greater concentrations for longer periods by virtue of the fenestrations in their vascular bed (Jacobs et al., 1976). Penetration into the CNS appears to be somewhat slower than into other tissues (Huston and Martin, 1955), while there seems to be little barrier into peripheral nerve (Webb, 1966). Since synthesis of new lipoate to replace that inactivated in the axon must come from the perikaryon, the more distal regions of the longer axons will be greatest at risk to sustained deprivation, particularly if the cell body mechanisms are also somewhat prejudiced (Cavanagh, 1979).

Given, therefore, these threads of circumstantial evidence we can knit them into a reasonable hypothesis to explain the clinical signs and symptoms of arsenic intoxication of nervous tissue. The concomitant reduction in growth of hair and nails, to produce in the latter Mees lines, are also a product of the high energy demands of these growing tissues and supports the idea of the energy-dependant nature of the neuropathy. Until a reproducible animal model is produced for further study, we may have to continue to live with this hypothesis as it stands at present.

THALLIUM INTOXICATION

Thallium is still used in many countries as a rodenticide despite it's evident dangers to children, pets and conserved wild animals. As with arsenic, it is a general biological poison and adversely affects plants and animals equally.

Entrance and Excretion

Thallium salts are readily soluble in water and are considered tasteless and odourless, though victims of poisoning have occasionally noted a metallic taste in retrospect. It is readily absorbed from the gut, but its intake is sometimes associated with vomiting and often with diarrhoea, both probably expressions of direct toxic effects on the mucosal cells. The monovalent thallium ion has many interactions, both chemically and biologically, with potassium ions (Schoer, 1984)(Table 2) . Thus, it has a similar ionic radius (1.33 A,K^+ -1.44 A) and enters cells through K^+ channels. Its pathways of absorption and excretion follow those of potassium and we see it excreted by the salivary glands, in the bile, and by the gut and the kidneys (Gehring and Hammond, 1966). Much of that which has passed into the gastro-intestinal tract is subsequently re-absorbed and the task of the pysician is to prevent this by giving suitable chemicals that render the ion insoluble.

Table 2. Some Metabolic Interactions of Thallous Ions

Size : hydrated ionic radius 0.144 nm.
c.f. K^+ 0.133 nm, & $NH4^+$ 0.143 nm.
Entrance : to cell through K^+ channels
Can replace K^+ ions in K^+ activated enzymes
a. 3 X the affinity of K^+ in (Na^+ + K^+)-activated ATP ase
b. up to 10 X affinity of K^+ ions for many others
c. K^+ions in some ribosomal functions
d. K^+ions in electrically excitable membranes
Excretion : mainly along K^+ion channels
a. salivary glands
b. gut epithelium
c. biliary tract
d. kidney
e. protein detritus, eg. hair, scales, nails,etc.

Once inside the animal body, it rapidly enters cells and concentrates in tissues. Normal subjects show uniformly low levels ($<$ 5 ppb), but after intoxication in Man and in experimental animals, kidney, salivary gland, liver and muscle show the greatest concentrations (Table 3) . In nervous tissue it is the grey matter with it's greater concentration of cells that has distinctly higher amounts than white matter or peripheral nerve. High concentrations are also found in hair (Cavanagh et al., 1974).

Inside the cell Tl^+ ions will replace K^+ ions in many K^+– dependant enzyme reactions (Gehring and Hammond, 1967), the avidity of the former being often substantially greater for the enzyme than the latter. It is not known, however, whether this replacement really makes much difference to the functions of the enzymes in the cell, e.g. the excitability of muscle or the electrogenic potential of nerve fibres.

Table 3 . Concentrations of Thallium in Tissues from one case of poisoning

(from Cavanagh et al., 1974)

Source of specimen	Thallium concentration (microgram / gram
Urine	5.9
Blood	3.4
Kidney	20.0
Heart	13.3
Brain (grey matter)	10.0
Skin	6.0
Liver	5.0
Bone	5.0
Muscle	5.0
Brain (white matter)	3.0
Lung	1.8
Gall-bladder	1.1
Sciatic nerve	1.0
Kidney after paraffin embedding	2.2

Toxic effects in tissues (Table 4)

Toxic doses in Man are greater than 8 mg/kg for this was the dose used to produce epilation in the treatment of ringworm of the scalp (Heyroth, 1947). This dose caused about 10% of the cases to develop peripheral neuropathy. In dogs the calculated LD_{50} is about 12 mg/kg (Greving and Gegel, 1929), in rat about 5 mg/kg and in mice about 7 mg/kg (Hart and Adamson, 1971). Cases dying of thallium intoxication may show fatty changes in the liver and kidney, and cell proliferation generally is inhibited in both plant and animal tissues. Thus, onion root tips are markedly affected (Truhaut, 1959). Testicular cells are inhibited and sperm production stopped and so also are bone marrow cells and gut epithelial cells. Quantitative studies on hair follicles in the neonatal rat have shown that there is a steady loss of mitoses at the base of the follicle over 48 hours following a single dose of thallium salt. This leads to varying degrees of necrosis of the base of the follicle where the cells are made, and the effect on the hair is to produce marked narrowing of the hair shaft as it subsequently emerges in time from the follicle which is responsible for the subsequent loss of hair (Cavanagh and Gregson, 1978). The damage to the hair is, therefore, similar in principle though not in exact mechanism to the hair loss caused by anti-mitotic agents. There are suggestions from in vitro work that thallium may have an inhibiting action on ribosomal function by displacing K^+ ions, but the concentrations used in mice, were rather high, namely 100 - 150 mg/kg, which is 30 - 50 times the LD_{50} (Hultin and Naslund, 1974).

Table 4 . Some Biological Effects of Thallous Ions

Interferes with oxidative phosphorylation by a number of possible mechanisms
Inhibits cell division probably through effects on cell respiration
Thus damages - gut epithelium
- bone marrow
- skin and appendages, eg. hair & nails
- testis and sperm production
- ascites tumour cells
Binds, but not avidly, to -SH groups, eg. hair proteins
Renders riboflavin insoluble and produces a syndrome similar to riboflavin deficiency
Causes "dying back" degeneration of long peripheral sensory and motor axons

On the other hand, tissue culture studies have suggested that the mitochondria may be adversely affected before the onset of the axonal degeneration (Spencer et al., 1973). This finding, perhaps, relates to the observations of Truhaut (1959) that the respiration of yeast is inhibited at low concentration of thallium and that ox heart preparations, made according to Keilin and Hartree, are also significantly inhibited at 2 - 4 mMol levels.

Action of Thallium on Nervous Tissue

Very few species appear to be sensitive to the neuropathic effects of thallium and apart from Man only cats and dogs have been reported (Kennedy and Cavanagh, 1976; Zook et al., 1967, 1968). Most of our information is, thus, based on human studies. Intoxication is usually by a single, relatively large dose rather than by chronic intake. Vomiting occurs early accompanied by diarrhoea. The first nervous symptoms are pain and tingling in the feet and fingers. Within a day or so distal weakness occurs which may spread proximally if the dose is large enough. In severe poisoning respiratory muscles and cranial nerves may be affected in the few days before death and the pulse rate will be increased probably due to vagal denervation. In milder cases the weakness may not spread more proximally than the knees and elbows and recovery will take place with time as the denervated axons regrow.

Epilation or hair loss regularly occurs with thallium poisoning but it rarely is seen before the 14th day (Heyroth, 1947) and, unless the hair is deliberately pulled, it may not be noticed until after the neurological illness is fully developed. It is not, therefore, a reliable sign of thallium poisoning. Since the hair follicles are only affected when they are mitotically active, those hairs that are not growing, or growing only slowly, such as lanugo hair and pubic and axillary hair, are much less affected. On recovery, the hair may be abnormally curly or otherwise misshapen for some time until the follicle has completely returned to normal.

In the nervous system, there is widespread distal degeneration of axons which may be almost total in many distal nerves in severe cases of poisoning. More proximal nerves, however, may be well preserved. The dorsal root ganglion cells and the anterior horn cells will show chromatolysis. This is a repair response that indicates that the cell body is attempting to repair the damaged axons. Lesser degrees of change will be found in nerves with shorter axons, such as the cranial nerves, and the wallerian degeneration seen there will be in an earlier stage of development. Except for severe degeneration of the dorsal columns (Scharrer, 1933; Kennedy and Cavanagh, 1976), which is secondary to the changes in the spinal ganglion cells, no other region of the nervous system shows stuctural changes. The bizarre psychiatric disturbances reported by Reed et al. (1963) which occurred some months after thallium treatment for ringworm have no explanation to date unless they are related in some way to the action of thallium on potassium functions.

Mechanism of Toxicity

This has been discussed earlier (Cavanagh, this volume) in some detail in relation to the degeneration of long axons in PNS and CNS, and there are strong circumstantial reasons for believing that energy deprivation of the nerve cells with distal effects upon the axons is responsible. This is hypothesised as coming about through the precipitating action of thallium upon riboflavin (Kuhn et al., 1933) and riboflavin deficiency produced in the monkey has many features that resemble thallium intoxication, especially the peripheral neuropathy and the skin and hair changes (Penstchew and Garro, 1969). Moreover, there are no other known actions of thallium that have the capacity to act upon the energy–producing mechanisms with such selectivity as to produce a neurological syndrome so closely resembling arsenical intoxication.

MERCURY INTOXICATION

Widely used in organic forms since historical times in the treatment of many diseases, especially syphilis, mercury has really become of general interest since the environmental hazards of methyl mercury were demonstrated in Japan in the 1950's. In fact methyl mercury intoxication is now synonymous with Minamata disease. There is still great uncertainty, however, as to how the underlying cellular changes are brought about, not only by organic mercury but also by inorganic mercury poisoning. I would like to emphasise here that the three types of mercury poisoning met with seem, on careful inspection, to show essentially the same effects within cells and the real differences between them are quantitative rather than qualitative (Table 5). If we are to interpret the much more complex changes in the developing brain correctly we must be certain of the underlying cellular pathology. The brain possesses no great toxicological mysteries, other than having a complex structure and an even more complex developmental sequence than any other tissue.

Absorption, Excretion and Tissue Concentration

It is now well established from numerous studies that the form in which mercury enters the body, and thus it's capacity to pass cell membranes, is an important part of the toxic process (Magos, 1975). Kidney/brain ratios are markedly related as to whether the mercury is in a divalent state or not. With mercurous salts or after inhalation of mercury vapour, the kidney/brain ratios are almost one tenth of that found after injection of divalent mercury. Both Hg and methyl mercury are able to enter the brain more rapidly than divalent mercury, despite the greater general toxicity of the latter. Methyl mercury, by comparison with the inorganic forms, has a longer biological half-life and is only slowly degraded to inorganic mercury in the tissues. Not only does methyl mercury tend to accumulate in nervous tissue, possibly by virtue of the large number of lipid membranous systems, but it is readily transferred by placenta and the milk to the dependant developing infant. This cumulative feature of methyl mercury, which is much less seen with the inorganic and the readily degradable phenyl forms, is without doubt the most important factor in determining the severity of the changes that it produces.

Clinical Effects of the Different Forms of Mercury

The striking feature of methyl mercury intoxication which presented itself to the earlier observers, who had had previous experience of inorganic mercury poisoning, was the irreversibility of the signs and symptoms (Hunter et al., 1940).

Table 5. Features that the three forms of mercury intoxication have in common. The severity of the intoxication is greatest in alkyl mercury poisoning and least in mercuric poisoning

	Alkyl mercury	Mercuric salts	Mercurous salts
Higher centres	Cortical and subcortical cell death	Mental changes and tremor -reversible	Irritability "Pink Disease -reversible
Cerebellum	Severe granule cell death	Focal granule cell death (rats)	Granule cell degeneration (man)
Peripheral neuropathy	Sensory (all species)	Sensory (rats)	Sensory(infant) (Pink Disease)
Selective damage to	Small cells and peripheral ganglion cells	Small cells and peripheral ganglion cells	Small cells and peripheral ganglion cells
Metabolic change	Protein synthesis inhibited	Protein synthesis inhibited	?

Inorganic mercury poisoning clinically shows evidence of mental disturbance (erethism) and tremors as well as drowsiness by day and insomnia by night. No structural basis for these symptoms has ever been shown and indeed they tend to disappear on withdrawal from exposure. By contrast, methyl mercury, whether from industrial exposure or by uptake from the environment, produces signs and symptoms that are irreversible and have a characteristically selective pattern. The three principal areas of the nervous system affected are the cerebral cortex, the cerebellum and the sensory ganglia. The cerebellum shows loss of the small granule cells (Figure 2) with relative sparing of the larger Purkinje cells. The cerebral cortex shows cell loss, especially in the visual, auditory and sensory cortex, three sites where the concentration of small neurons are greatest, and here too there is sparing of the larger cells. The so-called "agranular" cortex tends to be spared either partially or completely (Hunter and Russell, 1954; Takeuchi et al., 1962). Sometimes, however, the cell loss may be so massive as to obscure these important topographical points (Takeuchi et al., 1962). In peripheral nerve there is marked sensory nerve loss (Hunter et al., 1942; Eto and Takeuchi, 1977).

The changes in mercurous chloride poisoning, as seen in Pink Disease in infants (Patterson and Greenfield, 1923-1924) and in adults after long sustained intake of calomel (Davies et al., 1962) is a faint reflection of this pattern of neurological effects. There are in both conditions mental disturbances and peripheral neuropathy, and pathologically we see loss of granule cells in the cerebellum and degeneration of peripheral nerves.

Experimental Studies

The large number of experimental studies on many different species has clearly shown that the changes are essentially similar in the pattern of nerve cells affected and lost to that first observed in man (Hunter and Russell, 1954). Small granule cells in the cerebellum and small neurons in the cerebral cortex are especially at risk, while the cells of the sensory ganglia are also seriously affected.

In chronic mercuric chloride intoxication, we also see focal loss of cerebellar granule cells (Enders and Noetzel, 1955) and lesions of the same type as seen with methyl mercury are also present in the sensory ganglion cells (Jacobs et al., 1975b). It would thus appear from this kind of evidence that the same type of change is found regardless of the form of mercury given. Only in the severity of the effects and the number of dying neurons do we see a marked difference.

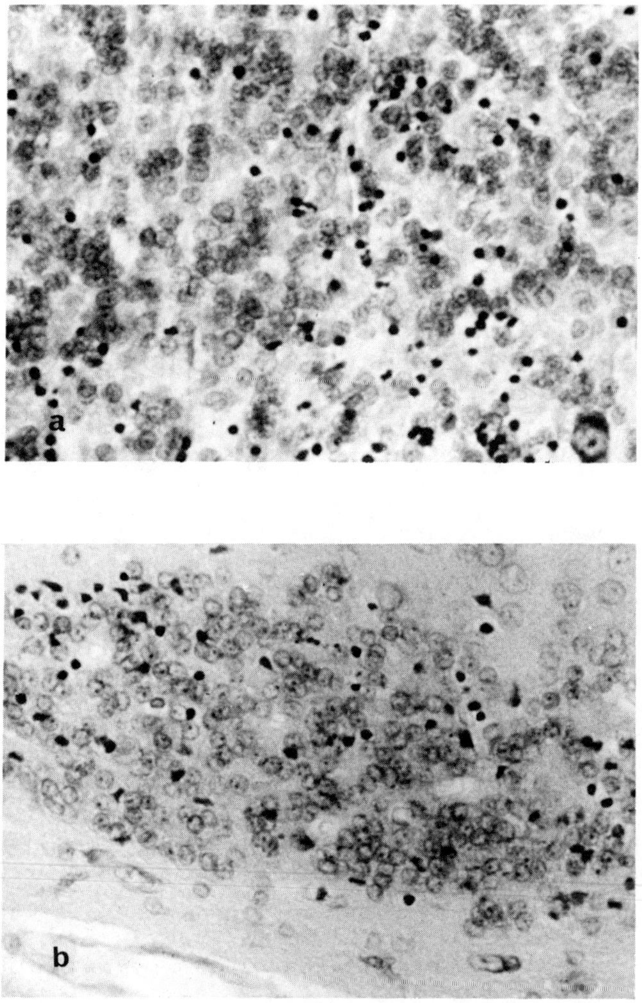

Fig.2. Rabbit tissues 7 days after four doses of 7.5 mg/kg methyl mercury (X 500)

a. Cerebellum showing diffuse loss of granule cells with pyknosis of their nuclei.

b. Cluster of small cells from the islands of Calleja in the base of the frontal lobe. Necrosis of these small neurons, as representative of the small neurons of the cerebrum, are almost as frequent as similar sized neurons in the cerebellum.

Cellular Mechanisms of Mercury Intoxication

There have been remarkably few detailed studies of the cellular changes in mercury poisoning. Chang and Hartman (1972) noted vacuolation of the dorsal root ganglion cells (DRG) as an early feature and in another study (Chang et al., 1972) they found changes in the state of the RNA. Herman et al. (1973) showed a number of intracellular changes, but the chronicity of the study made it difficult to be sure which change was primary and which was a reactionary response. Jacobs et al. (1975a) found distinct foci of ribosome loss and dispersion as early as 48 hours after beginning a course of 8 daily injections of 5.0 mg/kg Me-HgCl, which was almost a week before the onset of degenerative changes in the peripheral nerves. The areas of ribosomal clearing became more marked both with time and with increased dose to 7.5 mg/kg/day, when neuronal degeneration also occasionally occurred. Severe wallerian degeneration followed these changes in the perikaryon and also followed a striking reduction in the capacity of the tissues to incorporate amino acids into proteins (Cavanagh and Chen, 1971; Omata et al., 1980). Analogous changes were also noted in the cerebrum and in the cerebellum of both rats and rabbits (Jacobs et al., 1976) and it was noteworthy in these latter tissues that in the small neurons all ribosomes were often quite destroyed in the period just before abundant nerve cell necrosis occurred. The conclusions from these studies were that small neurons were probably killed because their content of polyribosomes and rough E.R., being normally very few in amount, were completely destroyed by the entrance of methyl mercury into the cell. Larger cells were able to survive this incursion simply because of their greater original content of these organelles. While there may well be other metabolic lesions in nerve cells caused by the entrance of methyl mercury, this sequence of events seen after relatively high doses of mercury, seemed to provide an explanation for most of the features seen in neurons in methyl mercury poisoning, and at the same time to explain the peculiar selective pathology found. There is the additional factor that puts the sensory nerve cells at greater risk, by comparison with anterior horn cells, for instance, which is the presence of fenestrations (Jacobs et al., 1976b) in the vascular bed of the sensory ganglia which would allow free access to plasma constituents containing methyl mercury directly to the surface of these cells. This lack of protection by a blood-nerve barrier must play as important role here as it undoubtedly does in the systemic toxic neuropathies. Certainly if we are to attempt a rational explanation of the selective vulnerability of the brain regions that are found in Minamata Disease then we must consider the importance of these secondary factors.

LEAD INTOXICATION

The literature of the putative effects of lead on the nervous system is voluminous and difficult to interpret. It only begins to become meaningful if we treat with the problem at two levels of lead body burden. To argue from one experimental system to another, without regard to the doses being given to the animals and the consequence on the blood levels, only leads to confusion of thought. There is no doubt that lead is a toxic ion. It has no role, however, in any known biological system and it, thus, may well interfere with other more important and more metabolically active ions such as calcium. It may well also be toxic by interaction with radicals such as -SH groupings. This we do not yet know, but what do know is that man and experimental animals both show significant pathological changes in nervous tissue when the blood lead levels are raised above 100 µg/dl for any length of time. If blood lead levels remain below this figure, then the classical changes of lead poisoning are not seen, but we are left with a body of evidence derived largely from behavioural studies which suggests that there may be adverse effects on certain regions of brain function. However, it must be stated that not only have these effects not been proven, but even if they do in fact exist their significance is very much in doubt, especially as to their relevance to human behaviour. This is a big toxicological problem and at present we only stand on the threshold of it, for the techniques are difficult to perform and even more difficult to interpret; in view of these facts serious doubts must remain as to the validity of the results of such tests. For the present we will look at the some of the mechanisms underlying the more conventional aspects of lead intoxication for we still have a lot to learn before we can begin to understand even these fairly gross changes. By so doing we may also gain a more balanced attitude towards these putative low-level effects.

Absorption, Transport and Excretion of Lead

Lead tends to follow calcium pathways in the tissues and is absorbed through the same channels as this ion. Calcium and lead compete with each other for facilitated transport mechanisms in the gut (Aungst and Fung, 1981) and for calcium binding protein (Barton et al., 1978). The protein, lipid and iron content of the diet, as well as it's vitamin D content all influence the intake of lead as they do on calcium. Age is also a very important factor for neonatal rats may absorb 50% of a given lead dose by comparison with only 1% in an adult animal (Kostial et al., 1971).

On absorption, lead passes to the blood where 95-99% is bound to the red cell. This binding is loose, however, and is readily reversed by the right conditions (Mortenson and Kellogg, 1944). Lead may have some influence on the $Na^+ + K^+$-ATPase activity of red cells, and may diminish the red cells energy reserves, thereby, leading to mild haemolysis (Joyce et al., 1954). The relationship between brain lead content and blood lead concentration is important (Table 6), and from the numerous careful studies available, it would seem that the relationship is virtually linear, the brain lead rising and falling in parallel with the blood lead changes (Grant et al., 1980; Kimmel et al., 1980; Collins et al., 1982; Mykannen et al., 1982). There is little reason for believing that lead accumulates in brain as we see mercury accumulating, for the two metal ions behave quite differently in every way. The principal sites of storage of lead are in the bones and in the kidneys. Because of the lability of the calcium pools in bones, which may readily respond to stressful situations, the presence of large quantities of lead in bones could act as an ever present threat to the individual.

Effects of High Levels of Lead on Nervous Tissue

By high levels in this context is meant blood concentrations greater than 100 µg/dl sustained over many days or weeks. In animals this is induced by intake in the food of 1000 ppm or more. Below this level of intake it is very doubtful, except perhaps in unusual circumstances, whether any significant structural changes occur in the adult or the neonatal nervous system.

Encephalopathy

With high lead intake, clinical signs of drowsiness, headache, and vomiting coupled with papilloedema and perhaps paralysis of the external recti muscles, are sure signs that cerebral oedema has developed, a state which might easily precipitate seizures. Both the brain swelling itself as well as the fits are capable of producing brain damage with permanent sequelae. The primary brain changes appear to be focal in nature and show themselves as local areas of intense vascular leakiness with petechial haemorrhages (Blackman, 1937; Smith et al., 1960). Similar areas of focal oedema and haemorrhage have been produced in the jersey bull calf by regular dosing with lead salts over 2 to 3 weeks (Wells et al., 1976).

Table 6 . Mean blood and brain concentrations of lead at various times after dosing from conception with lead in the maternal and weaned pups' water
Blood as ug/100 ml. Brain as µg/g tissue, in paren - theses. Variations from animal to animal were considerable (up to 100%). Estimates by atomic absorption spectroscopy (from Grant et al., 1980)

Age	Control	5 ppm	25 ppm	50 ppm	250 ppm
day 11	3(0.01)	13(0.01)	22(0.03)	35(0.07)	-
1 month	6(0.04)	16(0.04)	18(0.11)	48(0.22)	-
2 months	2(0.02)	9(0.06)	29(0.24)	30(0.33)	-
3 months	2(0.03)	10(0.05)	18(0.14)	47(0.18)	-
6 months	4(0.02)	14(0.05)	25(0.10)	37(0.18)	-
9 months	5(0.02)	11(0.03)	21(0.07)	26(0.24)	67(0.67)

There is no evidence for believing that the nerve cells are specifically attacked in the way we have seen, for instance, in mercury poisoning. Unfortunately, brain swelling of this magnitude together with the seizures are likely to lead to permanent sequelae of varying degrees of severity, and these were noted by Byers (1959) and by Perlstein and Attala (1966) in their long-term follow up studies.

There is no doubt that the developing brain is more susceptible to the effects of raised blood lead levels, though the reasons for this are not understood. The experimental model introduced by Pentschew and Garro (1966) makes use of this susceptibility of the rapidly growing cerebellum, which shows very marked vascular and haemorrhagic changes by comparison with the spinal cord and cerebrum of the same animals which show very few lesions. Here again the vascular lesions dominate the pathology and determine in large part the neuron and glial responses. In addition, there is the further factor of diminished maternal food intake due to the lead content and the effects that this also has on the brain growth and the neuronal maturation. Unfortunately, dietary lead even below 1000 ppm which gives blood lead levels of less than 100 ug/dl still produces evidence of general body growth deficiency (Fowler, 1980), and it is not possible, therefore, even at this dose level to be certain of the significance of any changes that there might be in neuronal maturation.

Peripheral Neuropathy

This condition is classically found in adults who have been chronically exposed to lead in the course of their work, e.g. lead painters. Clinically it is not a symmetrical peripheral neuropathy of the type found in other toxic conditions, such as we have seen with thallium and arsenic, by contrast one limb or even part of a limb is involved more than other regions. Also fatigue plays an important part in the occurrence of weakness and wasting (Hunter, 1955). Wrist drop is characteristic among manual workers, but other muscles of the arm are also affected. The few postmortem studies that there are have shown that there is in fact a general nerve involvement but that this is greatest in the part showing the most weakness. There is always marked slowing of the conduction velocity in such subjects.

Experimentally exactly the same patterns of changes are found and the same slowing of the conduction velocity (Fullerton, 1966), the axons showing both denervation as well as segmental demyelination. The most significant change, so far as the pathogenesis of the changes go, is the observation of Ohnishi et al.(1977) in rats given 4% lead in their diet for 3 months or more that there is profound oedema of the nerve which seems to be excessive for the amount of degeneration in progress. It is unclear, however, how much the oedema is responsible for the axon and Schwann cell changes by increasing endoneurial pressure in some way. Nor is it clear how this comes about for the demonstrable increase in permeability of the vascular bed to tracers seems to follow rather than to precede the loss of myelin (Poduslo et al., 1982). Some even believe that the vascular changes are an epiphenomenon. Lead accumulation in the nerve does, however, increase markedly and may be as much as ten times that in the blood (Windebank et al., 1980). One must conclude from the evidence so far that in the nerve, as in the brain, the vascular bed is an important site for the effects of lead, though the details of the actual toxic process on the peripheral nerve have yet to be resolved.

Cellular Mechanisms of Lead Toxicity

We do not yet know how lead adversely affects cells and leads to the changes that we see in lead intoxication. Stumpf et al.(1980) have shown by autoradiography that there is an early tendency for the lead to concentrate in the endothelial cells of the vascular bed of the brain, but the metabolic lesion it produces there is unknown. The effects on general cellular metabolism that have been found are relatively minor and unconvincing as the cause of the changes. It could, however, be capable of displacing calcium ions in some important cellular role or perhaps by binding to -SH groups interfere with some sensitive pathway. These possible actions have yet to be shown and at present we have no real knowledge as to what these might be.

REFERENCES

Aungst,B.J. and Fung,H.-L., 1981, Kinetic characterisation of in vitro lead transport across rat small intestine,Toxicol. Appl.Pharmacol., 61:39

Barton,J.C., Conrad,M.E., Harrison, L. and Nuby,S., 1978, Effects of calcium on the absorption and retention of lead, J.Lab.Clin.Med., 91:366

Blackman,S.S., 1937, The lesions of lead encephalitis in children, Bull.Johns Hopkins Hosp., 61:1

Byers,R.K., 1959, Lead poisoning: a review and report of 45 cases, Pediatrics, 23:585

Cavanagh,J.B. and Chen, F.C.-K., 1971, Amino acid incorporation into protein during the "silent phase" before organomercury and p-bromophenylacetylurea neuropathy in the rat, Acta Neuropathol.(Berl), 19:216

Cavanagh,J.B., Fuller,N.H., Johnson,H.R.M. and Rudge,P., 1974, The effects of thallium salts with particular reference to the nervous system changes, Q.J.Med., 43:293

Cavanagh,J.B. and Gregson, L., 1978, Some effects of a thallium salt on the proliferation of hair follicle cells, J.Pathol., 125:179

Chang,L.W. and Hartmann,H.A., 1972, Ultrastructural studies of the nervous system after methyl mercury poisoning, Acta Neuropathol.(Berl), 20:122

Chang,L.W., Desnoyers,P.A. and Hartmann,H.A., 1972, Quantitative cytochemical studies of RNA in experimental mercury poisoning, J.Neuropathol.Exp.Neurol., 31:489

Collins,M.F., Hrdina,P.D., Whittle,E. and Singal,R.L., 1982, Lead in blood and brain regions of rats chronically exposed to low levels of the metal, Toxicol.Appl.Pharmacol., 65:314

Crecelius,E.A., 1977, Changes in the chemical speciation of arsenic following ingestion in man, Environ.Health Perspect., 19:147

Cavanagh,J.B., 1979, The "dying back" process: a common denominator in many naturally occurring and toxic neuropathies, Arch.Pathol.(Chicago), 103:659

Davis,L.E., Nands,J.R., Weiss, S.A., Price,D.L. and Girling, E.F., 1974, Central Nervous System intoxication from mercurous chloride laxatives, Arch.Neurol(Chicago), 30:428

Enders,A. and Noetzel,H., 1953, Spezifische veranderungen im kleinhirn bei chronischer oraler vergiftung mit sublimat, Arch.Exp.Pathol.Pharmakol., 225:346

Eto,K. and Takeuchi,T., 1977, Pathological changes of human sural nerve in Minamata Disease (Methyl mercury poisoning), Virchows Arch.,B. Cellular Pathology, 23:109

Fowler,B A , Kimmel C.A., Woods,J.G , McConnell E.E. and Grant,L.D., 1980, Chronic low level lead toxicity in the rat. III.An integrated assessment of long term toxicity with special reference to the kidney, Toxicol.Appl.Pharmacol., 56:59

Fullerton.P.M., 1966, Chronic peripheral neuropathy produced by lead poisoning in guinea pigs J.Neuropathol.Exp.Neurol., 25:214

Greving,R. and Gegel,O., 1929, Pathologisch-anatomische befunde und Nervensystem nach experimenteller Thalliumvergiftung Z.Gesamte Neurol.Psychiatrie, 120:805

Gehring,P.C. and Hammond,P., 1967, Mechanisms for the increase in thallium excretion during administration of potassium, Pharmacologist, 8:218P

Gehring,P.C. and Hammond,P., 1967, The interrelationship between thallium and potassium in animals, J.Pharmacol. Exp. Ther., 155:187

Globus,J.H. and Ginsburg,S.W., 1933, Pericapillary encephalorrhagia due to arsphenamine, Arch.Neurol.Psychiatry(Chicago), 30:1226

Glaser,M.A., Immerman,C.P. and Immerman,S.W., 1935, So-called haemorrhagic encephalitis and myelitis secondary to intravenous arsphenamine, Am.J.Med.Sci., 189:64

Grant,L.D., Kimmel,C.A., West,G.L., Martinez-Vargez,C.M. and Howard,J.L., 1980, Chronic low level lead toxicity. II. Effects on the postnatal physical and behavioural development, Toxicol.Appl.Pharmacol., 56:42

Herman,S.P., Klein,R., Talley,F.A. and Krigman,M.R., 1973, An ultrastructural study of methyl mercury induced primary sensory neuropathy, Lab.Invest., 28:104

Hunter,D., 1955, Disease of Occupations, Oxford University Press

Hunter,D. and Russel,D.S., 1954, Focal cerebral and cerebellar atrophy in a human subject due to organic mercury compounds, J.Neurol.Neurosurg.Psychiatry, 17-235

Hunter,D., Bomford,R.R. and Russell,D.S., 1940, Poisoning by methyl mercury compounds, Q.J.Med., 9ns:193

Huston,M.J. and Martin,A.W., 1955, Effect of in vivo administration of dinitrophenol and sodium arsenite on respiration of tissue in contact with oxygen, Arch.Int.Pharmacodyn.Ther. 101:349

Hart,M.M. and Adamson,R.T.H., 1971, Anti-tumour activity and toxicity of salts of inorganic group.IIIa: aluminium, indium, gallium and thallium, Proc.Natl.Acad.Sci.USA, 68:1623

Heyroth,F.F., 1947, Thallium: a review and summary of the medical literature, U.S. Public Health Service, Public Health Rep., Suppl. 147

Hultin,T. and Naslund,P., 1974, Effects of thallium(I) on the structure and function of mammalian ribosomes,Chem.Biol. Interact., 8:315

Jacobs,J.M., Carmichael,N. and Cavanagh,J.B., 1975a, Ultrastructural changes in the dorsal root and trigeminal ganglia of rats poisoned with methyl mercury, Neuropathol. Appl. Neurobiol., 1:1

Jacobs,J.M., Cavanagh,J.B. and Carmichael,N., 1975b, Effects of chronic dosing with mercuric chloride on the dorsal root and trigeminal ganglia in rats, Neuropathol.Appl.Neurobiol., 1:321

Jacobs,J.M., Carmichael,N. and Cavanagh,J.B., 1976a, Ultrastructural changes in the nervous system of rabbits poisoned with methyl mercury, Toxicol.Appl.Pharmacol., 39:249

Jacobs,J.M., McFarlane,R.M. and Cavanagh,J.B., 1976b, Vascular leakage in the dorsal root ganglia of the rat studied with horseradish peroxidase, J.Neurol.Sci., 29:95

Jenkins,R.B., 1966, Inorganic arsenic and the nervous system, Brain, 89:479

Joyce,C.R.B., Moore,H. and Weatherall,M., 1954, The effects of lead, mercury and gold on potassium turnover of rabbit red blood cells, Br.J.Pharmacol., 9:463

Kennedy,P. and Cavanagh,J.B., 1976, Spinal changes in the neuropathy of thallium poisoning: a case with neuropathological studies, J.Neurol.Sci., 29:295

Kimmel,C.A., Grant,L.D., Sloan,C.S. and Gladen,B.C., 1980, Chronic low level lead toxicity in the rat.I.Maternal toxicity and perinatal effects, Toxicol.Appl.Pharmacol., 56:28

Kostial,K., Simonovic,I. and Pisonic,M., 1971, Lead absorption from the intestine in new-born rats, Nature(London), 233:564

Kuhn,R., Rudy,H. and Wagner-Jauregg,T., 1933, Ueber lactoflavin Ber.Deutsche Chemische Ges., 66:1950

LeQuesne,P.M. and McLeod,J.G., 1977, Peripheral neuropathy following a single exposure to arsenic. J.Neurol.Sci, 32:437

Longley,B.J., Clausen,N.M. and Tatum,A.L., 1942, The experimental production of optic atrophy in monkeys by administration of organic arsenic compounds, J.Pharmacol.Exp.Ther.,76:202

Magos,L., 1975, Mercury and mercurials, Br.Med.Bull., 31:241

Mortenson,R.A. and Kellog,K.E., 1944, The uptake of lead by blood cells as measured with a radioactive isotope, J.Comp. Physiol., 23:11

Murphy,M.J., Lyon,L.W. and Taylor,J.W., 1981, Subacute arsenic neuropathy, J.Neurol.Neurosurg.Psychiatry, 44:896

Mykkanen,H.M., Lancaster,M.C. and Dickerson,J.W.T., 1982, Concentration of lead in soft tissues of male rats during a long-term dietary exposure, Environ.Res., 28:147

Ohta,M., 1970, Ultrastructure of the sural nerve in a case of arsenical neuropathy, Acta Neuropathol.(Berl), 16:233

Omata,S., Sakimura,K., Tsubaki,H. and Sugano,H., 1978, In vivo effect of methyl mercury on protein synthesis in brain and liver of the rat, Toxicol.Appl.Pharmacol., 44:367

Ohnishi,A., Schilling,K., Brimijoin,W.S., Lambert,E.H., Fairbanks,V.F. and Dyck,P.J., 1977, Lead neuropathy . I. Morphometry, nerve conduction and acetyl transferase transport : new findings of the endoneurial edema associated with segmental demyelination, J.Neuropathol.Exp.Neurol., 36:499

Paterson,D. and Greenfield,J.G., 1923-1924, Erythroedema polyneuritis (The so-called Pink Disease), Q.J.Med., 17:6

Pentschew,A. and Garro,F., 1966, Lead encephalomyelopathy of the suckling rat and its implications in the porphyrinopathic nervous diseases, Acta Neuropathol.(Berl), 6:266

Pentschew,A. and Garro,F., 1969, Thallium encephalopathy in monkeys, J.Neuropathol.Exp.Neurol., 28:163P

Perlstein,M.A. and Attala,R., 1966, Neurologic sequelae of plumbism in children, Clin.Pediat., 5:292

Poduslo,J.F., Low,P.A., Windebank,A.J., Dyck,P.J., Berg,C.J. and Schmelzer,J.D., 1982, Altered blood-nerve barrier in experimental lead neuropathy assessed by changes in endoneurial albumen concentrations, J.Neurosci., 2:1507

Reed,D., Crawley,J., Faro,S.N., Pieper,S.J. and Kurland,L.T., 1963, Thallotoxicosis : acute manifestations and sequelae , J.Am.Med.Assoc., 183:515

Reynolds,E.S., 1901, An account of the epidemic outbreak of arsenical poisoning occurring in beer drinkers in the North of England and the Midlands in 1900, Lancet i:166

Scharrer,E., 1933, Histologische befunde in Zentralnervensystem bei Thalliumvergiftung, Z.Gesamte Neurol.Psychiatrie. 145:454

Schoer,J., 1984, Thallium, in "Handbook of Environmental Chemistry", O.Hutzinger,ed.,vol.3,part C, Springer-Verlag , Berlin

Smith,J.F., McLaurin,R.L., Nichols,J.R. ans Asbury,A., 1960, Studies in cerebral oedema and cerebral swelling.I. The changes in lead encephalopathy in children compared with those in alkyltin poisoning in animals, Brain, 83:411

Spencer,P.S., Peterson,E.R., Madrid,R.A. and Raine,C.S., 1973, Effects of thallium salts on neuronal mitochondria in organotypic cord-ganglion-muscle cultures,J.Cell Biol.,59:79

Stumpf,W.E., Sar,M. and Grant,L.D., 1980, Autoradiographic localisation of ^{210}Pb and its decay products in rat forebrain, Neurotoxicology, 1:593

Takeuchi,T., Morikawa,N., Matsumoto,H. and Shiraishi,Y., 1962, A pathological study of Minamata Disease in Japan , Acta Neuropathol.(Berl), 2:40

Truhaut,R., 1959, Recherches sur la toxicologie du thallium, Institut National Securite' pour la Prevention des Accidents de Travail, Paris

Va'konen,S., Savolainen,H. and Jarvisolo,J., 1983, Arsenic distributions and neurochemical effects in peroral sodium arsenite exposure of rats,Bull.Environ.Contam.Toxicol.,30:303

Webb,J.L., 1966, Enzyme and Metabolic Inhibitors, vol.iii, Academic press, New York

Wells,G.A.H., Howell,J.M.C. and Gopinath,C., 1976, Experimental lead encephalopathy in calves. Histological observations on the nature and distributions of the lesions, Neuropathol. Appl.Neurobiol., 2:605

Weston Hurst,E., 1955, The lesions produced in the central nervous system by certain organic arsenical compounds , J.Pathol.Bacteriol., 77:523

Windebank,A.J., McCall,J.T., Hunder,H.G. and Dyck,P.J., 1980, The endoneurial content of lead related to onset and severity of segmental demyelination, J.Neuropathol.Exp.Neurol., 39:692

Zook,B.C. and Gilmore,C.E., 1967, Thallium poisoning in dogs, J.Am.Vet.Med.Assoc., 151:204

Zook,B.C., Holdsworth,J. and Thornton,G.W., 1968, Thallium poisoning in cats, J.Am.Vet.Med.Assoc., 153:285

ORGANOPHOSPHORUS COMPOUNDS

Lucio G. Costa

Department of Environmental Health, SC-34
University of Washington
Seattle, Washington 98195, U.S.A.

Organophosphorus insecticides account for some 40% of the registered pesticides in the United States and their world market, already in the order of $1.5 billion, is projected to increase (Ecobichon, 1982a). Several books and reviews have been published on their chemistry, metabolism, toxicology and mechanism of action (O'Brien, 1960; 1967; Heath, 1961; Koelle, 1963; Casida, 1964; Karczmar et al., 1970; O'Brien and Yamamoto, 1970; Eto, 1974; Matsumura, 1975; Hayes, 1975; 1982; Wilkinson, 1976; Murphy, 1980; Aldridge, 1981). Organophosphorus compounds have diverse effects on both the central and peripheral nervous system (Davies, 1963; Davis and Richardson, 1980; Ecobichon, 1982b). Most of them are due to inhibition of acetylcholinesterase, the enzyme which hydrolizes the neurotransmitter acetylcholine. The biochemical mechanisms of acute cholinergic poisoning have been examined in many reviews and will be only briefly discussed. On the other hand, other aspects of the nervous system toxicity of organophosphates, such as their potential noncholinergic interactions, will be discussed in more detail.

HISTORICAL DEVELOPMENT OF ORGANOPHOSPHATES

Shortly before World War II, German chemists, urged to decrease the cost of importing nicotine and rotenone, developed the first organophosphates for use as insecticides. The first organophosphate insecticide used was tetraethylpyrophosphate (TEPP), which was soon abandoned because its chemical instability. In 1944 Gerhard Schrader synthetized parathion which had a wide range of insecticidal activities and low volatility and was rather stable in water. Parathion has been extensively used in agriculture and, although many less acutely toxic insecticides have been later developed, it is still one of the five most used organophosphates in the United States (Lerman et al., 1984). Together with insecticidal organophosphates, related extremely toxic compounds such as sarin and tabun were secretly developed in those years. Their high volatility and toxicity made them potentially suitable as chemical warfare agents. These compounds have been called "nerve gases", because their effects are predominantly on the nervous system. Some organophosphorus esters have also found useful applications as flame retardants, fuel additives, plasticizers and lubricants (Fisher and Van Wazer, 1961).

CHEMISTRY

The term organophosphate is used generically to indicate toxic organic compounds containing phosphorus. The nature of the atoms attached to the phosphorus allows a first subdivision of organophosphates; the names of the basic structures of organophosphorus compounds are given in Figure 1. Although this nomenclature, which was the result of an Anglo-American agreement reached in 1952 (Anonymous, 1952), is now followed by most scientists, several compounds are referred to with a variety of chemical names. In particular, when the side chains attached to the phosphorus are very complex, the naming of the side chain has often priority on the basic chemical moiety.

PHYSICAL AND CHEMICAL REACTIVITY

Factors that can alter or modify the structure of organophosphorus compounds are light, temperature, air and solvents (Dauterman, 1971). Ultraviolet light can be responsible for oxidations, isomerizations and hydrolysis. For example, parathion can be converted by UV light to paraoxon and S-ethyl parathion, while chlorpyrifos is hydrolized, in the presence of water, to 3,5,6-trichlo-2-pyridinol (Dauterman, 1971). Temperature is also known to cause isomerization while exposure to air, in the absence of UV light, can oxidize the P=S group to P=O. The S-side chain isomers, formed during the synthesis of phosphorothionate at elevated temperature, are usually their major contaminants and are responsible for the unpleasant odor and the direct anticholinesterase activity.

Various solvents have effects on the stability and toxicity of organophosphorus compounds. All organophosphates can be hydrolized and the rate of hydrolysis is directly related to the alkalinity. In fact, the mechanism of hydrolysis involves an attack on the phosphorus by an OH^-, i.e. a nucleophilic attack of a negatively charged group OH^- on the relatively positive site, the phosphorus (O'Brien, 1967). The more positive the site, the more effective is the attack. The rate of hydrolysis is determined by the properties of the group attached to the phosphorus which, by being more or less electrophylic, can make the phosphorus more or less positive. For example, since =O is more electrophylic than =S, paraoxon is 22-fold more susceptible to hydrolysis than parathion (O'Brien, 1967). Hydrolysis with a strong base is common laboratory procedure for inactivating organophosphates before their proper disposal.

BASIC STRUCTURES OF ORGANOPHOSPHORUS COMPOUNDS

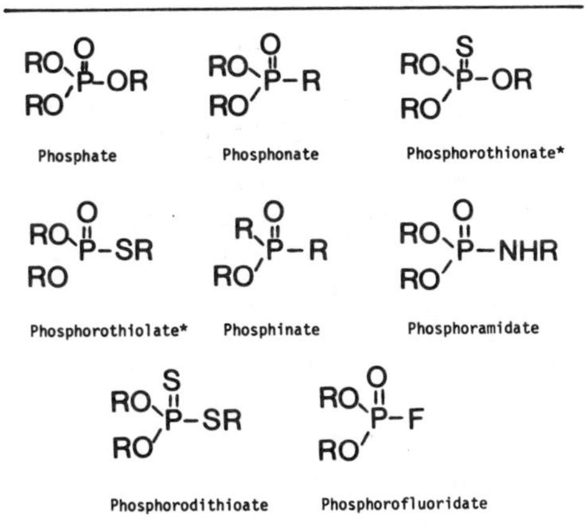

* Many authors do not distinguish a thiono sulfur,=S, from a thiolo sulfur,-S-, and refer to both these types as phosphorothioates.

Figure 1

METABOLISM

The metabolism of organophosphates has been extensively investigated and has been the subject of several reviews. In addition to various chapters in the books mentioned in the introduction, reviews by Fukuto and Metcalf (1969), Dauterman (1971), Ahmad and Forgash (1976), Kulkarni and Hodgson (1980), and Motoyama and Dauterman (1980) have covered different aspects of the biotransformation of organophosphates.

Organophosphate metabolism is usually divided into activative and degradative (O'Brien, 1967), the former being that which converts a compound from a poorer to a stronger anticholinesterase and the latter, the reverse. The four major reactions which activate an organophosphate are: oxidative desulfuration (conversion of P=S to P=O); thioether oxidation (formation of a sulfoxide, S=O, followed by the formation of a sulfone, O=S=O); hydroxylation; and cyclization (Figure 2). These reactions are catalyzed by a group of enzymes called mixed-function oxidases which are present in the microsomal fraction of liver and other tissues and utilize the coenzyme reduced nicotinamide adenine dinucleotide phosphate (NADPH) and molecular oxygen. The oxidative desulfuration of parathion and many other organophosphates has been demonstrated in insect, plants and mammals both in vitro and after in vivo administration (Dauterman, 1971). In mammals, it occurs primarily in the liver, however, extrahepatic activation, such as in lung and brain tissue (Norman and Neal, 1976) may play an important role in organophosphate toxicity. Certain compounds, such as disulfoton, in addition to undergoing oxidative desulfuration, are also subject of oxidation of the thioether moiety to the correspective sulfoxide and sulfone. Both metabolites are more potent inhibitors of acetylcholinesterase than the parent compound (Metcalf et al., 1957; Bull, 1965). The flavin adenine dinucleotide (FAD)-dependent monooxygenase in mammalian hepatic microsomes plays a major role in the oxidation of disulfoton to its corresponding sulfox-

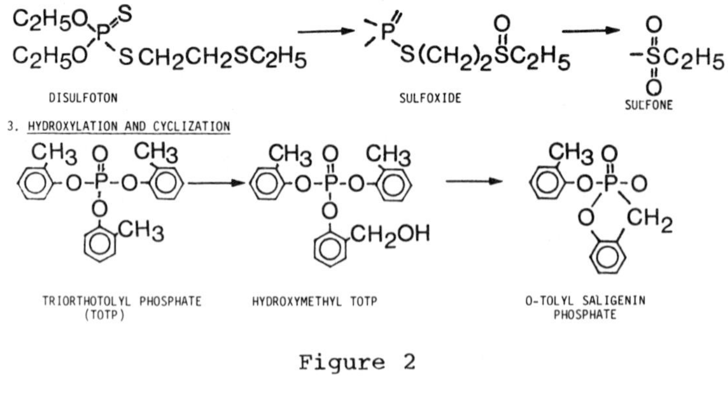

Figure 2

ide, but not to the sulfone (Hajjar and Hodgson, 1980). Recently, a flavin containing monooxygenase activity catalyzing the formation of sulfoxides has been identified in microsomes from rat corpus striatum (Duffel and Gillespie, 1984).

The compound triorthotolylphosphate (TOTP) is activated by hydroxylation on the o-methyl group to form hydroxymethyl TOTP. This intermediate is cyclized to form o-tolyl saligenin phosphate which is the metabolite responsible for the delayed neurotoxic effects of TOTP (Eto et al., 1967). These reactions are catalyzed by hepatic mixed function oxidases but plasma albumin can also act as a catalyst in cyclization of TOTP (Eto et al., 1967).

Many biochemical reactions lead to a decrease in the toxicity of organophosphates. These detoxication reactions are summarized in Figure 3. Oxidative dearylation and O-dealkylation occur with several organophosphates; an oxidative N-dealkylation catalyzed by mixed function oxidases has also been reported; this reaction can result in an increase, decrease or little change in toxicity (Dauterman, 1971). Diisopropylfluorophosphate (DFP) was the first organophosphorus compound for which the enzymatic hydrolysis of the P-F bond was demonstrated (Mazur, 1946). This "DFP-ase" also hydrolizes some structurally similar compounds, such as Tabun and Sarin (Hoskin, 1971). Paraoxonase is a serum and tissue esterase which hydrolizes paraoxon (Aldridge, 1953) and has generated great interest in the past decades since its activity in the human population is bimodally distributed, genetically determined and interethnically variable (Playfer et al., 1976). Carboxyamidases have been implicated in the metabolism of a number of organophosphorus insecticides containing carboxyamide groups such as dimethoate or dicrotophos (Dauterman, 1971). Carboxylesterase plays a major role in the detoxication of malathion in mammals and its rather selective insecticidal action is due to a relative lack of these hydrolytic enzymes in insects (Murphy, 1980). Inhibition of this detoxication pathway by another organophosphate greatly potentiates the toxicity of malathion (Murphy, 1969). Various insecticides can be detoxified by glutathione S-transferases (Motoyama and Dauterman, 1980). These enzymes are present in multiple forms and in extrahepatic tissues including the brain (Das et al., 1981; Costa and Murphy, 1984a), and appear to be a major metabolic pathway *in vivo* for the methoxy compounds, such as methylchlorpyrifos, fenithrothion or methyl parathion (Motoyama and Dauterman, 1980).

SITE OF ACTION

It is generally recognized that the biological activity of organophosphorus insecticides is due to their reaction with the enzyme acetylcholinesterase (AChE) and other cholinesterases. As mentioned in a previous section, organophosphates can be hydrolyzed by a mechanism involving an attack on the phosphorus by OH ions. A similar

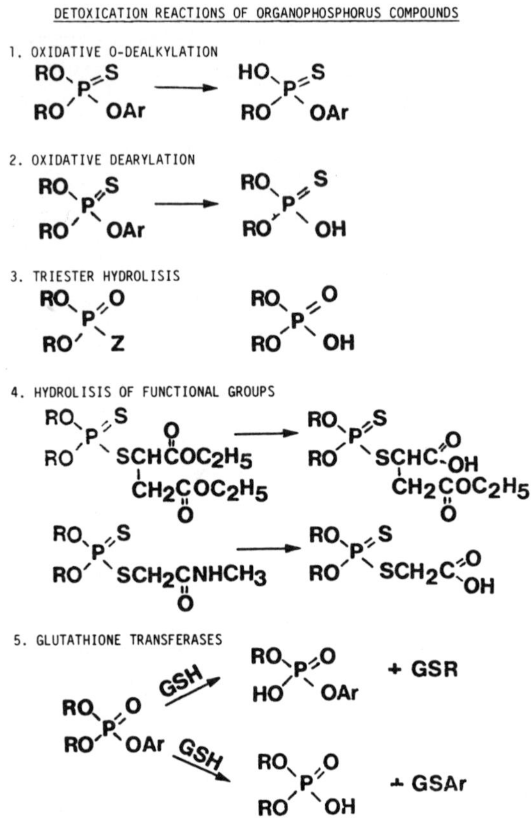

Figure 3

reaction occurs when an OH group on a serine residue in the cholinesterase reacts with the organophosphate (O'Brien, 1967). The serine involved is at the active site of cholinesterase and is essential for the functioning of the enzyme. The overall reaction can be schematically described as:

$$E + IX \underset{k_{-1}}{\overset{k_1}{\longrightarrow}} (EI)^R \underset{X^-}{\overset{k_2}{\longrightarrow}} (RI)^I$$

where E and I represent free enzyme and inhibitor, respectively. $(EI)^R$ is a reversible enzyme-inhibitor complex and $(EI)^I$ is the irreversibly phosphorylated enzyme. The formation of the complex is regulated by an affinity constant Ka (equal to k_{-1}/k_1), while k_2 is the phosphorylation constant, Kp (Main, 1964). The phosphorylated enzyme can undergo a further reaction:

$$(EI)^I \xrightarrow[H_2O]{k_3} E + I^-$$

which reactivates the enzyme. The most critical step for organophosphates is k_3, which is very low, so that $(EI)^I$ accumulates and the enzyme can be considered almost irreversibly inhibited (see O'Brien, 1967; Aldridge, 1971 and Karczmar et al., 1970 for more details on the mechanisms and kinetics of cholinesterase inhibition). The spontaneous reactivation of cholinesterase after inhibition by an organophosphate is very slow. However, great differences exist among organophosphates both *in vitro* and after *in vivo* administration (Karczmar et al. 1970). For example, the rate of reactivation *in vitro* for mouse brain and diaphragm cholinesterase after *in vivo* inhibition, was five to ten times greater for methylparathion and azinphosmethyl than for their ethyl analogs (Levine and Murphy, 1977).

Certain chemicals are able to accelerate the hydrolysis of the phosphorylated enzyme to regenerate active AChE. The reactivator in most common use is 2-PAM (2-pyridine aldoxime methiodide; pralidoxime) which is the treatment of choice for organophosphorus poisoning. The rate of reactivation by oximes is also dependent upon the chemical nature of the organophosphate. The diethoxy-phosphorylated enzyme is readily reactivated while diisopropoxy-phosphorylated cholinesterase is somewhat resistant to reactivation by oximes (Kerczmar et al., 1970; Murphy, 1980). With certain organophosphates a phenomenon occurs, called "aging", which is a process in which the inhibited enzyme becomes refractory to reactivation. The term aging has been applied to this process since the amount of inhibited (phosphorylated) enzyme refractory to reactivation increases with time. The rate of aging depends on the phosphoryl group but not on the leaving group and the process involves a dealkylation (Karczmar et al., 1970). When aging occurs, recovery of cholinesterase activity is dependent solely on synthesis of new enzyme molecules.

SIGNS AND SYMPTOMS OF ORGANOPHOSPHATE POISONING

Acetylcholine is a major neurotransmitter in the central and peripheral nervous system. Unlike other neurotransmitters, such as norepinephrine or GABA, which have more than one way to be removed from the synaptic cleft, acetylcholine is entirely dependent upon AChE for its inactivation. Hence, inhibition of AChE by an organophosphate causes a rapid accumulation of acetylcholine at cholinergic synapses. Signs and symptoms of acute poisoning with an organophosphorus insecticide, summarized in Table 1, may be classified into muscarinic (parasympathetic), nicotinic (sympathetic and motor) and central nervous system manifestations, according to the site of action (Namba et al., 1971). The time interval between the exposure and onset of symptoms varies with the route and degree of exposure and the chemical nature of the organophosphate.

Table 1

Peripheral Signs and Symptoms of Organophosphate Poisoning

1.	Muscarinic manifestations	
	Gastrointestinal system	Nausea, vomiting, abdominal tightness and cramps, diarrhea, tenesmus fecal incontinence
	Exocrine glands	Increased lacrimation, salivation and sweating
	Eyes	Miosis, blurring of vision
	Bladder	Urinary frequency and incontinence
	Respiratory tract	Increased bronchial secretion, bronchospasm and bronchoconstriction, cough, dyspnea, tightness in the chest
	Cardiovascular system	Bradycardia, decrease in blood pressure
2.	Nicotinic manifestations	
	Skeletal muscles	Muscle twitching, fasciculation, cramps, diminished tendon reflexes, weakness in peripheral and respiratory muscles, paralysis, flaccid or rigid tone
	Sympathetic ganglia	Tachycardia, pallor, increase in blood pressure

From: Namba et al. (1971) and Ecobichon (1982b).

According to a recent retrospective study on 236 patients acutely poisoned with organophosphates, more than 90% of the cases showed peripheral muscarinic symptoms (Hirshberg and Lerman, 1984; Lerman, et al., 1984). Among these, miosis was the most prevalent specific sign. Forty percent of the patients had CNS symptoms but only 17% presented a combination of muscarinic, nicotinic and CNS signs. Since only 15% of all cases were judged to be severe, that is, the patients required assisted ventilation, it appears that all symptoms and signs described in Table 1, are present only in severe poisoning (Lerman et al., 1984).

The central nervous system effects of organophosphates may result from an action of acetylcholine on brain muscarinic and nicotinic receptors and from the possible interactions with other neurotransmitter and neuropeptide systems. The central cholinergic system is involved in a variety of physiological and behavioral functions. Reviews on the role of cholinergic transmission in behavior have been published by Russell (1969; 1978; 1982), Karczmar (1969; 1975), Bignami (1976), Seiden and Dykstra (1977) and Aquilonius (1977), to cite only a few. Cholinergic mechanisms play an important role in memory (Deutsch, 1973; Moss and Deutsch, 1975; Davis and Yamamura, 1978), in mental disorders and various neuropsychiatric syndromes (Weiss et al., 1976; Davis et al., 1978a), sleep (Jouvet, 1975), temperature regulation (Clark and Clark, 1980) and central regulation of cardiovascular (Philippu, 1981) and respiratory (Brimblecombe, 1977) functions. Innumerable studies in experimental animals have investigated the effects of cholinergic stimulation, via a direct acting cholinergic agonist or a cholinesterase inhibitor, on various biochemical, physiological and behavioral functions. The relevance of some of these studies to the CNS effects of organophosphates have been recently reviewed (Karczmar, 1984). Table 2 lists the effects of acute poisoning with organophosphates on CNS functions as summarized by various reports on human intoxication. These effects usually disappear within a few days or weeks in coincidence with the gradual recovery of cholinesterase activity. Following acute poisoning, however, delayed effects are often observed. The time-lapse between what seems to be a recovery from the acute poisoning to the appearance of the delayed effects can vary from a few days to months. These delayed effects, are commonly limited to the central nervous system but might include ventricular arrhythmias (Kiss and Fazekas, 1979) and also death (Lerman et al., 1984). Certain phosphorothioates (for example O,O,S-trimethyl phosphorothioate) can cause a delayed toxic effect, apparently noncholinergic in nature, which is characterized by progressive weight loss and significant liver damage (Hammond et al., 1982). Hirshberg and Lerman (1984) observed that EEG abnormalities (diffuse delta and theta activity) and neuropsychiatric symptoms (depression, confusion, agitation, insomnia, motor weakness) were still present up to three months after acute poisoning.

Table 2

Effects of acute poisoning with organophosphates on CNS functions

Anxiety	Giddiness
Apathy	Headache
Cheney-Stoke respiration	Hypothermia
Confusion	Impaired ability to concentrate
Convulsions	Indifference to the environment
Depersonalization	Irritability
Depression of respiratory and circulatory centers	Restlessness
Drowsiness	Tension
Emotional lability	Tremors
Excessive dreaming	Slowness of recall
Generalized weakness	Slurred speech

From: Grob and Harvey, 1953; Dille and Smith, 1964; Bowers et al., 1964; Namba et al., 1971; Karczmar, 1984.

the central nervous system. A study showing that administration of acetylcholine to schizophrenic patients had improved their condition (Fiamberti, 1946), led Rowntree et al. (1950) to test DFP in 17 cases of schizophrenic and nine cases of manic depressive psychosis. However, in six schizophrenics the psychosis was activated by repeated DFP administration and the patients' general mental status was aggravated instead of improved. A correlation between chronic organophosphate exposure and psychiatric disorders was later reproposed by Gershon and Shaw (1961) in a paper describing a series of central nervous system effects (summarized in Table 3), which they found in 16 workers exposed for 1.5 to 10 years to organophosphorus insecticides. The most persistent symptoms were schizophrenic and depressive reactions, severe memory impairment and difficulty in concentration. This paper, which claimed to have established a connection, if not a casual relationship, between exposure to organophosphorus insecticides and the development of psychiatric disturbances, generated much concern and controversy. Particularly, the choice of the title "Psychiatric sequelae of chronic exposure to organophosphorus insecticides" led J.M. Barnes to comment that".....surely it is incumbent upon both authors and journals to take more care at least in choosing the title of their papers if it is felt necessary to publish observation of doubtful significance"(Barnes, 1961).

Table 3

Effects of organophosphates on the central nervous system

Impaired Memory	Impaired Concentration
Severe Depression	Nightmares
Schizophrenic Reactions	Paranoia
Headache	Apathy
Irritability	Somnambulism
Fatigue	Speech Difficulties
Auditory Hallucinations	Aggression
Dullness	

From: Gershon and Shaw (1961).

In the same year three letters to the editor were published in The Lancet criticizing the study (Barnes, 1961; Bidstrup, 1961; Golz, 1961). Two other studies, a few years later, were also critical of Gershon and Shaw's report (Stoller et al. 1965; Durham et al. 1965). The main criticisms regarded a lack of information on the degree of organophosphate exposure, since no blood cholinesterase levels were reported and that only four cases were described in more detail. Also, the alleged conclusion that organophosphates activate a tendency towards schizophrenic or depressive illness was confuted, and clinical and epidemiological studies were reported, which showed no association between organophosphates and such psychiatric disorders (Bidstrup, 1961; Stoller, 1965; Durham, 1965).

Although this particular study (Gershon and Shaw, 1961) might have overstated its conclusions, there are many other reports in the literature describing the effects of chronic organophosphate exposure on the central nervous system. Holmes and Gaon (1957) reported that 25 of 600 patients with acute poisoning had persistent symptoms including confusion, decreased mental concentration, instability and forgetfulness, whereas the main features in a group of 37 cases of multiple exposure were forgetfulness and irritability. Dille and Smith (1964) reported on two cases of aerial-applicator pilots with a long history of exposure to organophosphates. Their main symptoms were anxiety, uneasiness, depression, dizziness and emotional lability. In a study of 56 workers chronically exposed to organophosphates, Metcalf and Holmes (1969) found various electroencephalographic, neurologic and psychologic alterations. One of the main symptoms was forgetfulness, reported by 53% of the patients (Table 4). Memory defects had been also observed by Gershon and Shaw (1961). On the other hand, Korsak and Sato (1977) failed to find any memory impairment in 59 organophosphate-exposed workers. The same patients, however, showed significant deficits in performance of various neuro-

Table 4

Comparison of Control and Exposure Groups*

Symptoms Reported on Psychiatric Interviews

	CONTROL GROUP		EXPOSURE GROUP	
	Number Reporting Symptom (N = 22)		Number Reporting Symptom (N = 56)	
Irritable and impatient	11	50%	35	60%
Forgetfulness	5	20%	29	53%
General fatigue	1	5%	19	35%
Change in sexual desire - decrease	6	25%	14	23%
Increased dreaming	4	18%	10	18%
Trouble sleeping	2	10%	5	10%
Difficulty in thinking tasks	1	5%	6	12%
Lethargy, "Don't give a damn"	0	0%	4	7%
GI distress	7	30%	11	21%
Visual difficulty	0	0%	14	30%
Headaches	2	10%	7	14%
Muscular aches and pains	0	0%	6	12%
Increased perspiration	0	0%	2	4%

*Average: 38.3 years; average time of employment: 77.68 months or 6.47 years.

Adapted from: D.R. Metcalf and J.H. Holmes, Ann. N.Y. Acad. Sci. 160, 357 (1969).

psychological tests which the authors attributed to dysfunction of the left frontal brain hemisphere. They also suggested that organophosphate exposure might be another etiologic factor in the production of the minimal brain dysfunction syndrome in children (Korsak and Sato, 1977). Although there are no other solid data to validate such a hypothesis, developing organisms are undoubtedly at high risk for possible deleterious effects of organophosphates, in particular because of the higher susceptibility of the developing nervous system to external insult, and the presence of underdeveloped detoxifying mechanisms. It is therefore surprising that a review of the literature indicated that studies on the effects of pre- and post-natal developmental exposure to organophosphates on the nervous system are very few and inconclusive.

Depression and anxiety were among the CNS symptoms present in 38 patients with chronic organophosphate poisoning (Perold and Bezuidenhout, 1980). Anxiety was also the major behavioral symptom in two other groups of workers chronically exposed to organophosphates (Levin, 1974; Levin et al., 1976). One study (Davis et al., 1978b) reports on the development of parkinsonism in a 48 year old patient with a history of chronic organophosphate exposure. The authors suggested the existence of a possible relationship between chronic organophosphate exposure and alterations in central cholinergic or dopaminergic activity, but also prudently indicated that the patient's parkinsonism and chronic exposure to organophosphates may have been coincidental.

EEG abnormalities have been reported by several investigators after acute or chronic exposure to organophosphates. In many cases these EEG changes were still present six months to one year following cessation of exposure (Metcalf and Holmes, 1969; Dille and Smith, 1964; Holmes and Gaon, 1957). A study in monkeys receiving either one symptomatic exposure or a series of subclinical exposures to sarin, revealed the presence of alterations in the EEG frequency spectrum for up to a year (Burchfiel et al., 1976). A subsequent study in workers occupationally exposed to the same organophosphate, found similar EEG changes (particularly increase in beta activity) as well as disturbances in REM sleep (Duffy et al., 1979). Alteration of EEG was also observed in rats fed the organophosphate malathion for three months (Farkas et al., 1976).

A target particularly sensitive to the toxicity of organophosphorus compounds is the visual system. Apart from acute symptoms (e.g. miosis, blurred vision) several other long lasting effects have been reported after acute or chronic exposure. Chronic exposure to organophosphates produces pathological changes in the ciliary muscle and in the optic nerve of both animals and humans (Uga et al., 1977; Ishikawa, 1973) and can cause the development of myopia (Ishikawa and Miyata, 1980). A single exposure to an organophosphate in rats can cause abnormalities of the electroretinogram persisting for more than two months (Imai, 1975), and decreases in retinal sensitivity have been reported in human following chronic organophosphate exposure (Ohto, 1974). A recent study reported functional and histological changes in chronically fenthion-exposed rats (Imai et al., 1983). Blurred vision, discomfort while reading and photophobia were the main symptoms in a group of farm workers, four months after an acute exposure to mephinvos and phosphamidon (Whorton and Obrinsky, 1983). Another recent study (Misra et al., 1982) reported visual impairment (night blindness, black dots in front of the eyes, blurring vision) and macular degeneration in workers exposed for several years to organophosphates.

Certain organophosphates such as paraoxon can produce a dose-dependent necrosis in rat skeletal muscle (Wecker and Dettbarn, 1976).

This myopathy can be prevented by transection of the given motor nerve and can be markedly modified by hemicholinium, suggesting that the muscle fiber necrosis is the result of excessive acetylcholine (Fenichel et al., 1972). For this subacute myopathy to occur, AChE activity has to be inhibited by at least 85% over a period of two hours (Wecker et al., 1978).

TOLERANCE TO ORGANOPHOSPHATES

During a chronic feeding study with the organophosphorus insecticide parathion, Barnes and Denz (1951) noticed that rats had clearly diminished signs of toxicity after two months on the diet. Although animals in this group failed to gain as much weight as controls, and occasionally still had tremors, severity of other signs (which included fasciculation, lacrimation and salivation) continued to diminish during the third month of feeding, and were virtually absent during the remainder of the year that the rats were exposed. This and several other studies confirmed that the development of tolerance, as evidenced by marked decreases and disappearance of a behavioral and physiological symptoms of toxicity, after chronic treatment with organophosphates, is a reproducible phenomenon and does not depend upon the organophosphate used, the route of administration or the animal species (Bignami et al., 1975; Clark, 1971; Russell et al., 1975; Costa et al., 1982a). On the other hand, the development of tolerance is dependent upon certain factors such as the dose of the organophosphate, the sex and other genetic variables and the behavioral test utilized (Bignami et al., 1975; Russell, 1982; Russell et al., 1983).

Most of these studies have employed high doses or dietary concentrations of organophosphates that initially produced the typical cholinergic signs of toxicity. From a practical standpoint it is, however, important to determine whether tolerance would develop in the absence of an initial period of signs of acute toxicity. In fact, if workers were exposed on a regular basis to these compounds and if they developed signs of acute toxicity they would, it is hoped, interrupt their exposure. However, if they escaped acute signs, they might not interrupt exposure and might ultimately develop tolerance (Murphy et al., 1982). Development of tolerance in the absence of acute signs of toxicity was demonstrated in rats repeatedly injected with a low dose of DFP (Chippendale et al., 1972) or fed the insecticide disulfoton for two months (Schwab and Murphy, 1981). These observations suggest that tolerance might be inducible under exposure conditions that could prevail in an occupational setting. Tolerance to organophosphates can develop in humans as well (Sumerford et al., 1953; DeRoeth et al., 1965). A tolerance to the effects of anticholinesterase compounds is also observed in patients treated for myasthenia gravis (Munsat, 1984).

Since AChE activity was highly inhibited and acetylcholine levels were elevated in brain from organophosphate-tolerant animals (Bombinski and DuBois, 1958), it was suggested that tolerance permitted animals to tolerate higher concentrations of acetylcholine at neuroeffector sites. Experiments demonstrating subsensitivity of various behavioral and physiological effects of cholinergic agonists in organophosphate-tolerant animals led to the hypothesis that a refractoriness of cholinergic receptors to acetylcholine might be involved in the development of tolerance (Brodeur and DuBois, 1964; Russell et al, 1975; and references in Costa et al., 1982a). Decreases in the density of muscarinic cholinergic receptors have been found in the brain and some peripheral organs of organophosphate-tolerant animals (Costa et al. 1981; Ehlert et al. 1980; and references in Costa et al., 1982a). These alterations of cholinergic receptors are probably responsible for the development of tolerance and subsensitivity to cholinergic agonists, however, other mechanisms might be also involved in this phenomenon. For example, pre-synaptic muscarinic receptors involved in the release of acetylcholine may be modified in tolerant animals (Raiteri et al., 1981; Russell et al., 1981). No receptor alterations were found in cardiac tissue of organophosphate-tolerant animals, in spite of a subsensitivity to agonists, suggesting the existence of other mechanisms distal to ligand recognition sites or removed from the receptor complex (Schwab et al., 1983). Furthermore, in studies on the development of tolerance to behavioral effects of organophosphates, there is evidence of a behaviorally augmented component, when animals are treated and tested on a chronic basis (Bignami et al., 1975; Giardini et al., 1982).

Tolerance might, on one hand, be considered a protective mechanism by which the organism normalizes function despite challenge from the external environment. However, the possibility that the biochemical modifications involved in this process might alter certain brain functions and/or the response to other external agents should be considered. For example, while the response to cholinergic agonist is decreased, a pharmacological supersensitivity to antagonists has been described in chronic organophosphate-treated animals (Chippendale et al., 1972; Russell et al., 1971; Fernando et al., 1984a). This poses the potential for an exaggerated reaction to atropine or to other compounds able to interact with the muscarinic receptor, such as antidepressants or neuroleptics. Furthermore, it has been shown that while the toxic effects of an organophosphate are diminished following chronic exposure to the same compound, cross-tolerance to other insecticides is not always present. For example, animals tolerant to the organophosphate disulfoton were cross-tolerant to chlorpyrifos but more sensitive than controls to the toxicity of malathion and of the carbamate propoxur (2-isopropoxy-phenyl-methylcarbamate; Costa and Murphy, 1983).

A decreased density of muscarinic receptors is present in the striatum of chronically organophosphate-treated animals (Ehlert et al., 1980; Costa and Murphy, 1982). Recently, Olianas et al. (1984) showed that chronic AChE inhibition by DFP reduced the capacity of acetylcholine to inhibit basal and dopamine-stimulated adenylate cyclase activity in homogenates from rat striatum. Since in vivo a fraction of the dopamine-sensitive adenylate cyclase may be tonically inhibited by muscarinic imput, chronic organophosphate exposure should theoretically result in facilitation of dopaminergic transmission at the level of adenylate cyclase (Olianas et al., 1984). Interestingly, symptoms of central dopaminergic hyperactivity, such as schizoaffective disorders have been observed in human following chronic organophosphate exposure (see previous section).

Memory deficits in aged animals have been associated with a decreased number of brain muscarinic receptors (Lippa et al., 1980). Since forgetfulness and memory impairment had been reported in workers chronically exposed to organophosphates (Metcalf and Holmes, 1969; Gershon and Shaw, 1961) and a decreased density of muscarinic receptors is present in brain from organophosphate-tolerant animals (Costa et al., 1982a), a few studies investigated if tolerant animals would exhibit memory impairment in a passive-avoidance test. Reiter et al. (1973) and Costa and Murphy (1982) did not find any alteration in retention in a one-trial passive avoidance test in animals repeatedly treated with parathion and disulfoton, respectively. On the other hand, rats made tolerant to DFP were reported to have a reduced retention of a passive avoidance response as compared to controls (Gardner et al., 1984). The reasons for this discrepancy are not apparent and need to be further investigated.

In conclusion, while it is tempting to think of tolerance to anticholinesterases as a protective phenomenon or an annoying loss of therapeutic action, possible harmful sequelae cannot be ruled out. Further work on one of the mechanisms postulated (cholinergic receptor loss) and others not yet elucidated certainly warranted to make interpretation of the biological significance of tolerance more precise.

NON-CHOLINERGIC EFFECTS OF ORGANOPHOSPHATES

Although inhibition of AChE is considered the main mechanism of action of organophosphates and cholinergic intoxication is the cause of acute toxicity and death, there is growing evidence that these compounds may have actions independent of cholinesterase inhibition and/or that cholinesterase inhibition may lead to interactions with systems other than the cholinergic (O'Neill, 1981). For example, DFP and Sarin have been shown to cause EEG desynchronization and subsequent EEG seizures in the rabbit, which could not be solely attributed to accumulation of acetylcholine (Van Meter et al., 1978).

The remainder of this chapter will discuss some of such non-cholinergic effects of organophosphates. Some of these interactions may offer an explanation for effects such as the delayed neurotoxicity induced by certain organophosphates, or the potent convulsant activity of bicyclic phosphorus esters. Some interactions, in particular those with other neurotransmitter systems and neuropeptides, may be involved in certain acute and/or chronic effects of organophosphate exposure. Whereas the cholinergic mechanisms involved in organophosphate toxicity are well established, other possible effects have not been extensively investigated. Although the following sections may not offer strong evidence or conclusive answers for new mechanisms of neurotoxicity, they might hopefully serve as a stimulus for more research in new areas, which might lead to a better understanding of certain effects of organophosphates on the nervous system.

INTERACTIONS OF ORGANOPHOSPHATES WITH "CLASSICAL" NEUROTRANSMITTERS

A few reports have examined the interactions of organophosphorus compounds with "classical" neurotransmitters, other than acetylcholine, in the nervous system.

Certain organophosphates have been shown to cause convulsions. Although the central cholinergic system is involved in the mechanism of seizures (Karczmar, 1974; Olney et al., 1983), there is some evidence that acetylcholine may not be the only neurotransmitter involved in organophosphate-induced seizures. For example, atropine reduces the increase in brain acetylcholine levels induced by organophosphates but does not significantly alter the convulsions. Since convulsions and seizure activity are often related to altered metabolism of GABA (Wood, 1975), the effects of organophosphates on this neurotransmitter have been investigated. Kar and Matin (1972) reported that the injection of a convulsive dose of paraoxon decreased the brain content of GABA in addition to increasing acetylcholine levels. Administration of drugs such as aminooxyacetic acid, which increase brain GABA levels, protected against paraoxon induced seizures, while having no effect on the increased acetylcholine content (Matin and Kar, 1973).

Various benzodiazepines terminated or prevented seizure activity in the monkey following administration of Soman (Lipp, 1973). Benzodiazepines also antagonized the increase in cerebellar cyclic GMP induced by soman in rats as well as blocking convulsions, while atropine had no significant effect on soman-induced increase in cGMP concentrations nor on convulsive activity (Lundy and Magor, 1978). Subsequent studies by the same investigators, however, failed to find any alteration of glutamic acid decarboxylase (GAD), GABA transaminase and GABA levels in soman-intoxicated rats (Lundy et al.,1978). On the other hand, Sivam et al. (1983a) found that DFP increased the number of GABA receptors in rat striatum after both acute and chronic treatment. DFP also increased GABA levels, and decreased the uptake and spontaneous release of GABA while it had no effect on GAD and GABA-transaminase (Sivam et al., 1983b).

Although some effects on the GABAergic system are apparent, these studies do not clarify the interactions of organophosphates with this system, nor its role in soman- or paraoxon- induced convulsions. Furthermore, it is not known if the increase in cerebellar cGMP content induced by soman is due to stimulation of muscarinic receptors (Lee et al., 1972), to an interaction with the GABA system (Mao et al., 1974) or to a generalized CNS excitation via the action of some other neurotransmitters (Lundy and Shaw, 1983). It is also noteworthy that in spite of the importance of cyclic nucleotides in the regulation of several brain functions (Nathanson, 1977), very few studies on the effects of organophosphates on cyclic nucleotides have been published (reviewed by Bodnaryk, 1982).

An interaction of organophosphates with the dopaminergic, serotoninergic and noradrenergic systems has also been reported. DFP markedly inhibited the spontaneous and potassium-stimulated release of endogenous dopamine from rat striatum in vitro (Kant et al., 1984). At high concentrations, DFP appeared to inhibit dopamine release to a greater extent which can be explained by the presence of excess acetylcholine, suggesting that the effect of DFP was not entirely cholinergic (Kant et al., 1984). An interesting observation was that of Freed et al. (1976), who found that mipafox and leptophos, two organophasphates which cause delayed neuropathy, decrease the level of dopamine in the striatum, whereas fenitrothion neither produced motor dysfunction nor changed the level of striatal dopamine. Since brain dopamine is associated with certain motor dysfunctions, these authors suggested that a reduction of dopamine in the corpus striatum may be partly involved in the delayed neurotoxic effects of certain organophosphorus compounds. The effect on dopamine content also appeared to be unrelated to the degree of cholinesterase inhibition (Freed et al., 1976). However, alterations in catecholamine levels or turnover rates have been reported after the administration of cholinesterase inhibitors that do not cause delayed neuropathy,such as parathion and disulfoton, as well as after leptophos, when administered at doses eliciting no motor deficits in rats (Fiscus and Van Meter, 1977; Holt and Hawkins, 1978; Aldous et al., 1982). Thus any relationship between alterations of catecholamine systems, particularly dopamine, and delayed neuropathy, remains to be established.

Possible interactions of organophosphates with alpha$_2$-adrenoceptor are suggested by two studies reporting alterations of [^{3}H]-clonidine binding in various brain areas of TOTP-treated rats (Hollingsworth et al., 1982) and a protective effect of clonidine against the toxicity of cholinesterase inhibitors (Buccafusco, 1982).

DFP, soman, paraoxon, sarin and tabun caused an increase in the turnover of 5-hydroxytryptamine in the rat striatum (Koehn and Karczmar, 1978; Prioux-Guyonneau et al., 1982; Fernando et al., 1984b). Although there is disagreement on whether this effect is a consequence of acetylcholine accumulation (Fernando et al., 1984b) or if it is unrelated to AChE inhibition (Prioux-Guyonneau et al., 1982), an increased turnover of 5-hydroxytryptamine could facilitate the tremors and hind-limb abduction caused by anticholinesterase organophosphates (Fernando et al., 1984).

ORGANOPHOSPHATES AND NEUROPEPTIDES

Since it was first suggested that the cholinesterases play an important role in the destruction of choline esters in the body (Dale, 1914), these enzymes have been the subject of innumerable studies (see Augustinsson, 1963; 1971; Koelle, 1963; Silver, 1974; Holmstedt, 1971; Massoulie and Bon, 1982; Brimijoin, 1983, for reviews). One of these enzymes was found to be particularly enriched at cholinergic synapses and to inactivate acetylcholine released at the synapse and was therefore named acetylcholinesterase. For many years AChE has been used as a marker of cholinergic neurons (Burcher, 1978). However, it has become apparent that AChE is not a specific marker labeling only cholinergic neurons, since the enzyme is present in different populations of monoaminergic neurons and in non-neural structures (Silver, 1974; Burcher, 1978; Lehman and Fibiger, 1979). On the other hand, the acetylcholine-synthetizing enzyme cholineacetyltransferase (ChAT) appears to be a more useful and valid marker for cholinergic neurons (Fonnum, 1975).

A recent study by Eckenstein and Sofroniew (1983) has examined the neurons in the rat central nervous system for their content in AChE, measured histochemically, and ChAT measured by an immunohistochemical method. The main conclusion of this study was that all neurons containing ChAT also contained AChE, but that in many neurons containing the acetylcholine-degrading enzyme, ChAT is absent. Brain areas containing intensely AChE- positive neurons (in the absence of ChAT) included the substantia nigra, the lateral posterior hypothalamus, the hypothalamic arcuate and dorsomedialis nuclei, the zona incerta, the medial septum and the nucleus of the diagonal band of Broca (Eckenstein and Sofroniew, 1983). There appear to be two possible explanations for the presence of noncholinergic, AChE containing neurons. These neurons may be cholinoceptive, that is, contain cholinergic receptors, and/or AChE may be involved in activities other than hydrolysis of acetylcholine (Eckenstein and Sofroniew, 1983). In the substantia nigra of various animal species, AChE is released from dopaminergic neurons (Greenfield et al., 1980). Although these neurons appear to be cholinoceptive, acetylcholine receptors play no part in the release of AChE. On the other hand, there is evidence that in the substantia nigra, AChE is closely related to dopaminergic transmission (see references in Greenfield et al., 1984). It has been recently shown that AChE secreted in the substantia nigra has a functional significance (induction of rotational behavior) in the rat, independent from cholinergic transmission (Greenfield et al., 1984). Indeed, a role of AChE as a neuropeptide transmitter has been suggested (Chubb et al, 1983a). The distribution of AChE also suggests that other endogenous substrates, in addition to acetylcholine, may be hydrolized by this enzyme. In particular, since studies on its esterase activity have not proved fruitful in the past, recent research has addressed the hypothesis that AChE could act also as a peptidase and hydrolize peptide bonds.

During the past decade remarkable progress has been made in the discovery of new neuropeptides, both opioid and nonopioid and in the study of their synthesis, degradation and functions. The following reviews cover several aspects of their biology and pharmacology: Iversen, 1983; Meites and Sonntag, 1981; Bloom, 1983; Akil et al., 1984; Buck et al., 1982; Moss and Dudley, 1984; Emson, 1979; Hokfelt, 1980; Gilbert and Emson, 1983; Graf and Kastin, 1984; Krieger, 1983.

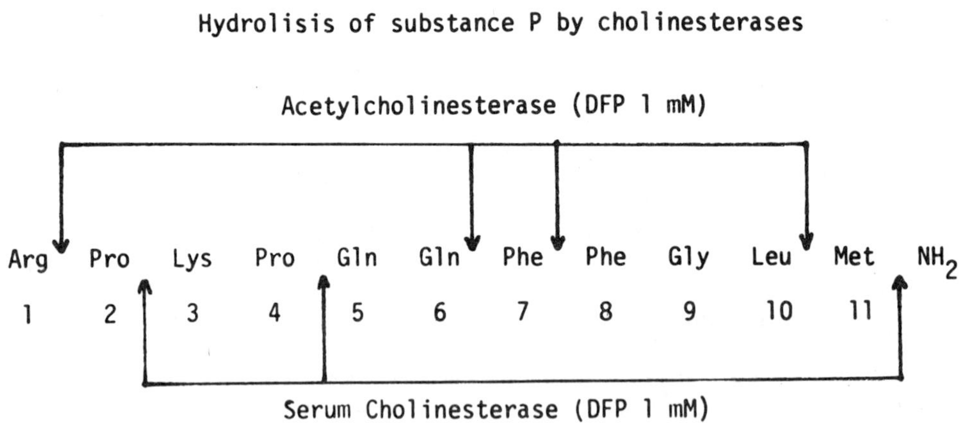

From: Chubb et al., Neuroscience 6, 2065 (1980)
Lockridge, J. Neurochem. 39, 106 (1982)

Figure 4

The first evidence that AChE is capable of hydrolizing a peptide bond in addition to ester bonds, came from the work of Chubb et al. (1980). One of the areas where AChE is concentrated, but ChAT and acetylcholine are absent, are the dorsal horn of the spinal cord and associated spinal ganglia. The most likely neurotransmitters released by sensory neurones are neuropeptides, especially substance P, somatostatin, VIP, bombesin, cholecystokinin and angiotensin II (Buck et al., 1982). Chubb et al. (1980) investigated whether AChE had the ability to degrade one of them, substance P, *in vitro.* AChE purified from electric eel and from fetal bovine serum was found to hydrolize substance P *in vitro* by attacking the Leu^{10}-$Met^{11}.NH_2$ and the Arg^1-Pro^2 bonds (Figure 4). There was also an excellent correlation between the distribution of AChE and that of substance P in the chicken spinal cord, suggesting that AChE may be able to hydrolize substance P *in vivo* (Chubb et al., 1980). High concentrations of acetylcholine inhibited the hydrolysis of substance P and likewise inhibited the esterase activity of AChE (Silver, 1974). Physostigmine and edrophonium were unable to inhibit the hydrolysis of substance P, while concentrations of DFP 100-fold greater than those required to prevent the breakdown of acetylcholine, were required to block the hydrolysis of substance P by AChE (Chubb et al., 1980). These two observations suggest that the peptidase center of AChE differs from its anionic site and that it is accessible to the organophosphate DFP but not to the two carbamates.

The same group of investigators recently showed that purified AChE is also able to hydrolize leu- and met- enkephalin but not other neuropeptides such as beta-endorphin, bombesin, oxytocin, angiotensin II and vasopressin *in vitro* (Figure 5; Chubb et al. 1983b). This enkephalin-hydrolizing activity was inhibited by acetylcholine, by DFP (1.0 mM) but not by physostigmine, edrophonium, or the aminopeptidase inhibitor puromycin (Chubb et al., 1983b). Both the amino- and the carboxy-terminal amino acid of the enkephalins were liberated. The conclusions suggested by this study are similar to the previous ones: AChE appears to have two separate active centers, one with esterase activity and the other displaying peptidase activity, and the latter appears to be affected only by high concentrations of DFP.

The physiological roles of acetylcholinesterase in the erythrocyte and of plasma cholinesterase remain unknown, although their activities serve as useful parameters of the degree of exposure to organophosphorus insecticides (Holmstedt, 1971). Recently Lockridge (1982) showed that purified human serum cholinesterase (pseudo- or butyryl-cholinesterase) was also able to hydrolize substance P (Figure 4). The sites cleaved by serum cholinesterase (Pro^2-Lys^3; Pro^4-Gln^5; Met^{11}-NH_2) are different from those cleaved by AChE (Chubb et al., 1980) but the peptidase activity was similarly inhibited by DFP (Lockridge, 1982). Since butyryl-cholinesterase is present in nervous tissue, in addition to serum, it might also be involved in the physiological regulation of substance P.

Effect of Acetylcholinesterase on enkephalins

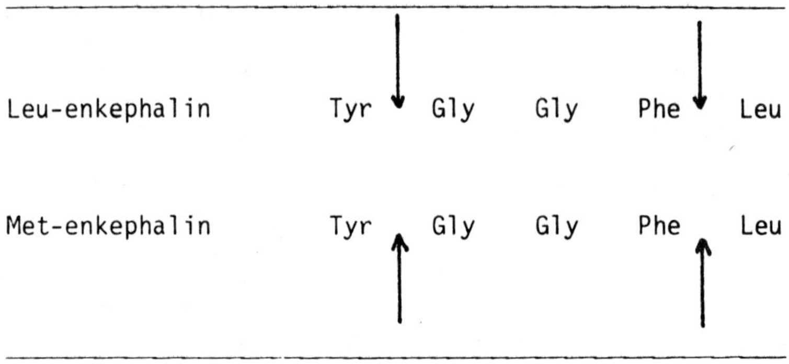

DFP (10^{-3}M) inhibits the hydrolisis. Physostigmine has no effect.

From: Chubb et al., Neuroscience 10, 1369 (1983).

Figure 5

Many peptidase activities have been studied using various peptides as substrates and many specific enzymes have been purified. The activities of some of them are not inhibited by the organophosphate DFP. For example,DFP is inactive toward a membrane-bound substance P-degrading enzyme purified from human brain (Lee et al., 1981), toward endopeptidase-24.11, present in caudate membranes and able to hydrolize substance P and leu-enkephalin (Matsas et al., 1983), and toward enkephalinase (enkephalin dipeptidylcarboxypeptidase; Schwartz et al., 1981). However, DFP was found to inhibit, at micromolar concentrations, dipeptidylaminopeptidase IV isolated from pig kidneys (Barth et al., 1974) and 1 mM DFP also inhibited the inactivation of substance P by cultured human endothelial cells (Johnson and Erdos, 1977). In particular,DFP strongly inhibits a prolyl endopeptidase which hydrolizes substance P, with an IC_{50} value of 10^{-6}M (Kato et al., 1980). Inhibition of prolyl endopeptidase by DFP appears to be worth further investigations since (1) Its activity is inhibited by rather low concentrations of DFP (at 10^{-5}M DFP causes more than 90% inhibition Kato et al., 1980); and (2) many biologically active peptides such as substance P, neurotensin, TRH, angiotensin II, as well as precursors like alpha-neo-endorphin, contain a proline residue and could therefore serve as its substrates.

The serine protease inhibitor phenylmethylsulfonyl fluoride (PMSF) is often used instead of DFP for characterizing the activities of various peptidases. However, these two compounds do not always have the same effect, as for example in case of prolyl endopeptidase which is only weakly inhibited by PMSF (Kato et al., 1980). Therefore, observations made with PMSF are not always directly transferable to DFP or other organophosphates. It is interesting, however, that PMSF is an inhibitor of enkephalinase A_2 which hydrolizes leu-enkephalin to give the Tyr- Gly- Gly fragment (Gorenstein and Snyder, 1980).

If inhibition of such peptidase activities would occur after in vivo administration of DFP, and possibly other organophosphates, one would expect a prolongation and/or potentiation of the effects of several neuropeptides. There is no evidence in fact that the action of neuropeptides is terminated by other means, such as presynaptic uptake, other than degradation by peptidases. Furthermore peptidases are responsible for generating various neuropeptides by cleavage of larger precursor molecules. Recently, it has been also shown that AChE is able to increase the enkephalin and substance P content in the chick retina, possibly by hydrolizing their precursors (Millar and Chubb, 1984). Inhibition of such peptidase activities by organophosphates would therefore cause a decrease in the formation of certain neuropeptides. Since the known biological and behavioral actions of neuropeptides are several and various (Moss and Dudley, 1984), an effect of organophosphates on the processes of formation and/or degradation of neuropeptides might account for many of their adverse effects which cannot be attributed to accumulation of acetylcholine (O'Neill, 1981).

The potential interactions of organophosphates with neuropeptides have not been investigated, hence any inference on their role in certain in vivo effects of organophosphorus compounds is only speculative. However, a series of studies conducted with DFP and Soman, suggest that these compounds might interact in vivo with a class of neuropeptides, the endogenous opioids. These studies will be reviewed in more detail.

DFP has been shown to have an antinociceptive effect both in rats, in the hot-plate test, and in mice, in a tail-immersion test (Koehn and Karczmar, 1978; Koehn et al., 1980; Zorn et al., 1983). Antinociception is antagonized by centrally active muscarinic antagonists, such as atropine or scopolamine and by the opiate antagonist naloxone (Koehn and Karczmar, 1978; Koehn et al. 1980, Zorn et al., 1983). This latter finding suggests that in addition to a cholinergic mechanism, the opiate system might play a role in DFP-antinociception. Cholinergic drugs, such as the muscarinic agonist oxotremorine, nicotine, or the carbamate cholinesterase inhibitor physostigmine also induce antinociception, however this is usually not antagonized by naloxone (Ireson, 1970; Sahley and Berutson, 1979; Zorn, et al., 1983).

DFP-induced antinociception is dose-dependent and long lasting and can be separated from the effects of DFP on locomotor activity and body temperature, in that the latter two are not antagonized by naloxone (Koehn et al. 1980; Zorn et al., 1983; Costa and Murphy, 1984b). In addition, antinociception induced by both morphine and DFP is antagonized stereospecifically, confirming that naloxone is blocking antinociception by acting on stereospecific receptors and not by a nonspecific action (Koehn et al., 1980).

To establish possible mechanisms of DFP-induced antinociception, its ability to directly interact with the opiate receptor *in vitro* and to alter endogenous opioid levels after *in vivo* adminstration, were investigated (Zorn et al., 1984). DFP did not inhibit the binding of [^{3}H]-dihydromorphine to μ-receptors in mouse brain *in vitro*, suggesting that it does not interact with the opiate receptor directly. When administered to mice at the dose of 6.0 mg/kg, DFP caused an 80% increase of met-enkephalin content in the striatum (Zorn et al., 1984). On the other hand, a maximal antinociceptive dose of physostigmine (0.425 mg/kg) did not cause any elevation of met-enkephalin content (Zorn et al., 1984). Two other organophosphates, soman and sarin, were also shown to have an antinociceptive effect in mice (Clement and Copeman, 1984). Similarly to DFP, this analgesia was antagonized by atropine and naloxone, although the latter did not completely reverse the antinociceptive effect. Furthermore, soman did not affect the binding of [^{3}H]-naloxone to opiate receptors *in vitro* (Clement and Copeman, 1984). The serine protease inhibitor PMSF was also shown to cause antinociception in mice and to potentiate the analgesic effect of beta-endorphin given centrally (Pinsky et al., 1982). PMSF-induced analgesia was antagonized by naloxone but not by atropine, suggesting a lack of the cholinergic component in its effect.

Further studies have investigated the effect of naloxone toward DFP-antinociception at two dose levels, 3 and 6 mg/kg (Costa and Murphy, 1984c). Naloxone antagonized the antinociception induced by the highest dose of DFP, confirming previous results, but not that caused by the 3 mg/kg dose. Furthermore, reaction time had returned to control values 24 h after 3 mg/kg DFP, whereas the antinociceptive effect of 6 mg/kg was still present 24 h after administration. This residual antinociception was reversed by naloxone but not by atropine, suggesting that it was due to the non-cholinergic component of DFP-antinociception. High doses of soman and sarin were also shown to cause a long-lasting analgesia which, at 24 h after dosing, was reversed by naloxone but not by atropine (Clement and Copeman, 1984). These data suggest that antinociception induced by low doses of DFP is due solely to a cholinergic action, while higher doses might affect also the opiate system. The recovery that occurs 24 h after administration of 3 mg/kg DFP might be due to short-term desensitization of muscarinic receptors, as previously reported (Costa et al., 1982b). On the other hand, the residual antinociception present 24 h after high doses of DFP, soman and sarin, might be due solely to a reduced destruction of endorphins and/or enkephalins, since it was sensitive to naloxone but not to atropine. All together these data offer the first experimental evidence suggesting an involvement of neuropeptides in one action of organophosphates. Although the biochemical and molecular mechanism of sucn interaction have yet to be explored DFP, soman and sarin might reduce the catabolism of endogenous opioids or other peptides (e.g. substance P) involved in pain control, possibly by inhibiting certain peptidase activities. Interestingly, this involvement of neuropeptides appears to be evident only with high doses of organophosphates administered acutely. This seems to be in agreement with the greater concentrations of DFP required *in vitro* to inhibit the peptidase activity of AChE than its esterase activity. In addition, a carbamate AChE inhibitor, such as physostigmine, appears to induce a solely cholinergic antinociception, again in agreement with its lack of inhibition of peptidase activity *in vitro*. DFP, soman and sarin are not used as insecticides and are very potent phosphorylating agents. Further studies are needed to determine whether other insecticidal organophosphates are capable of inhibiting the peptidase activity of AChE and other enzymes, both *in vitro* and after acute and chronic administration. It also needs to be determined whether carbamates are devoid of anti-peptidase action. Because of the potential role of neuropeptides as neurotransmitters and/or co-transmitters, and their involvement in several biological and behavioral functions, these studies will hopefully shed light on some of the still unexplained effects of organophosphates on the nervous system.

ORGANOPHOSPHATE-INDUCED NARCOSIS

The organophosphate dimethoate can produce a deep narcosis after oral administration to rats, rabbits and guinea pigs (Casida and Sanderson, 1963). The onset of narcosis preceded the cholinergic signs that are typical of the anticholinesterase action of dimethoate by at least one hour, and the animals had usually recovered from narcosis when cholinergic signs began. A similar narcotic effect was observed by Vandekar (1957) after iv injection of a series of eight organic phosphates which included three inhibitors of cholinesterase. Brown and Murphy (1971) investigated more in detail the narcosis produced by dimethoate, triethyl phosphate and triethyl phosphorothioate. Their results indicated that the narcotic action of dimethoate is independent from its anticholinesterase action, which is consistent with the findings that the sensitivity of male and female rats and of rats and mice to the lethal cholinergic effects is inversely correlated with their sensitivity to narcosis. The mechanism of this narcotic effect is, however, still unknown and the only hypothesis is that of Heath (1961) who suggested that narcosis may be induced by blockage of nerve conduction at the axon, due to interference with sodium transport.

ORGANOPHOSPHATE-INDUCED DELAYED NEUROPATHY

Certain organophosphorus compounds cause a specific syndrome characterized by a delay of one to three weeks after intoxication before clinical effects are manifested, thus the term "delayed" neuropathy. The clinical signs are numbness of the limbs which progresses to ataxia and paralysis. Morphologically, organophosphate-induced delayed neuropathy (OPIDN) consists of symmetrical degeneration of primarily long, large diameter axons in peripheral nerves and in the spinal cord. No necrosis of muscle fibers is observed. This particular axonal degeneration is described as a distal (dying-back) axonopathy, since the general pattern of a distal to proximal degeneration is present (Davis and Richardson, 1980).

A series of reviews which deal primarily with the pathological aspects of OPIDN have been published (Davies, 1963; Cavanagh, 1964; 1973; Hopkins, 1975; LeQuesne, 1975; Abou-Donia, 1981; Baron, 1981). OPIDN has been recognized since the 1920s , when more than 20,000 people developed paralysis after consumption of a beverage adulterated with TOTP (Smith et al., 1930) and many outbreaks of poisoning have occurred in various countries (Davis and Richardson, 1980). The recovery from OPIDN is usually poor and there is no treatment for this neuropathy (Davis and Richardson, 1980). Adult hens are the models for human intoxication by organophosphates that cause delayed neuropathy (Johnson, 1982).

Earlier studies indicated that neither inhibition of AChE nor of butyryl-cholinesterase were involved in OPIDN (Abou-Donia, 1981). The systematic investigations of Johnson, who followed an early suggestion by Aldridge that an esterase might be the target of OPIDN, have led to the identification of a target protein. Phosphorylation of this protein, which has been characterized as an esterase and is referred to as "neurotoxic esterase" or "neuropathic target esterase" (NTE), is believed to be the initial biochemical event in OPIDN. There is a good correlation between phosphorylation of NTE, inhibition of its esterasic activity and genesis of the disease. Several reviews have been published on the involvement of NTE in OPIDN (Johnson 1975 a, b; 1980 a,b; 1982; Davis and Richardson, 1980; Lotti et al., 1984) and a chapter of this volume is devoted to this subject.

Two conditions must be present for inhibition of NTE resulting in clinical signs of poisoning. There is a threshold for inhibition (at least 70 to 80% of NTE activity needs to be inhibited after a single-dose in the hen) and the inhibited enzyme must undergo aging (Johnson, 1982; Lotti et al., 1984). Structure-activity studies have shown that some compounds (e.g. phosphinates), which are able to inhibit NTE but do not age, do not cause neuropathy and are able to afford protection from a susequent challenging dose with, for example, a phosphate (Johnson, 1975a; 1982; Lotti et al. 1984).

Studies on tissue, regional and subcellular distribution of NTE have not given any indication on the possible relation between this enzyme and the development of a delayed neuropathy. NTE activity has been found in lymphatic tissue (Dudek and Richardson, 1982) but no good evidence exists for involvement of immune processes in the development of organophosphate neuropathy (Johnson, 1982). Although the processes of development of neuropathy after initiation are not yet known, the identification of NTE as the initial biochemical target allows the use of its catalytic activity for practical purposes. Rules are available to predict possible neurotoxic hazard to humans from in vitro studies with NTE, and exposure to neurotoxic compounds can be monitored (Johnson, 1982; Lotti et al., 1984). However, many questions on OPIDN remain partially or totally unanswered. Among them: (1) Why are some species (hen, human) very susceptible to OPIDN while others (Japanese quail, rat) are rather insensitive? (2) Why is there an age difference for susceptibility? (3) What is the physiological role of NTE or its endogenous substrate(s)? (4) What are the events leading to axonal degeneration? (5) What is the significance of the "aging" process? These and many other questions (Johnson, 1982) which need to be addressed in order to gain a better understanding of OPIDN offer a challenge not only to pesticide toxicologists but particularly to scientist from other biomedical disciplines.

NEUROTOXICITY OF BICYCLIC PHOSPHORUS ESTERS

Certain bicyclic organophosphorus compounds (Figure 6) first described by Bellet and Casida (1973), are very potent neurotoxicants. The ethyl-(EPTBO) and isopropyl-(IPTBO) derivatives have LD_{50} values (ip in mice) of 1.0 and 0.18 mg/kg, respectively, and produce tonic-clonic convulsions and death within a few minutes after injection

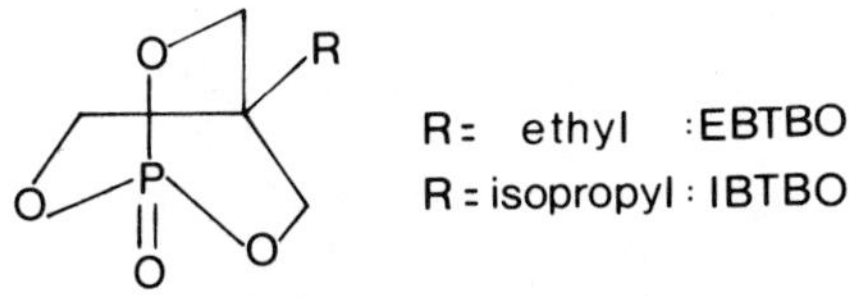

4-Alkyl-1-phospha-2,6,7-trioxabicyclo [2.2.2] octane-1-oxide

Figure 6

(Bellet and Casida, 1973). The finding that such compounds can be formed during the thermal decomposition of polyurethane foams treated with fire retardants containing phosphorus (Petajan et al., 1974) led to further studies investigating their mechanism of action. Despite their similarity to other organophosphates, the toxic signs of bicyclic phosphorus compounds in mice and rats do not resemble the characteristic manifestations of poisoning by anticholinesterase agents, i.e. there is no indication of parasympathetic stimulation or inhibition of brain or blood cholinesterase activity even after a lethal dose (Bellet and Casida, 1973). A recent study (Ozoe et al., 1982) showed that these compounds are very poor inhibitors of bovine erythrocyte and housefly head acetylcholinesterase. This lack of inhibitory activity is due to a low affinity for AChE and a poor phosphorylating ability. Another serine-containing enzyme, alpha-chimotrypsin, was also poorly phosphorylated by these compounds (Ozoe et al., 1982). Since the signs of poisoning resemble those induced by GABA antagonists, such as bicuculline and picrotoxin, Bowery et al. (1976) investigated the effect of IPTBO and EPTBO on the neuronal firing and on the ganglionic depolarization induced by GABA. In both experiments, the bicyclic phosphorus esters were able to antagonize the effects of GABA, with a potency comparable to that of other GABA antagonists. IPTBO was also found to antagonize the depressant action of glycine, although to a lesser degree than GABA (Bowery et al., 1976). A subsequent study showed that convulsive and subconvulsive doses of EPTBO and IPTBO increase the levels of cyclic GMP in the cerebellum (Mattson et al., 1977). Levels of cyclic AMP and of cyclic GMP in cerebral cortex and subcortical tissues were not affected. Diazepam decreased the acute toxicity of EPTBO and antagonized the increase in cerebellar cyclic GMP content induced by both compounds, while atropine had no significant effect (Mattson et al., 1977). *In vitro* binding studies showed that bicyclic phosphorus esters do not interact with the GABA binding site (Ticku and Olsen, 1979). However, they inhibit the binding of [^{3}H]-dihydropicrotoxin to its binding site on the GABA/ionophore receptor complex, suggesting that their neurotoxic action is due to a picrotoxin-like effect.

NON NERVOUS SYSTEM EFFECTS OF ORGANOPHOSPHATES

Organophosphorus compounds have been reported to exert various non-nervous system toxic effects. Certain organophosphates are teratogenic in chick embryos, an action apparently unrelated to cholinesterase inhibition and possibly attributable to an imbalance of NAD metabolism (Proctor et al., 1976). However, data on teratogenic effects in mammals are mostly negative and/or inconclusive. Some organophosphates are mutagenic in various bacterial tests (Moriya et al., 1983), while others can alkylate DNA (Wooder and Wright, 1981). Effects of organophosphates on hepatic microsomal enzymes have also been reported (Stevens et al., 1972).

CONCLUSIONS

The study of the biological properties of organophosphates has not only elucidated many aspects of their toxicity, but has also brought important contributions to the understanding of the biological systems themselves. Although their main mechanism of action and the antidotal treatment for intoxication were discovered soon after they were synthetized, organophosphates have been the object of a great deal of interest and research over the years. Despite these efforts many of the effects of organophosphates on the nervous system have not been clarified. Three areas in particular appear to deserve further investigation: (1) The interaction of organophosphates with components of the nervous system other than the cholinergic such as neuropeptides offers the potential for many interesting studies and discoveries; (2) the effects of developmental exposure to organophosphates has been surprisingly neglected, and potential neurochemical and behavioral alterations following pre- and/or post natal exposure should be investigated; and (3) despite great progress, an input of new ideas is needed in the study of the mechanism of organophosphate-induced delayed neurotoxicity. These and other areas of research will help clarify the neurotoxic effects of organophosphates and their mechanisms and allow a better understanding of their potential hazards to humans.

ACKNOWLEDGMENTS

The author thanks Dr. Sheldon D. Murphy for introducing him to the field of organophosphate toxicology and for his continuous advice and support. Experimental work by the author described herein was supported by Grant ES 03424 from the National Institute of Environmental Health Sciences. Mrs. Ruth Larsen patiently typed this manuscript.

REFERENCES

Abou-Donia, M.B. Organophosphorous ester-induced delayed neurotoxicity. Ann. Rev. Pharmacol. Toxicol. 21: 511-548 (1981).

Ahmad, S. and Forgash, A.J. Nonoxidative Enzymes in the Metabolism of Insecticides. Drug Metal. Rev. 5: 141-164 (1976).

Akil, H., Watson, S.J., Young, E., Lewis, M.E., Kuachaturian, H. and Walker, J.M. Endogenous opioids: Biology and Function. Ann. Rev. Neurosci. 7: 223-255 (1984).

Aldous, C.N., Farr, C.H. and Sharma, R.P. Effects of leptophos on rat brain levels and turnover rates of biogenic amines and their metabolites. Ecotoxicol. Environm. Safety 6: 570-576 (1982).

Aldridge, W.N. An enzyme hydrolysing diethyl p-nitrophenyl phosphate (E600) and its identity with the A-esterase of mammalian sera. Biochem. J. 53: 117-124 (1953).

Aldridge, W.N. The nature of the reaction of organophosphorus compounds and carbamates with esterases. Bull. Wld. Hlth. Org. 44: 25-30 (1971).

Aldridge, W.N. Organophosphorus compounds: molecular basis for their biological properties. Sci. Prog. Oxf. 67: 131-147 (1981).

Anonymous. Nomenclature of compounds containing one phosphorus atom. Chem. Eng. News 30: 4515-4526 (1952).

Aquilonius, S.M. Role of acetylcholine in the central nervous system. In "Metabolic and deficiency diseases of the nervous system", Part III, Handbook of Clinical Neurology vol. 29 (P.J. Vinken and G.W. Bruyn, Eds), North Holland, Amsterdam, 1977, pp.435-458.

Augustinsson, K.B. Classification and comparative enzymology of the cholinesterases and methods for their determination. In: "Handbook der Experimentellen Pharmakologie", vol. 15, (G.B. Koelle,Ed.), Springer-Verlag, Berlin, pp. 89-128, 1963.

Augustinsson, K.B. Comparative aspects of the purification and properties of cholinesterase. Bull. Wld. Hlth, Org. 44: 81-89 (1971).

Barnes, J.M. and Denz, F.A. The chronic toxicity of p-nitrophenyl diethyl thiophosphate (E.605). J. Hyg. 49: 430-441 (1951).

Barnes, J.M. Psychiatric sequelae of chronic exposure to organophosphorus insecticides. Lancet II: 102-103 (1961).

Baron, R.L. Delayed neurotoxicity and other consequences of organophosphate esters. Ann.Rev.Entomol. 26: 29-48 (1981).

Barth, A., Schulz, H. and Neubert, K. Untersuchunger zur Reinigung and Charakterisierung der Dipeptidylaminopeptidase IV. Acta Biol. Med. Germ. 32: 157-174 (1974).

Bellet, E.M. and Casida, J.E. Bicyclic Phosphorus Esters: High toxicity without cholinesterase inhibition. Science 182: 1135-1136 (1973).

Bidstrup, P.L. Psychiatric sequelae of chronic exposure to organophosphorus insecticides. Lancet II: 103 (1961).

Bignami, G. Behavioral Pharmacology and Toxicology. Ann. Rev. Pharmacol. Toxicol. 16: 329-366 (1976).

Bignami, G., Rosic, N., Michalek, H., Milosevic, M., and Gatti, G.L. Behavioral toxicity of anticholinesterase agents: methodological, neurochemical and neuropsychological aspects. In: "Behavioral Toxicology" (B. Weiss and V.G. Laties, Eds.), Plenum Press, NY, 1975, pp.155-215.

Bloom, F.E. The Endorphins: A growing family of pharmacologically pertinent peptides. Ann. Rev. Pharmacol. Toxicol. 23: 151-170 (1983).

Bodnaryk, R.P. The effects of pesticides and related compounds on cyclic nucleotide metabolism. Insect Biochem. 12: 589-597 (1982).

Bombinski, T.J. and Dubois, K.P. Toxicity and mechanism of action of Di-Syston. Arch. Ind. Hlth. 17: 192-199 (1958).

Bowers, M.B., Goodman, E. and Sim, V.M. Some behavioral changes in man following anticholinesterase administration. J. Nerv. Ment.Dis. 138: 383-389 (1964).

Bowery, N.G., Collins, J.F. and Hill, R.G. Bicyclic phosphorus esters that are potent convulsants and GABA antagonists. Nature 261: 601-603 (1976).

Brimblecombe, R.W. Drugs acting on central cholinergic mechanisms and affecting respiration. Pharmacol. Ther. 3: 65-74 (1977).

Brimijoin, S. Molecular forms of acetylcholinesterase in brain, nerve and muscle: nature, localization and dynamics. Prog. Neurobiol. 21: 291-322 (1983).

Brodeur, J. and Dubois, K.P. Studies on the mechanism of acquired tolerance by rats to O,O-diethyl S-2 (ethylthio) ethyl phosphorodithioate (Disyston). Arch. Int. Pharmacodyn. 149: 560-570 (1964).

Brown, D.R. and Murphy, S.D. Factors influencing dimethoate and triethyl phosphate-induced narcosis in rats and mice. Toxicol. Appl. Pharmacol. 18: 895-906 (1971).

Buccafusco, J.J. Mechanism of the clonidine-induced protection against acetylcholinesterase inhibitor toxicity. J. Pharmacol. Exp. Ther. 222: 595-599 (1982).

Buck, S.H., Walsh, J.H., Yamamura, H.I. and Burks, T.F. Neuropeptides in sensory neurons. Life Sci. 30: 1857-1866 (1982).

Bull, D.L. Metabolism of Di-Syston by Insects, Isolated Cotton Leaves and Rats. J. Econ. Entomol. 58: 249-254 (1965).

Burchfiel, J.L., Duffy, F.H. and Sim, V.M. Persistent effect of sarin and dieldrin upon the primate electroencephalogram. Toxicol. Appl. Pharmacol. 35: 365-379 (1976).

Burcher, L.L. Recent advances in histochemical techniques for the study of central cholinergic mechanisms. In: "Cholinergic Mechanisms and Psychopharmacology", (D.J. Jenden, Ed.), Plenum Press, NY, 1978, pp. 93-124.

Casida, J.E. Esterase inhibitors as pesticides. Science 146: 1011-1017 (1964).

Casida, J.E. and Sanderson, D.M. Reaction of certain phosphorothioates with alcohols and potentiation by breakdown products. J. Agr. Food Chem. 11: 91-96 (1963).

Cavanagh, J.B. The significance of the "Dying-Back" process in experimental and human neurological disease. Int. Rev. Exp. Path. 3: 219-267 (1964).

Cavanagh, J.B. Peripheral neuropathy caused by toxic agents. CRC, Crit. Rev. Toxicol. 2: 365-417 (1973).

Chippendale, T.J., Zawolkow, G.A., Russell, R.W. and Overstreet, D.H. Tolerance to low acetylcholinesterase levels: modification of behavior without acute behavioral change. Psychopharmacologia (Berl.) 26: 127-139 (1972).

Chubb, I.W., Hodgson, A.J. and White,G.H. Acetylcholinesterase Hydrolizes Substance P. Neurosci. 5: 2065-2072 (1980).

Chubb, I.W., Greenfield, S.A. and Hodgson, A.J. Is acetylcholinesterase the biggest "neuropeptide" of them all? Neurosci. Lett Suppl. 11: S6-S7 (1983b).

Chubb, I.W., Ranieri, E., White, G.H. and Hodgson, A.J. The enkephalins are amongst the peptides hydrolized by purified acetylcholinesterase. Neurosci. 4: 1369-1377 (1983).

Clark,G. Organophosphate insecticides and behavior: A Review Aerosp. Med. 42: 735-740 (1971).

Clark, W.G. and Clark, Y.L. Changes in body temperature after administration of acetylcholine, histamine, morphine, prostaglandins and related agents. Neurosci. Biobehav. Rev. 4: 175-240 (1980)

Clement, J.G. and Copeman, H.T. Soman and Sarin induce a long-lasting naloxone-reversible analgesia in mice. Life Sci. 34: 1415-1422 (1984).

Costa, L.G. and Murphy, S.D. Passive avoidance retention in mice tolerant to the organophosphorus insecticide disulfoton. Toxicol. Appl. Pharmacol. 65: 451-458 (1982).

Costa, L.G. and Murphy,S.D. Unidirectional cross-tolerance between the carbamate insecticide propoxur and the organophosphate disulfoton in mice. Fund. Appl. Toxicol. 3: 483-488 (1983).

Costa, L.G. and Murphy, S.D. Interaction between acetaminophen and organophosphates in mice. Res. Comm. Chem. Pathol. Pharmacol. 44: 389-400 (1984a).

Costa, L.G. and Murphy, S.D. Tolerance to DFP-induced antinociception: lack of cross-tolerance to morphine. Toxicologist 4(1): 15 (1984b).

Costa, L.G. and Murphy, S.D. Cholinergic and opiate involvement in the antinociceptive effect of diisopropylfluorophosphate. Soc. Neurosci. Abst. 10: (1984c).

Costa, L.G., Schwab, B.W., Hand, H. and Murphy, S.D. Reduced [^{3}H]-quinuclidinyl benzilate binding to muscarinic receptors in disulfoton-tolerant mice. Toxicol. Appl. Pharmacol. 60: 441-450 (1981).

Costa, L.G., Schwab, B.W. and Murphy, S.D. Tolerance to anticholinesterase compounds in mammals. Toxicology 25: 79-97 (1982a).

Costa, L.G., Schwab, B.W. and Murphy, S.D. Differential alterations of cholinergic muscarinic receptors during chronic and acute tolerance to organophosphorus insecticides. Biochem. Pharmacol. 31: 3407-3413 (1982b).

Dale, H.H. The action of certain esters and ethers of choline and their relation to muscarine. J. Pharmacol. Exp. Ther. 6: 147-190 (1914).

Das, M., Dixit, R., Seth, P.K. and Mukhtar, H. Glutathione-S-Transferase activity in the brain: Species, Sex, Regional and Age Differences. J. Neurochem. 36: 1439-1442 (1981).

Dauterman, W.C. Biological and Nonbiological Modifications of Organophosphorus Compounds. Bull. Wld. Hlth. Org. 44: 133-150 (1971).

Davies, D.R. Neurotoxicity of organophosphorus compounds. In: "Handbuch der Experimentellen Pharmakologie", vol. 15, (G.B. Koelle, Ed.) Springer-Verlag, Berlin, pp. 860-882 (1963).

Davis, K.L. and Yamamura, H.I. Cholinergic underactivity in human memory disorders. Life Sci. 23: 1729-1734 (1978).

Davis, K.L., Berger, P.A., Hollister, L.E. and Barchas, J.D. Cholinergic involvement in mental disorders. Life Sci. 22: 1865-1872 (1978a).

Davis, K.L., Yesavage, J.A. and Berger, P.A. Possible organophosphate-induced Parkinsonism. J. Nerv. Ment. Dis. 166: 222-225 (1978b).

Davis, C.S. and Richardson, R.J. Organophosphorus Compounds. In: "Experimental and Clinical Neurotoxicology" (P.S. Spencer and H.H. Schaumburg, Eds), Williams & Wilkins, Baltimore, pp. 527-544 (1980).

DeRoeth, A., Dettbarn, W.D., Rosenberg, P., Wilensky, J.G. and Wong, A. Effect of phospholine iodide on blood cholinesterase levels of normal and glaucoma subjects. Am. J. Ophtalm. 59: 586-592 (1965).

Deutsch, J.A. The cholinergic synapse and the site of memory. In: "The physiological basis of memory" (J.A. Deutsch, Ed.), Academic Press, NY, pp. 59-76 (1973).

Dille, J.R. and Smith, P.W. Central nervous system effects of chronic exposure to organophophate insecticides. Aerospace Med. 35: 475-478 (1964).

Dudek, B.R. and Richardson, R.J. Evidence for the existence of neurotoxic esterase in neural and lymphatic tissue of the adult hen. Biochem. Pharmacol. 31: 1117-1121 (1982).

Duffel, M.W. and Gillespie, S.G. Microsomal flavin-containing monooxygenase activity in rat corpus striatum. J.Neurochem. 42: 1350-1353 (1984).

Duffy, F.H.,Burchfiel, J.L., Bartels, P.H., Gaon, M. and Sim, V.M. Long term effects of an organophosphate upon the human electroencephalogram. Toxicol. Appl. Pharmacol. 47: 161-176 (1979).

Durham, W.F., Wolfe, H.R. and Quinby, G.E. Organophosphorus insecticides and mental alertness. Arch. Environm. Hlth. 10: 55-66 (1965).

Eckenstein, F. and Sofroniew, M.V. Identification of central cholinergic neurons containing both choline acetyltransferase and acetylcholinesterase and of central neurons containing only acetylcholinesterase. J. Neurosci. 3: 2286-2291 (1983).

Ecobichon, D.J. Environmental dynamics and toxicokinetics of pesticides. In: "Pesticides and Neurological Diseases" (D.J. Ecobichon and R.M. Joy, Eds), CRC Press, Boca Raton, FL, pp. 15-52 (1982a).

Ecobichon, D.J. Organophosphorus ester insecticides. In: "Pesticides and Neurological Diseases" (D.J. Ecobichon and R.M. Joy, Eds.), CRC Press, Boca Raton, FL, pp. 151-203 (1982b).

Ehlert, F.J.,Kokka, N. and Fairhurst, A.S. Altered [^{3}H]-quinuclidinyl benzilate binding in the striatum of rats following chronic cholinesterase inhibition with diisopropylfluorophosphate. Mol. Pharmacol. 17: 24-30 (1980).

Emson, P.C. Peptides as neurotransmitter candidates in the mammalian CNS. Prog. Neurobiol. 13: 61-116 (1979).
Eto, M. Organophosphorus pesticides: Organic and Biological Chemistry. CRC Press, Boca Raton, FL. (1974).
Eto, M., Oshima, Y. and Casida, J.E. Plasma albumin as a catalyst in cyclization of diaryl o-(alpha-hydroxy)tolyl phosphates. Biochem. Pharmacol. 16: 295-308 (1967).
Farkas, I.,Desi, I. and Dura, G. Differences in the acute and chronic neurotoxic effects of chlorinated hydrocarbon, organophosphate and carbamate pesticides. In: "Adverse Effects of Environmental Chemicals and Psychotropic Drugs", vol. 2,(M.Horvath, Ed.), Elsevier, pp. 201-213 (1976).
Fenichel, G.M., Kibler, W.B., Olson, W.H. and Dettbarn, W.D. Chronic inhibition of cholinesterase as a cause of myopathy. Neurology 22: 1026-1033 (1972).
Fernando, J.C.R., Hoskins, B. and Ho, I.K. Behavioral super-sensitivity to atropine following treatment with organophosphate cholinesterase inhibitors. Fed. Proc. 43: 565 (1984a).
Fernando, J.C.R., Hoskins, B.H. and Ho, I.K. A striatal serotoninergic involvement in the behavioral effects of anticholinesterase organophosphates. Eur. J. Pharmacol. 98: 129-132 (1984b).
Fiamberti, A.M. Riv. Pat. Nerv. Ment. 66: 1 (1946).
Fiscus, R.R. and Van Meter, W.G., Effects of parathion on turnover and endogenous levels of norepinephrine and dopamine in rat brain. Fed. Proc. 36: 951 (1977).
Fisher, E.B. and Van Wazer, J.R. Uses of organic phosphorus compounds. In: "Phosphorus and its compounds", vol.II (J.R. Van Wazer, Ed.), Interscience Publishers, NY, pp. 1897-1936, (1961).
Fonnum, F. Review of recent progress in the synthesis, storage and release of acetylcholine. In: "Cholinergic Mechanisms" (P.G. Waser, Ed.), Raven Press, NY, pp. 145-160 (1975).
Freed, V.H., Matin, M.A., Fang, S.C. and Kar, P.P. Role of striatal dopamine in delayed neurotoxic effects of organophosphorus compounds. Eur. J. Pharmacol. 35: 229-232 (1976).
Fukuto, T.R. and Metcalf, R.L. Metabolism of insecticides in plants and animals. Ann. N.Y. Acad. Sci. 160: 97-113 (1969).
Gardner, R., Ray, R., Frankenheim,J., Wallace, K., Loss, M. and Robichaud, R. A possible mechanism for diisopropylfluorophosphate-induced memory loss in rats. Pharmacol. Biochem. Behav. 21: 43-46 (1984).
Gershon, S. and Shaw, F.H. Psychiatric sequelae of chronic exposure to organophosphorus insecticides. Lancet I: 1371-1374 (1961).
Giardini, V. Meneguz, A., Amorico, L., DeAcetis, L. and Bignami, G. Behaviorally augmented tolerance during chronic cholinesterase reduction by paraoxon. Neurobehav. Toxicol. Teratol. 4: 335-345 (1982).

Gilbert, R.F.T. and Emson, P.C. Neuronal coexistence of peptides with other putative transmitters. In: "Handbook of Psychopharmacology", vol. 16 (L.L. Iversen, S.D. Iversen and S.H. Snyder, Eds.), Plenum Press, NY, pp. 519-556, (1983).

Golz, H.H. Psychiatric sequelae of chronic exposure to organophosphorus insecticides. Lancet II: 369-370 (1961).

Gorenstein, C. and Snyder, S.H. Enkephalinases. Proc. R. Soc. Lond. B 210: 123-132 (1980).

Graf, M.V. and Kastin, A.J. Delta-Sleep-Inducing Peptide (DSIP): A Review. Neurosci. Biobehav. Rev. 8: 83-93 (1984).

Greenfield, S.A., Cheramy, A., Leviel, V. and Glowinski, J. In vivo release of acetylcholinesterase in the cat substantiae nigrae and caudate nuclei. Nature 284: 355-357 (1980).

Greenfield, S.A., Chubb, I.W., Grunewald, R.A., Henderson, Z., May, J., Portnoy, S., Weston, J. and Wright, M.C. A non-cholinergic function for acetylcholinesterase in the substantia nigra: behavioral evidence. Exp. Brain Res. 54: 513-520 (1984).

Grob, D. and Harvey, A.M. The effects and treatment of nerve gas poisoning. Am. J. Med. 14: 52-63 (1953).

Hajjar, N.P. and Hodgson, E. Flavin adenine dinucleotide-dependent monooxygenase: Its role in sulfoxidation of pesticides in mammals. Science 209: 1134-1136 (1980).

Hammond, P.S., Braunstein, H., Kennedy, J.M., Badawy, S.M.A. and Fukuto, T.R. Mode of action of the delayed toxicity of O,O,S-trimethyl phosphorothioate in the rat. Pest. Biochem. Physiol. 18: 77-89 (1982).

Hayes, W.J. Toxicology of Pesticides. Williams and Wilkins, Baltimore, pp. 580 (1975).

Hayes, W.J. Pesticides Studied in Man. Williams and Wilkins, Baltimore, pp.672 (1982).

Heath, D.F. Organophosphorus Poisons (Anticholinesterases and Related Compound), Pergamon Press, London, pp.338-339 (1961).

Hirshberg, A. and Lerman, Y. Clinical problems in organophosphate insecticide poisoning: the use of a computerized information system. Fund. Appl. Toxicol. 4: S209-S214 (1984).

Hokfelt, T., Johansson, O., Ljungdahl, A., Lundberg, J.M. and Schultzberg, M. Peptidergic neurones. Nature 284: 515-521 (1980).

Hollingsworth, P.J., Richardson, R.J. and Smith, C.B. Triorthocresyl phosphate increases $alpha_2$ adrenoceptors in specific areas of the rat brain. Toxicologist 2(2): 223 (1982).

Holmes, J.H. and Gaon, M.D. Observations on acute and multiple exposure to anticholinesterase agents. Trans. Am. Clin. Climat. Ass. 68: 86-103 (1957).

Holmstedt, B. Distribution and determination of cholinesterases in mammals. Bull. Wld. Hlth. Org. 44: 99-107 (1971).

Holt, T.M. and Hawkins, R.K. Rat hippocampal norepinephrine response to cholinesterase inhibition. Res. Comm. Chem. Pathol. Pharmacol. 20:239-251 (1978).

Hopkins, A.P. Peripheral neuropathy due to industrial agents. In: "Peripheral Neuropathy" (P.J. Dyck, P.K. Thomas and E.H. Lambert, Eds.), W.B. Sanders, Philadelphia, pp. 1207-1226 (1975).

Hoskin, F.C.G. Diisopropylphosphofluoridate and Tabun: Enzymatic hydrolisis and nerve function. Science 172: 1243-1245 (1971).

Imai, H. Toxicity of organophosphorus pesticide (Fenthion) on the retina. Correlative study especially on its residue action on the retina, liver and blood cholinesterase activities and on electroretinogram. Acta. Soc. Ophthalmol. Japon. 79: 1067-1076 (1975).

Imai, H., Miyata, M., Uga, S. and Ishikawa, S. Retinal degeneration in rats exposed to an organophosphate pesticide (Fenthion). Env. Res. 30: 453-465 (1983).

Ireson, J.D., A comparison of the antinociceptive actions of cholinomimetic and morphine-like drugs. Br. J. Pharmacol. 40: 92-101 (1970).

Ishikawa, S. Chronic optico-neuropathy due to environmental exposure of organophosphate pesticides (Saku disease). Clinical and experimental study. Acta Soc. Ophthalmol. Japon. 77-1835-1886 (1973).

Ishikawa, S. and Miyata, M. Development of myopia following chronic organophosphate pesticide intoxication: an epidemiological and experimental study. In: "Neurotoxicity of the Visual System" (W.H. Merigan and B. Weiss, Eds.), Raven Press, NY, pp. 233-254 (1980).

Iversen, L.L. Nonopioid neuropeptides in mammalian CNS. Ann. Rev. Pharmacol. Toxicol. 23: 1-27 (1983).

Johnson, A.R. and Erdos, E.G. Inactivation of substance P by cultured human endothelial cells. In: "Substance P" (U.S von Euler and B. Pernow, Eds.) Raven Press, NY, 1977, pp. 253-260.

Johnson, M.K. Organophosphorus esters causing delayed neurotoxic effects: Mechanism of action and structure/activity studies. Arch. Toxicol. 34:259-288 (1975a).

Johnson, M.K. The delayed neuropathy caused by some organophosphorous esters: Mechanism and challenge. CRC, Crit. Rev. Toxicol. 3: 289-316 (1975b).

Johnson, M.K. The mechanism of delayed neuropathy caused by some organophosphorous esters: using the understanding to improve safety. J. Environ. Sci. Health, B15: 823-841 (1980a).

Johnson, M.K. Organophosphate neuropathy: Progress in understanding. In: "Advances in Neurotoxicology" (L. Manzo, Ed.), Pergamon Press, Oxford, 1980, pp. 223-235.

Johnson, M.K. The target of initiation of delayed neurotoxicity by organophosphorous esters: Biochemical studies and toxicological applications. In: "Reviews in Biochemical Toxicology", vol. 4 (E. Hodgson, J.R. Bend and R.M. Philpot, Eds), Elsevier, NY, 1982, pp. 141-212.

Jouvet, M. Cholinergic mechanisms and sleep. In: "Cholinergic Mechanisms" (P.G. Waser, Ed.), Raven Press, NY, pp. 455-476 (1975).

Kant, G.J., Kenion, C.C. and Meyerhoff, J.L. Effects of diisopropylfluorophosphate and other cholinergic agents on release of endogenous dopamine from rat brain striatum in vitro. Biochem. Pharmacol. 33: 1823-1825 (1984).

Kar, P.P. and Matin, M.A. Possible role of gamma-aminobutyric acid in paraoxon-induced convulsions. J. Pharm. Pharmacol. 24: 996-997 (1972).

Karczmar, A.G. Is the central cholinergic nervous system overexploited? Fed. Proc. 28: 147-157 (1969).

Karczmar, A.G. Brain acetylcholine and seizures. In: "Psychobiology of convulsive therapy" (M. Fink, S. Kety, J. McGaugh and T. A. Williams, Eds), John Wiley & Sons, New York, pp. 251-270 (1974).

Karczmar, A.G. Cholinergic influences on behavior. In "Cholinergic Mechanisms" (P.G. Waser, Ed.), Raven Press, NY, pp. 501-529 (1975).

Karczmar, A.G. Acute and long lasting central actions of organophosphorus agents. Fund. Appl. Toxicol. 4: S1-S17 (1984).

Karczmar, A.G., Usdin,E. and Wills, J.H. Anticholinesterase Agents. Pergamon Press, Oxford (1970).

Kato, T., Nakano, T., Kojima, K., Nagatsu, T. and Sakakibara, S. Changes in prolyl endopeptidase during maturation of rat brain and hydrolisis of substance P by the purified enzyme. J. Neurochem. 35: 527-535 (1980).

Kiss, Z. and Fazekas, T. Arrhythmias in organophosphate poisoning. Acta Cardiol. 34: 323-330 (1979).

Koehn, G.L. and Karczmar, A.G. Effect of diisopropyl phosphofluoridate on analgesia and motor behavior in the rat. Prog. Neuro-Psychopharmacol. 2: 169-177 (1978).

Koehn, G.L., Henderson, G. and Karczmar, A.G. Diisopropyl phosphofluoridate-induced antinociception: possible role of endogenous opioids. Eur. J. Pharmacol. 61: 167-173 (1980).

Koelle, G.B. (Ed.) Cholinesterases and Anticholinesterase Agents Springer Verlag, Berlin (1963).

Korsak, R.J. and Sato, M.M. Effects of chronic organophosphate pesticide exposure on the central nervous system. Clin. Toxicol. 11: 83-95 (1977).

Krieger, D. Brain Peptides: what, where and why? Science 222: 975-985 (1983).

Kulkarni, A.P. and Hodgson, E. Metabolism of insecticides by mixed function oxidase systems. Pharmacol. Ther. 8: 379-475 (1980).

Lee, C.M., Sandberg, B.E.B., Hanley, M.R. and Iversen, L.L. Purification and characterization of a membrane-bound substance P-degrading enzyme from human brain. Eur. J. Biochem. 114: 315-327 (1981).

Lee, T.P., Kuo, J.F. and Greengard, P. Role of muscarinic cholinergic receptors in regulation of guanosine 3'5'cyclic monophosphate content in mammalian brain, heart, muscle and intestinal smooth muscle. Proc. Natl. Acad. Sci. USA 69: 3287-3291 (1972).

Lehmann, J. and Fibiger, H.C. Acetylcholinesterase and the cholinergic neuron. Life Sci. 25: 1939-1947 (1979).

Lequesne, P.M. Neurotoxic substances. In: "Modern Trends in Neurology", Vol. 6 (D. Williams, Ed.), Butterworth, London, pp. 83-97 (1975).

Lerman, Y. Hirshberg, A. and Shteger, Z. Organophosphate and carbamate pesticide poisoning: the usefulness of a computerized clinical information system. Am. J. Ind. Med. 6: 17-26 (1984).

Levin, H.S. Behavioral effects of occupational exposure to organophosphate pesticides. In: "Behavioral Toxicology. Early detection of occupational hazards" (C. Xintaras, B.L. Johnson and I. deGroot, Eds.), US Department of Health, Education and Welfare, pp. 154-164 (1974).

Levin, H.S., Rodnitzky, R.L. and Mick, D.L. Anxiety associated with exposure to organophosphate compounds. Arch. Gen. Psychiat. 33: 225-228 (1976).

Levine, B.S. and Murphy, S.D. Esterase inhibition and reactivation in relation to piperonyl butoxidephosphorothionate interactions. Toxicol. Appl. Pharmacol. 40: 379-391 (1977).

Lipp, J.A. Effect of Benzodiazepine derivatives on Soman-induced seizure activity and convulsions in the monkey. Arch. Int. Pharmacodyn. 202: 244-251 (1973).

Lippa, A.S., Pelham, R.W., Beer, B., Critchett, D.J., Dean, R.L. and Bartus, R.T. Brain cholinergic disfunction and memory in aged rats. Neurobiol. Aging 1: 13-19 (1980).

Lockridge, O. Substance P hydrolyis by human serum cholinesterase. J. Neurochem. 39: 106-110 (1982).

Lotti, M., Becker, C.E. and Aminoff, M.J. Organophosphate polyneuropathy: pathogenesis and prevention. Neurology (Cleveland) 34: 658-662 (1984).

Lundy, P.M. and Magor, G.F. Cyclic GMP concentrations in cerebellum following organophosphate administration. J. Pharm. Pharmacol. 30: 251-252 (1978).

Lundy, P.M. and Shaw, R.K. Modification of cholinergically induced convulsive activity and cyclic GMP levels in the CNS. Neuropharmacol. 22: 55-63 (1983).

Lundy, P.M., Magor, G. and Shaw, R.K. Gamma Aminobutyric acid metabolism in different areas of rat brain at the onset of Soman-induced convulsions. Arch. Int. Pharmacodyn. Ther. 234: 64-73 (1978).

Main, A.R. Affinity and phosphorylation constants for the inhibition of esterases by organophosphates. Science 144: 992-993 (1964).

Mao, C.C., Guidotti, A. and Costa, E. The regulation of cyclic guanosine monophosphate in rat cerebellum: possible involvement of putative amino acid neurotransmitters. Brain Res. 79: 510-514 (1974).

Massoulie', J. and Bon, S. The molecular forms of cholinesterase and acetylcholinesterase in vertebrates. Ann. Rev. Neurosci. 5: 57-106 (1982).

Matin, M.A. and Kar, P.P. Further studies on the role of gamma-aminobutyric acid in paraoxon-induced convulsions. Eur. J. Pharmacol. 21: 217-221 (1973).

Matsas, R., Fulcher, I.S., Kenny. A.J. and Turner, A.J. Substance P and leu-enkephalin are hydrolized by an enzyme in pig caudate synaptic membranes that is identical with the endopeptidase of kidney microvilli. Proc. Natl. Acad. Sci. USA 80: 3111-3115 (1983).

Matsumura, F. Toxicology of Insecticides. Plenum Press, NY (1975).

Mattson, H. Brandt, K. and Heilbronn, E. Bicyclic phosphorus esters increase the cyclic GMP level in rat cerebellum. Nature 268: 52-53 (1977).

Mazur, A. An enzyme in animal tissues capable of hydrolyzing the phosphorus-fluorine bond of alkyl fluorophosphates. J. Biol. Chem. 164: 271-289 (1946).

Meites, J. and Sonntag, W.E. Hypothalamic hypophysiotropic hormones and neurotransmitter regulation: current views. Ann. Rev. Pharmacol. Toxicol. 21: 295-322 (1981).

Metcalf, D.R. and Holmes, J.H. EEG, psychological and neurological alterations in humans with organophosphorus exposure. Ann. NY Acad. Sci. 160: 357-365 (1969).

Metcalf, R.L., Fukuto, T.R. and March, R.B. Plant metabolism of Dithio-Systox and Thimet. J. Econ. Entomol. 50: 338-345 (1957).

Millar, T.J. and Chubb, I.W. Treatment of sections of chick retina with acetylcholinesterase increases the enkephalin and substance P immunoreactivity. Neurosci. 12: 441-451 (1984).

Misra, V.K., Nag, D., Misra, N.K. and Krishna Murti, C.R. Macular degeneration associated with chronic pesticide exposure. Lancet I: 288 (1982).

Moriya, M., Ohta, T., Watanabe, K., Miyazawa, T., Kato, K. and Shirasu, Y. Further mutagenicity studies on pesticides in bacterial reversion assay systems. Mutat. Res. 116: 185-216 (1983).

Moss, D.E. and Deutsch, J.A. Review of cholinergic mechanisms and memory. In: "Cholinergic Mechanisms" (P.G. Waser, Ed.), Raven Press, NY, pp. 483-492 (1975).

Moss, R.L. and Dudley, C. The challenge of studying the behavioral effects of neuropeptides. In: "Handbook of Neuropharmacology", vol. 18 (L.L. Iversen, S.D. Iversen and S.H. Snyder, Eds.), Plenum Press, NY, pp. 397-454 (1984).

Motoyama, N. and Dauterman, W.C. Glutathione S-transferases: their role in the metabolism of organophosphorus insecticides. In: "Reviews in biochemical Toxicology", vol. 2 (E. Hodgson, J.R. Bend and R.M. Philpot, Eds.), Elsevier, pp. 49-69 (1980).

Munsat, T.L. Anticholinesterase abuse in myasthenia gravis. J. Neurol. Sci. 64: 5-10 (1984).

Murphy, S.D. Mechanisms of pesticide interactions in vertebrates. Residue Rev. 25: 201-221 (1969).

Murphy, S.D. Pesticides. In: "Toxicology: The Basic Science of Poisons" (J. Doull, C.D. Klaassen and M.O. Amdur, Eds.), MacMillan, NY, pp. 357-408 (1980).

Murphy, S.D., Costa, L.G. and Schwab, B.W. Pesticide interactions and development of tolerance. In: "Effects of chronic exposures to pesticides on animal systems" (J.E. Chambers and J.D. Yarbrough, Eds.), Raven Press, NY, pp. 227-242 (1982).

Namba, T., Nolte, C.T. Jackrel, J. and Grob, D. Poisoning due to organophosphate insecticides. Acute and chronic manifestations. Am. J. Med. 50: 475-492 (1971).

Nathanson, J.A. Cyclic nucleotides and nervous system function. Physiol. Rev. 57: 157-256 (1977).

Norman, B.J. and Neal, R.A. Examination of the metabolism in vitro of parathion (diethyl p-nitrophenyl phosphorothionate) by rat lung and brain. Biochem. Pharmacol. 25: 37-45 (1976).

O'Brien, R.D. Toxic Phosphorus Esters. Academic Press, NY, pp. 434 (1960).

O'Brien, R.D. Insecticides: Action and Metabolism. Academic Press, NY, (1967).

O'Brien, R.D. and Yamamoto, I. (Eds.) Biochemical Toxicology of Insecticides. Academic Press, NY, (1970).

Ohto, K. Long term follow up study of chronic organophosphate pesticide intoxication (Saku disease) with special reference with retinal pigmentary degeneration. Acta Soc. Ophthalmol. Japon. 78: 237-243 (1974).

Olianas, M.C., Onali, P., Schwartz, J.P., Neff, N.H. and Costa, E. The muscarinic receptor adenylate cyclase complex of rat striatum: desensitization following chronic inhibition of acetylcholinesterase activity. J. Neurochem. 42: 1439-1443 (19 84).

Olney, J.W., DeGubareff, T. and Labruyere, J. Seizure-related brain damage induced by cholinergic agents. Nature 301: 520-522 (1983).

O'Neill, J.. Non-cholinesterase effects of anticholinesterases Fund. Appl. Toxicol. 1: 154-160 (1981).

Ozoe, Y., Mochida, K. and Eto, M. Reaction of toxic bicyclic phosphates with acetylcholinesterases and alpha-chimotrypsin. Agric. Biol. Chem. 46: 2527-2531 (1982).

Perold, J.G. and Bezuidenhout, D.J.J. Chronic Organophosphate Poisoning. S.A. Med. J. 57: 7-9 (1980).

Petajan, J.H. Vorhees, K.J., Packham, S.C., Baldwin, R.C., Einhorn, I.N., Grunnet, M.L., Dinger, B.G. and Birky, M.M. Extreme Toxicity from combustion products of a fire-retarded polyurethane foam. Science 187: 742-744 (1975).

Philippu, A. Involvement of cholinergic systems of the brain in the central regulation of cardiovascular functions. J. Auton. Pharmacol. 1: 321-330 (1981).

Pinsky, C., Dua, A.K. and La Bella, F.S. Phenylmethylsulfonyl fluoride (PMSF) given systemically produces naloxone-reversible analgesia and potentiates effects of beta-endorphin given centrally. Life Sci. 31: 1193-1196 (1982).

Playfer, J.R., Eze, K.C., Bullen, M.F. and Evans, D.A.P. Genetic polymorphism and interethnic variability of plasma paraoxonase activity. J. Med. Genet. 13: 337-342 (1976).

Prioux-Guyonneau, M., Coudray-Lucas, C., Coq, H.M., Cohen, Y. and Wepierre, J. Modification of rat brain 5-Hydroxytryptamine metabolism by sublethal doses of organophosphate agents. Acta Pharmacol. Toxicol. 51: 21982).

Proctor, N.G., Moscioni, A.D. and Casida, J.E. Chicken embryo NAD levels lowered by teratogenic organophosphorus and methylcarbamate insecticides in duck embryos. Biochem. Pharmacol. 25: 757-762 (1976).

Raiteri, M., Marchi, M. and Paudice, P. Adaptation of presynaptic acetylcholine autoreceptors following long-term drug treatment. Eur. J. Pharmacol. 74: 109-110 (1981).

Reiter, L., Talens, G. and Woolley, D. Acute and subacute parathion treatment: effects on cholinesterase activities and learning in mice. Toxicol. Appl. Pharmacol. 25: 582-588 (1973).

Rowntree, D.W., Nevin, S. and Wilson, A. The effects of diisopropylfluorophosphate in schizophrenia and manic depressive psychosis. J. Neurol. Neurosurg. Psychiat. 13: 47-62 (1950).

Russell, R.W. Behavioral aspects of cholinergic transmission. Fed. Proc. 28: 121-131 (1969).

Russell, R.W. Cholinergic substrates of behavior. In: "Cholinergic Mechanisms and Psychopharmacology" (D.J. Jenden, Ed.), Plenum Press, pp. 709-731 (1978).

Russell, R.W. Cholinergic system in behavior: the search for mechanisms of action. Ann. Rev. Toxicol. Pharmacol. 22: 435-463 (1982).

Russell, R.W., Vasquez, B.J., Overstreet, D.H. and Dalglish, F.W. Effects of cholinolytic agents on behavior following development of tolerance to low cholinesterase activity. Psychopharmacologia (Berl.) 20: 32-41 (1971).

Russell, R.W., Overstreet, D.H., Cotman, C.W., Carson, V.G., Churchill, L., Dalglis h, F.W. and Vasquez, B.J. Experimental tests of hypotheses about neurochemical mechanisms underlying behavioral tolerance to the anticholinesterase, diisopropyl fluorophosphate. J Pharmacol. Exp. Ther. 192: 73-85 (1975).

Russell, R.W., Carson, V.G., Booth, R.A. and Jenden, D.J. Mechanisms of tolerance to the anticholinesterase DFP: acetylcholine levels and dynamics in the rat brain. Neuropharmacol. 20: 1197-1201 (1981).

Russell, R.W., Overstreet, D.H. and Netherton, R.A. Sex-linked and other genetic factors in the development of tolerance to the anticholinesterase DFP. Neuropharmacol. 22: 75-81 (1983).

Sahley, T.L. and Berntson, G.G. Antinociceptive effects of central and systemic administration of nicotine in the rat. Psychopharmacol. 65: 279-283 (1979).

Schwab, B.W. and Murphy, S.D. Induction of anticholinesterase tolerance in rats with doses of disulfoton that produce no cholinergic signs. J. Toxicol. Env. Hlth. 8: 199-204 (1981).

Schwab, B.W., Costa, L.G. and Murphy, S.D. Muscarinic receptor alterations as a mechanism of anticholinesterase tolerance. Toxicol. Appl. Pharmacol. 71: 14-23 (1983).

Schwartz, J.C., Malfoy, B. and De La Baume, S. Biological inactivation of enkephalin and the role of enkephalin-dipeptidyl-carboxypeptidase ("enkephalinase") as neuropeptidase. Life Sci. 29: 1715-1740 (1981).

Seiden, L.S. and Dykstra, L.A. Acetylcholine and behavior. In: "Psychopharmacology: a biochemical and behavioral approach", Van Nostrand Reinhold Company, NY, pp. 213-242 (1977).

Silver, A. The biology of cholinesterases. Elsevier, pp. 596 (1974).

Sivam, S.P., Norris, J.C., Lim, D.K., Hoskins, B. and Ho, I.K. Effect of acute and chronic cholinesterase inhibition with diisopropylfluorophosphate on muscarinic, dopamine, and GABA receptors of the rat striatum. J. Neurochem. 40: 1414-1422 (1983a).

Sivam, S.P., Nabeshima, T., Lim, D.K., Hoskins, B. and Ho, I.K. Diisopropylfluorophosphate and GABA synaptic function: effect on levels, enzymes, release and uptake in the rat striatum. Res. Comm. Chem. Pathol. Pharmacol. 42: 51-60 (1983b).

Smith, M.I., Elvove, E. and Frazier, W.H. The pharmacological action of certain phenol esters, with special reference to the etiology of the so called ginger paralysis. Public Health Rep. 45: 2509-2524 (1930).

Stevens, J.T., Stitzel, R.E. and McPhillips, J.J. Effects of anticholinesterase insecticides on hepatic microsomal metabolism. J. Pharmacol. Exp. Ther. 181: 576-583 (1972).

Stoller, A., Krupinski, J., Christophers, A.J. and Blanks, G.K. Organophosphorus insecticides and major mental illness. An epidemiological investigation. Lancet I: 1387-1388 (1965).

Sumerford, W.T., Hayes, W.J., Johnston, J.M., Walker, K. and Spillane, J. Cholinesterase response and symptomatology from exposure to organic phosphorus insecticides. A.M.A. Arch. Ind. Hyg. Occup. Med. 7: 383-398 (1953).

Ticku, M.K. and Olsen, R.W. Cage convulsant inhibit picrotoxinin binding. Neuropharmacol. 18: 315-318 (1979).

Uga, S., Ishikawa, S. and Mukuno, K. Histophathological study of canine optic nerve and retina treated by organophosphate pesticide. Invest. Ophtalmol. 16: 877-881 (1977).

Vandekar, M. Anesthetic effect produced by organophosphorus compounds. Nature (London) 179: 155-156 (1957).

Van Meter, W.G., Karczmar, A.G. and Fiscus, R.R. CNS effects of anticholinesterases in the presence of inhibited cholinesterases. Arch. Int. Pharmacodyn. 231: 249-260 (1978).

Wecker, L. and Dettbarn, W.D. Paraoxon-induced myopathy: muscle specificity and acetylcholine involvement. Exp. Neurol. 51: 281-291 (1976).

Wecker, L., Kiauta, T. and Dettbarn, W.D. Relationship between acetylcholinesterase inhibition and the development of a myopathy. J. Pharmacol. Exp. Ther. 206: 97-104 (1978).

Weiss, B.L., Foster, F.G. and Kupfer, D.J. Cholinergic involvement in neuropsychiatric symdromes. In: "Biology of Cholinergic Function" (A.M. Goldberg and I. Hanin, Eds.), Raven Press, NY (1976).

Whorton, M.D. and Obrinsky, D.L. Persistence of symptoms after mild to moderate acute organophosphate poisoning among 19 farm field workers. J. Toxicol. Env. Hlth. 11: 347-354 (1983).

Wilkinson, C.F. (Ed.) Insecticide Biochemistry and Physiology. Plenum Press, NY (1976).

Wood, J.D. The role of gamma-aminobutyric acid in the mechanism of seizures. Prog. Neurobiol. 5: 77-95 (1975).

Wooder, M.F. and Wright, A.S. Alkylation of DNA by organophosphorus pesticides. Acta Pharmacol. Toxicol. 49 (Suppl. V): 51-55 (1981).

Zorn, S.H., Costa, L.G. and Murphy, S.D. Diisopropylfluorophosphate- and physostigmine-induced antinociception in mice. Toxicologist 3(1): 14 (1983).

Zorn, S.H., Costa, L.G. and Murphy, S.D. Interaction between diisopropylfluorophosphate and the opiate system in mice. Toxicologist 4(1): 171 (1984).

APPENDIX

Chemical names of the organophosphorus compounds mentioned in the text

Azinphosmethyl	O,O-dimethyl S-[(4-oxo-1,2,3-benzotriazin-3(4H)-yl) methyl phosphorodithioate
Chlorpyrifos	O,O-diethyl-O-(3,5,6-trichloro-2-pyridyl) phosphorothioate
Dicrotophos	3-(dimethoxyphosphinyloxy)-N,N-dimethyliso-crotonamide
Dimethoate	O,O-dimethyl S-(N-methylcarbamoyl methyl) phosphorodithioate
Disulfoton	O,O-diethyl S-2(ethylthio)-ethyl phosphoro-dithioate
DFP	Diisopropylfluorophosphate
Fenitrothion	O,O-dimethyl O-(4 nitro-m-tolyl) phosphoro-thioate
Fenthion	O,O-dimethyl-O-[4-(methylthio)-m-tolyl] phosphorothioate
Leptophos	O-4-Bromo-2,5-dichlorophenyl O-methyl phenyl-phosphonothioate
Malathion	O,O-dimethyl-S-(1,2-dicarbethoxyethyl) phos-phorodithioate
Mephinvos	2-Carbomethoxy-1-methyl-vinyl dimethyl phosphate
Methylchlorpyrifos	O,O-dimethyl-O-(3,5,6-trichloro-2-pyridyl) phosphorothioate
Methylparathion	O,O-dimethyl O-p-nitrophenyl phosphate
Mipafox	N,N'-Diisopropylphosphorodiamidic fluoride
Paraoxon	O,O-diethyl O-p-nitrophenyl phosphate
Parathion	O,O-diethyl O-p-nitrophenyl phosphorothioate
Phorate	O,O-diethyl S-[(ethylthio) methyl] phosphoro-dithioate
Phosphamidon	2-Chloro-2-diethylcarbamoyl-1-methylvinyl dimethyl phosphate
Sarin	Isopropyl methylphosphonofluoridate
Soman	Pinacolyl methylphosphonofluoridate
Tabun	Ethyl N-dimethyl phosphoroamidocyanidate
TEPP	Tetraethylpyrophosphate
TOTP	Triorthotolylphosphate

THE DELAYED POLYNEUROPATHY CAUSED BY SOME ORGANOPHOSPHORUS ESTERS

Marcello Lotti

Istituto di Medicina del Lavoro, Universita' degli Studi, Via Facciolati 71-PADOVA , Italy

Organophosphorus esters (OP) are used as pesticides, plasticizers, hydraulic fluids and flame retardants. They have diverse effects on both the central and peripheral nervous system including the well known acute cholinergic syndrome, as results from the inhibition of acetylcholinesterase (AChE) at nerve endings [1]. Some bicyclic phosphate esters cause convulsive seizures, not related to AChE inhibition, but possibly acting as γ-aminobutyrate antagonists [2,3]. Some cholinesterase inhibitors produce also a necrosis of rat skeletal muscle related to a critical inhibition of AchE over a short period of time [4,5].

Organophosphate induced delayed polyneuropathy (OPIDP) is a syndrome which is distinct from the above, is caused by some, but not all, organophosphates and is characterized by axonal degeneration of long fibers in susceptible species. Several extensive reviews about OPIDP have been recently published [6,7,8,9,10]. Therefore, the clinical features of this toxicity and the mechanism of initiation will be briefly summarized; some aspects of toxicity assessment, rationalized by the understanding of these mechanisms, will be also shortly reported.

In this paper the term neurotoxicity is defined as the delayed axonopathy caused by OP esters.

CLINICAL ASPECTS IN MAN

Several cases of delayed neurotoxicity have occurred in man [11,12,13,14,15], including outbreaks affecting thousands of patients [16,17]. Symptoms of OPIDP begin 1 to 3 weeks after acute exposure to the toxic substance, but less predictably after chronic exposure. The delay between exposure and onset of symptoms depends in part on the dose and the nature of the exposure. OPIDP due to pesticides generally follows acute cholinergic symptoms.

The findings on examination indicate a distal, symmetric, predominantly motor polyneuropathy, with wasting and flaccid weakness of distal limb muscles, especially in the legs. This is of variable severity, but there may be quadriplegia, with foot and wrist drop [10]. With time, there may be some functional recovery [18], but commonly pyramidal and other signs of central neurologic involvement become more evident [19]. The degree of pyramidal involvement may determine the ultimate prognosis for functional recovery [18,20]. Objective evidence of sensory loss is usually slight or completely lacking.

Electrophysiologic evaluation reveals partial denervation of affected muscles, with increased insertional activity, abnormal spontaneous activity (fibrillation potentials and positive sharp waves), and a reduced interference pattern; large polyphasic motor unit potentials to supramaximal stimulation of motor nerves are reduced in amplitude, and terminal motor latencies are delayed; maximal motor conduction velocity is usually normal or slightly reduced [10].

Characteristic neurophysiological changes sometimes may be found in exposed subjects, before any clinical deficit is apparent [21].

THE EXPERIMENTAL MODEL

Several species are susceptible to OPIDP and the experimental animal of choice is the adult hen [6]. Rodents are relatively resistant even though a rodent model of OPIDP has been recently reported [22]. The toxic response can be produced by a single dose of OP compound with a 10-14 day delay. Histopathologic findings reveal a distal axonopathy [23,24,25]. Abnormalities in the central nervous system have been also reported [22,26], especially degeneration of the anterior columns of the thoracic and lumbar spinal cord [23,27]. The vulnerability

of nerve fibers is directly related to axonal length and diameter, large diameter and long fibers being more susceptible than small and short ones[28].
Experimental neurophysiologic studies have indicated that in OPIDP there is functional damage of peripheral portions of the nerve fibers[29].

THE INITIATION MECHANISM

The mechanism of OPIDP was recently reviewed extensively by M.K. Johnson[8]. In brief, in the early 1970s, Johnson demonstrated that OPIDP is initiated by the phosphorylation of a protein in the nervous tissue designated Neuropathy Target Esterase (NTE). A second step is further required to produce the effect : the "aging" of the phosphoryl-enzyme complex. This is usually a rapid, non-enzymatic reaction, and involves the loss of a group attached to the phosphorus, leaving a negatively charged phosphorus group attached tot the protein; groups lost during aging might have a wide range of reactivity. It is unknown whether the negative charge itself or the lost group are involved in the pathogenesis of the disease. This aging process depends only on the chemistry of the OP. OP-NTE complexes that are able to age are those formed by phosphates, phosphonates and phosphoamidates : those formed by phosphinates, carbamates and sulphonates are not able to age. The former compounds might cause delayed neuropathy when the treshold of inhibition of NTE <u>in vivo</u> is reached, whereas the latter will never cause OPIDP.
Furthermore, recent evidence shows that "aging" depends also on the stereoisomery of the organophosphate : different optical isomers of the same organoposphate might age at extremely different speeds[30]. A high level (70-80%) of inhibition of NTE in the nervous system, soon after a single dose of a neurotoxic OP predicts the development of ataxia 2 weeks later in those that survive. This level might be lower in the case of chronic exposure.

When high inhibition of NTE is achieved in animals dosed with phosphinates, carbamates or sulphonates, no neuropathy occurs; however if similarly treated animals are dosed also with a high dose of a potent neurotoxic OP, neuropathy still fails to develop, because the catalytic site of NTE is already phosphorylated and there is no possibility of forming an aged NTE.

The physiological substrate for NTE is not known but its catalytic activity does not seem to be vital to the health of the neuron because it can be blocked by protective agents without overtly harming experimental animals. Furthermore, clinical symptoms develop despite restoration of NTE activity. This mechanism contrasts with that of acute toxicity: inhibition of AChE by OPs leads to accumulation of acetylcholine at nerve endings and thus to cholinergic symptoms.
The cascade of reactions which follows this two steps initiation mechanism, leading to the onset of clinical symptoms 2 weeks later, is unknown.

In a recent study the effect of OPs on axonal NTE and on cell body NTE was dissociated by means of intraarterial injection of the compound. The critical level of NTE inhibition must be reached in the axon to cause either neuropathy or protection. These results suggest that NTE is associated with some axonal functions which are relevant in maintaining the health of the neuron[31].
Several studies on distribution of NTE in neuronal and extra-neuronal tissues of both hen and humans have been performed[32,33,34,35]. NTE is present in nervous tissue, lymphatic tissue and testes in birds and in several organs including liver and kidney in man; these studies did not revealed possible physiological functions of NTE but have been exploited for in vivo monitoring of the effects of OPs (see below).

To summarize the actual level of biological understanding about the role of NTE in the development of OPIDP, it is not known which physiological functions are associated with this protein that have an experimentally useful but physiological irrelevant catalytic activity.

PRACTICAL GAINS FROM UNDERSTANDING THE MECHANISM OF INITIATION

a. Toxicity Testing.

The loss of esteratic activity of NTE can be measured as the graduate response to neurotoxic OP in brief screening tests. Johnson suggested recently a two-stage screening test for OP esters[36]. Preliminary stage: groups of hens are dosed at 4 dose-levels. Brain NTE should be measured in one bird per group within 2 days. Clinical observation should last for 3 weeks but no histopathology is required.

Main stage: dose ranges are adjusted in the light of the clinical and biochemical responses in stage 1 and increased to the point where atropine and oxime treatment is necessary for survival. Three dosing protocols are followed with larger groups of birds. NTE assays are done on brain, spinal cord and peripheral nerves [31,37] of dosed birds at specified intervals: survivors must be observed clinically throughout and histopathology is required 3 weeks after the final dose. Johnson considers that all informations necessary for evaluation of neurotoxic potential can be obtained from tests with a.Single doses ; b.4 consecutive daily doses; c.20 daily doses. Using this protocol he demonstrates that more useful information is obtained or is deducible than is gained from current prolonged tests.

b.Structure Activity Relationship

"Each early discovery of a structure-activity relationship seemed, to its contemporaries, to be a universal explanation of drug action, and it was not clear seen that, had this been true, drugs could evoke only one kind of biological effect. Nowadays, more correctly, we accept different explanations for different biological actions, but are still troubled by our nomenclature. Thus when we say 'structure', we mean 'constitution'; namely, all the information on physical and chemical properties that is stored in the chemical formula, or that can be discovered by measurement and experimentation. Also when we say 'activity' we mean the action on the drug receptor, but this effect, we know, is often connected to the desired physiological result only through a long chain of other reactions. It is only with reference to the action at the receptor that the constitution of the drug has any relevance" [38].

This long sentence taken from a classical textbook, highlights the definition of structure-activity studies. Structure-activity predictions are now possible for the biochemical and neurotoxic activity of many organophosphates and are based on NTE activity assays both <u>in vitro</u> and <u>in vivo</u> [39,40]. General rules for predicting neurotoxicity of tri-aryl-phosphates (plasticizer-type of OP with very low acute toxicity) are :

i. Esters having substituted rings in the ortho position are highly neurotoxic (via metabolic formation of cyclic derivatives). Neurotoxicity is higher in isomers having only one ortho-substituent compared with the symmetrical tri-ortho-ester. Further substitution in the ring containing the ortho-substituent or a larger and more branched ortho-substituent reduces neurotoxicity ;

ii. Esters having no ortho-substituents are less active (metabolism produces inactive inhibitors).

General rules for predicting neurotoxicity of pesticide-type OPs (at doses lower than the letal ones) are the following :

Phosphonates and phosphoroamidates are more neurotoxic than analogous phosphates. OPs with a longer chain or hydrophobic "R" groups are also more neurotoxic. Non planar "R" or acidic groups, nitrophenyl, heterocyclic and oximes acidic groups and thioether linkage of the acidic group, decrease the neurotoxic potential of OPs.

The practical application of these rules should lead to the design of OPs having low neurotoxic potential while retaining their desiderable physical and pesticidal properties.

c. *In vitro-in vivo* extrapolations

Several OPs have been tested *in vitro* against NTE and AChE to determine their inhibition power (I_{50}). I_{50} ratios (I_{50} AChE / I_{50} NTE) are very closed to the corresponding *in vivo* ratios (LD_{50} / neurotoxic dose). Therefore, once molecules of esterase inhibitor arrive in the nervous system, the particular toxic response which will occur is reflected by the compound's ability to inhibit one or other of the target enzymes [41]. Since this ability can be determined *in vitro* we have a useful predictive test. Comparison with similarly derived *in vitro* data with human enzymes reveals that there is never more than a four fold difference between the I_{50}s for either enzyme from the two sources. Therefore, the comparative sensitivity of the enzymes in human brain is the same as in the hen and we might deduce that the comparative acute/delayed toxicity will also be similar. Routine assay of new OP esters against NTE and AChE of hen and human brain will enable biochemical toxicologists to improve the standard of assessment at an earlier stage of product development.

d. Biochemical monitoring

Comprehensive studies of the occurrence of NTE in the tissues of hen and man showed that NTE was present in lymphatic tissue [32,35]. Dudek and Richardson suggested that if inhibition of NTE in blood lymphocytes correlates with inhibition of NTE in nervous tissue, it might be possible to monitor and assess the potential neurotoxic hazard after an exposure to OPs by measuring NTE activity in peripheral lymphocytes. In their study, inhibition of NTE in lymphocytes correlated highly with inhibition of NTE in brain of hens 4 hours after a single exposure [32]. However, this correlation was not evident at any other time in hens after an acute exposure or during a chronic exposure to OP in an earlier study [42].

Furthermore, lymphocytic NTE activity was characterized and measured in humans after both single and repeated exposures to different OPs [43,44,45,46].

From the acute poisoning cases due to potentially neurotoxic OPs, we learned that there is no likelyhood of development of OPIDP if lymphocyte NTE activity is not affected. Furthermore lymphocyte NTE activity correlates with that in peripheral nerves; however,this correlation is evident only over a limited period of time after the poisoning, confirming the same intriguing observation in the animal studies [47].

After subacute occupational exposure to a potentially neurotoxic OP, lymphocytic NTE activity was significantly affected (less than the 70% threshold required in the hen model) but there was no correlation with neuropathy; no neurological abnormalities were detected [46]. Because of the possible peculiar pharmacokinetics of the OP involved, a possible explanation is that the altered lymphocyte NTE activity might represent a false positive case.

It is also not yet known whether or not the percentage of inhibition of NTE necessary to initiate neuropathy in humans is different than that required in hens. This might be answered by <u>post-mortem</u> assay of both AChE and NTE in nervous tissue after OP intoxication [48]. This would help to build up a dat bank for comparison with observed clinical responses in non fatal cases. As more <u>post-mortem</u> and lymphocytic NTE data are published, it might be possible to assess the maximum inhibition of NTE that can be tolerated by humans without expectation of clinical neuropathic response.

This short review underlines the relevance of the understanding of the mechanism of action of OPs. The results in toxicity assessment and monitoring have been described, even though other gains like those in neurobiology and enzymology should not be forgotten.

REFERENCES

1. Taylor,P., 1980, Anticholinesterase Agents, in "The Pharmacological Basis of Therapeutics", A.G. Gilman L.S. Goodman eds., p.100, Macmillan, New York
2. Bellet,E.M., Casida,J.E., 1973, Bicyclic phosphorus esters high toxicity without cholinesterase inhibition, Science, 187:1135
3. Bowery,N.G., Collins,J.F., Hill,R.G., 1976,Bicyclic phosphorus esters that are potent convulsants and GABA antagonists, Nature, 261:601
4. Wecker,L., Dettbarn,W.D., 1976, Paraoxon-induced myopathy: muscle specificity and acetylcholine involvement, Exp. Neurol., 51:281
5. Wecker,L., Kianta,T., Dettbarn,W.D., 1978, Relationship between acetylcholinesterase inhibition and the development of a myopathy, J.Pharmacol.Exp.Therap., 206:97
6. Johnson,M.K., 1975, The delayed neuropathy caused by some organophosphorus esters: mechanism and challenge, CRC Crit.Rev.Toxicol., 3:289
7. Davis,C.S, Richardson,R.J., 1980, Organophosphorus Compounds in "Experimental and Clinical Neurotoxicology", P.S. Spencer and H.H. Schaumburg eds.,p.527, Williams & Wilkins, Baltimore,London
8. Johnson,M.K., 1982, The target for initiation of delayed neurotoxicity by organophosphorus esters: biochemical studies and toxicological applications, Rev.Biochem. Toxicol., 4:141
9. Lotti,M., 1983, Lymphocytic Neurotoxic Esterase, in "Neurobehavioural Methods in Occupational Medicine", Advances in Biosciences, vol.46, R. Gilioli et al. eds., Pergamon Press, New York
10. Lotti,M., Becker,C.E., Aminoff,M.J., 1984, Organophosphate polyneuropathy: pathogenesis and prevention, Neurology, 34:658
11. Bidstrup,P.L., Bonnel,J.A., Beckett,A.G., 1953, Paralysis following poisoning by a new organic phosphorus insecticide (mipafox): report on two cases, Br.Med.J., 1:1068
12. Hierons,R., Johnson,M.K., 1978, Clinical and toxicological investigations of a case of delayed neuropathy in man after acute poisoning by an organophosphorus pesticide Arch.Toxicol., 40:279

13. Jedrzejowska,H., Rowinska-Marcinska,K., Hoppe,B., 1980, Neuropathy due to phytosol (Agritox): report of a case, Acta Neuropathol.(Berl.), 49:163
14. Xintaras,C., Burg,J.R., Tanaka,S., 1978, Occupational exposure to leptophos and other chemicals, US Dept. of Health,Education and Welfare, p. 78,NIOSH Publ., Government Printing Office
15. Senanayake,N., Johnson,M.K., 1982, Acute polyneuropathy after poisoning by a new organophosphate insecticide, N.Engl.J.Med., 306:155
16. Valaer,P.J., 1930, Adulterated ginger responsible for recent paralysis epidemic, J.Am.Pharm.Assoc., 19:948
17. Smith,H.V., Spalding,J.M.K., 1959, Outbreak of paralysis in Marocco due to orthocresyl phosphate poisoning, Lancet, 2:1019
18. Sananayake,N., 1981, Tri-cresyl phosphate neuropathy in Sri Lanka: a clinical and neurophysiological study with a three years follow up, J.Neurol.Neurosurg.Psychiatry, 44:775
19. Morgan,J.P., Penovich,P., 1978, Ginger paralysis: forthy seven-year follow up, Arch.Neurol., 35:530
20. Vasilescu,C., 1979, Triortho cresyl phosphate neuropathy, Arch.Neurol., 36:455
21. LeQuesne,P.M., 1978, Neurophysiological investigations of subclinical and minimal toxic neuropathies, Muscle & Nerve, 1:392
22. Veronesi,B., 1984, The distribution of central and peripheral neuropathology in the rodent model of organophosphorus induced delayed neuropathy, The Toxicologist, 4:55
23. Hern,J.E.C., 1971, Some effects of experimental organophosphorus intoxication in primates, D.M. Thesis, Univ. of Oxford
24. Bouldin,T.W., Cavanagh,J.B., 1979, Organophosphorus neuropathy.I. A teased fiber study of the spatiotemporal spread of axonal degeneration, Am.J.Pathol., 94:241
25. Bouldin,T.W., Cavanagh,J.B., 1979, Organophosphorus neuropathy.II. A fine structural study of the early stages of axonal degeneration, Am.J.Pathol., 94:253
26. Ahmed,M.M., Glees,P., 1971, Neurotoxicity of tricresylphosphate (TCP) in slow loris (Nycticebus coucang coucang), Acta Neuropathol.(Berl.), 19:94

27. Abou-Donia,M.B., 1979, Delayed neurotoxicity of phenylphosphothionate esters, Science, 205:713
28. Spencer,P.S., Schaumburg,H.H., 1978, Pathobiology of neurotoxic axonal degeneration, in "Physiology and Pathobiology of Axons", S.G. Waxman ed., p. 265, Raven Press, New York
29. Baker,T., Lowndes,H.E., Johnson,M.K., Sanborg,I.C., 1980, The effects of phenylmethanesulphonylfluoride on delayed organophosphorus neuropathy, Arch.Toxicol., 46:305
30. Johnson,M.K., 1984, Private communication
31. Caroldi,S., Lotti,M., Masutti,A., 1984, Intraarterial injection of diisopropylfluorophosphate or phenylmethanesulphonylfluoride produces unilateral neuropathy or protection, respectively, in hens, Biochem.Pharmacol., 33:3213
32. Dudek,B.R., Richardson,R.J., 1982, Evidence for the existence of neurotoxic esterase in neural and lymphatic tissue of the adult hen, Biochem.Pharmacol., 31:1117
33. Lotti,M., Wei,E.T., Spear,R.C., Becker,C.E., 1984, Neurotoxic esterase in rooster testis, Toxicol.Appl.Pharmacol., in press
34. Lotti,M., Johnson,M.K., 1980, Neurotoxic esterase in human nervous tissue, J.Neurochem., 34:747
35. Moretto,A., Fassina,A., Lotti,M., 1983, Neurotoxic esterase in extranervous tissues of man, Second International Meeting on Cholinesterase : Fundamental and Applied Aspects, Bled, Yugoslavia, September 17-21,1983
36. Johnson,M.K., 1983, Delayed neurotoxicity tests of organophosphorus esters: a proposed protocol integrating neuropathy target esterase (NTE) assays with behavior and histopathology tests to obtain more information more quickly from fewer animals, International Conference on "Environmental Hazards of Agrochemicals in Developing Countries", A.H. El Sebae ed., vol.1, p.474, Alexandria, Egypt, November 8-12,1983
37. Caroldi,S., Lotti,M., 1982, Neurotoxic esterase in peripheral nerve: assay inhibition and rate of resynthesis, Toxicol.Appl.Pharmacol., 62:498
38. Albert,A., 1981, Selective Toxicity. The Physico-Chemical Basis of Therapy, p. 49, Sixth edition, Chapman & Hall, London,New York

39. Johnson,M.K., 1975, Structure-activity relationship for substrates and inhibitors of hen brain neurotoxic esterase, Biochem.Pharmacol., 24:797

40. Johnson,M.K., 1975, Organophosphorus esters causing delayed neurotoxic effects. Mechanism of action and structure-activity studies, Arch.Toxicol., 34:259

41. Lotti,M., Johnson,M.K., 1978, Neurotoxicity of organophosphorus pesticides: predictions can be based on in vitro studies with hen and human enzymes, Arch.Toxicol., 41:215

42. Lotti,M., Johnson,M.K., 1980, Repeated small doses of a neurotoxic organophosphate: monitoring of neurotoxic esterase in brain and spinal cord, Arch.Toxicol., 45:263

43. Bertoncin,D., Ruffolo,A., Caroldi,S., Lotti,M., 1984, Neuropathy target esterase in human lymphocytes, Arch. Environ.Hlth., in press

44. Caroldi,S., Lotti,M., Pegoraro,M., 1981, La NTE linfocitaria come test di monitoraggio per la neurotossicità da esteri organofosforici, 44o Congresso Nazionale della Società Italiana di Medicina del Lavoro ed Igiene Industriale, Padova, Italy, October 21-24,1981

45. Osterloh,J., Lotti,M., Pond,S., 1983, Toxicologic studies in a fatal overdose of 2,4-D,MCPP and Chlorpyrifos, J.Anal.Toxicol., 7:125

46. Lotti,M., Becker,C.E., Aminoff,M.J., Woodrow,J.E., Seiber, J.N., Talcott,R.E., Richardson,R.J., 1983, Occupational exposure to the cotton defoliants DEF and Merphos: a rational approach to monitoring organophosphorus-induced neurotoxicity, J.Occup.Med., 25:517

47. Dudek,B.R., 1979, Brain and leucocyte neurotoxic esterase as biomonitors of organophosphorus delayed neurotoxicity, PhD Thesis, The University of Michigan, Ann Arbor,USA

48. Lotti,M., Ferrara,S.D., Caroldi,S., Sinigaglia,F., 1981, Enzyme studies with human and hen autopsy tissue suggest omethoate does not cause delayed neuropathy in man, Arch.Toxicol., 48:265

CENTRAL NERVOUS SYSTEM EFFECTS OF LEAD: A STUDY MODEL IN NEURO-TOXICOLOGY

S. Govoni, F. Battaini, R.A. Rius, C. Fernicola*,
L. Coniglio*, and M. Trabucchi**

Institute of Pharmacological Sciences, University of Milan, *Occupational Health Unit, Brescia and **Chair of Toxicology, 2nd University of Rome, Italy

Interest in lead intoxication has grown significantly over the last decades as a consequence of the large use of this metal and of its diffusion in the environment. In spite of the concern about lead toxicity, occupational exposure is still present in small, low-technology factories.

Lead may act as a neurotoxin at very low doses so that its presence in the environment represents a threat to the health of large portions of the human population, chiefly those at increased risk for toxicity. In fact, both clinical and experimental studies indicate that developing and young organisms are more susceptible to lead neurotoxicity. At low doses the signs of lead neurotoxicity may be subtle, requiring the evaluation of complex behaviour and the completion of physiological tests to reveal mental impairment. In a recent survey of this subject, Needleman (1983) proposes guidelines to avoid methodological problems in such testing and shows that children exposed to lead (dentine lead 27 ppm) have an altered electroencephalographic pattern with an increase of slow delta waves (Needleman, 1983; Burchfiel, 1980). European studies (Winneke et al. 1983; Winneke and Kraemer, 1984) also indicate neurotoxic effects of low lead levels in children. These investigations have indicated that lead exposed children (as measured by tooth lead levels) present an impairment in visual motor integration and reaction performance, without deficits of general intelligence when the data are corrected with social background variables. In spite of the discrepancy between these findings and the U.S. studies concerning the effects on general intelligence, which may depend on the assessement of I.Q. and on the criteria chosen for discriminating between high and low exposure, all the studies agree that lead is an important neurotoxin and that children are particularly sensitive to it. To emphasize the extent of the phenomenon, recent epidemiological data (Mahaffey et al. 1982) available on the U.S. population indicate that if it is assumed that lead is neurotoxic at values above 20 mcg/100 ml of blood, three to four million children may suffer neurotoxic damage. In particular, it is important to note that 50.000 of them have a blood lead (PbB) over 39 mcg/dl.

In addition to the data on children, recent observations on occupationally lead exposed workers indicate that in absence of changes of biological indicators of toxicity, physiological dysfunctions and disturbances in subjective feelings of well being may be demonstrated (Grandjean et al. 1978; Arnvig et al. 1980; Hanninen et al. 1980).

The concern about the CNS effects of low-level lead exposure has stimulated the development of animal models of lead intoxication which, according to the available experimental data, provide a useful and reliable tool to understand the biochemical modifications elicited at central and peripheral levels by lead poisoning. Exposure of the rats during development to high lead levels produces encephalopathic lesions comparable to those observed in Man (Winder et al. 1983). Behavioral effects of lead, however, may precede and be manifest in absence of morphological damage of the CNS.

Behaviorally, the effect of lead is debated and many inconsistencies are present in the literature due to differences in the neurobehavioral test, animals, strains or exposure protocol. Many papers provide evidence for lead-induced disturbances of mechanisms of attention and hyperactivity (Silbergeld and Goldberg, 1973; Silbergeld and Goldberg, 1975; Golter and Michaelson, 1975; Maker et al. 1975; Grant et al. 1975), while others do not suggest this hypothesis (Gray and Reiter, 1977; Sobotka and Cook, 1974; Modak et al. 1975). In a recent paper Mc Carren (1983) testing the effect of lead at three different dose levels (543, 1363 and 2725 ppm in the drinking water of the lactating dam), observed an increase in activity at only a single dose (1363 ppm) and at a specific age (16 days). On the other hand, as indicated by Winneke et al. (1977, 1982), the effect of lead is complex resulting more precisely in an increase of behavioral reactivity and in a disrupted performance in complex discrimination tasks than solely in hyperkinesis. Moreover in studies using a battery of sensory-motor tests and pharmacological manipulations, Fox (1979) has shown that lead-exposed rats exhibit delayed maturation, altered developmental patterns and long-term CNS disturbances. Lead-exposed rats also exhibit altered drug responsivity. In particular, they present a paradoxical (decreased activity) or a reduced stimulatory response to amphetamine, methylphenidate and fenfluramine. A reduced sensitivity to the stimulus properties of amphetamine has been recently shown using a drug-discrimination learning paradigm by Zenick and Goldsmith (1981). Their results suggest also that the development of hyposensitivity depends primarily on the exposure of the animal during the neonatal period, since the deficit was seen also in animals which were not continued on lead after weaning.

Behavioral studies available on primates suggest that lead ingestion (daily ingestion in milk for one year, producing blood Pb levels of 30-100 μg/dl) alters the social development of infant rhesus monkeys (Bushnell and Bowman, 1979). The behavioral effects of lead have stimulated the search for the underlying neurochemical changes. The general biochemical effects of lead on the CNS include changes in protein or DNA concentrations and decreases in respiratory activity; however most of these changes occur at high levels of exposure. Other biochemical effects include changes in lipid composition, competition with calcium effects on enzyme systems, including catecholamine-synthesizing enzymes (for a review of the general biochemical effects of lead on the CNS, see Winder and Kitchen, 1984).

The neurochemical effects of lead seem to involve almost all the neurotransmitters that have been so far investigated (see the above quoted review by Winder and Kitchen, 1984). In particular, studies are avialble on the effect of lead on acetylcholine, catecholamine, gamma-amino butyric acid, serotonin and peptidergic transmitter (mostly met-enkephalin).

However, it is not known whether all these lead-induced changes in neurotransmitter function represent a primary effect of lead or whether some systems are more susceptible to the toxic action and then drive compensatory changes in other neurotransmitters.

A peculiar observation is that the effect of lead is area-specific. For example, in one study (Dubas and Hrdina, 1978), serotonin levels of lead-exposed rats at 8 weeks of age were found decreased in cortex and hypothalamus and unmodified in striatum and midbrain. Dopamine turnover is decreased in striatum and increased in nucleus accumbens of lead-exposed rats (Govoni et al. 1979). In the same animals, GABA-binding sites were found decreased in striatum, increased in cerebellum and unchanged in cortex and hypothalamus (Govoni et al. 1980; Memo et al. 1980b).

The selective action of lead may reflect either a different accumulation of the metal within distinct anatomical regions or differences in the mechanisms regulating synthesis, release and uptake of the involved neurotransmitter in the various brain areas. Experimental data support both the possibilities. In fact, Collins et al. have observed in their experiments that the hippocampus accumulates lead (Collins et al. 1984) confirming an earlier report (Fjerdungstad et al. 1974) of selective lead accumulation in this brain region. However, the reason for this preferential storage (vascular, biochemical, neurochemical) is presently unclear. On the other hand, as shown in the following paragraphs, the differential effect of lead on dopaminergic transmission in striatum with respect to nucleus accumbens may be explained on the basis of a different mechanism regulating dopamine uptake in the two areas. Although data and theories on the neurochemical substrate involved in lead toxicity abound, several reports consistently indicate that lead induces alterations in the dopaminergic transmission. This view is supported also by behavioral data (Zenick and Goldsmith, 1981). In the present paper the evidences for the involvment of dopaminergic transmission in lead neurotoxic action will be reviewed in detail. In addition a paragraph will be devoted to the discussion of some recent result we obtained studying the interaction lead-calcium as investigated by measuring the binding of ^{3}H-nitrendipine, a ligand supposed to label Ca^{++} channels.

LEAD EXPOSURE

The exposure protocol employs lead acetate (2.5 and or 0.04 g liter, corresponding to 1350 and 218 ppm, respectively, of lead) in the drinking water; pregnant rats (day 16 of pregnancy) receive this solution as the only source of water. After birth the offspring receive the same drinking solution and at 5 weeks of age they are all tested for locomotor activity; an increased in motor activity without loss of weight compared to control unexposed animals is considered sign of intoxication (details of the exposure protocol, blood and brain Pb levels are reported in the quoted papers). The exposure to lead through the drinking water seems to be a suitable model, also in view of recent literature data suggesting that lead in water may substantially contribute to elevate blood lead levels (Elwood, 1984).

NIGROSTRIATAL AND MESOLIMBIC DOPAMINERGIC SYSTEM

Since an activation of mesolimbic dopaminergic system is reported to evoke locomotor hyperactivity (Pijnenburg et al. 1976) the turnover of dopamine in various brain areas rich in dopamine was examined first; a different pattern of action is observed according to the area examined. In fact, while there is no modification in substantia nigra, an increase is apparent in nucleus accumbens and a decrease is observed in striatum and frontal cortex (Table 1). The functional state of adenylate cyclase, either basal or dopamine stimulated, is not affected in any of the areas examined after lead intoxication; the receptors for dopamine, labeled by ^{3}H-spiroperidol are unaffected as well (Govoni et al. 1979), although in vitro lead may inhibit this binding (Bondy and Agrawal, 1980).

TABLE 1
LEAD INDUCED CHANGES IN CENTRAL DOPAMINERGIC TRANSMISSION

Prameter measured	Striatum	Accumbens
Dopamine turnover*	decrease	increase
Adenylate cyclase: Basal	no change	no change
Dopamine stimulated	no change	no change
Dopamine receptor density (using ^{3}H-Sulpiride)	increase	decrease
Dopamine uptake	increase	decrease
Na^{+} dependent ^{3}H-Cocaine binding	increase	----
Na^{+} independent ^{3}H-Cocaine binding	no change	no change

*measured as DOPAC concentration decay after dopamine synthesis inhibition; in the same animals no change were observed in S. Nigra and a decrease in Frontal cortex.

It was later recognized that dopamine receptors as labeled by ^{3}H-sulpiride are differentially affected according to the area examined; ^{3}H-sulpiride labels preferentially D_2 dopamine receptors (not linked to the adenylate cyclase system) (Spano et al. 1980). Lead exposure decreased the density of dopamine receptors in nucleus accumbens while inducing an increase in striatum; no modification in the affinity was detected in both areas (Lucchi et al. 1981). These results are consistent with the changes in dopamine turnover; in fact receptor supersensitivity may occur as a consequence of the reduced dopaminergic activity observed at striatal levels following lead exposure. Oppositely, in nucleus accumbens, an increased synthesis of dopamine is followed by receptor subsensitivity. The observation that in substantia nigra, where dopamine is released from dendrites of neurons projecting axons to the striatum, dopamine turnover is unmodified by lead, may suggest that the target of the intoxication is not on cell bodies of nigrostriatal dopaminergic neurons but may be located at a striatal level. It was then interesting to examine the utilization of dopamine in the dopaminergic areas more directly influenced by lead poisoning. Release and uptake of dopamine were investigated in striatum and nucleus accumbens slices of lead-exposed rats. The release of endogenous dopamine in our experimental conditions is not affected by lead in both striatum and nucleus accumbens either under basal or depolarized conditions; the uptake for dopamine, on the other hand, is decreased in striatum (-44%) and increased (+55%) in nucleus accumbens, measured as maximal capability to transport the neurotransmitter, while no change is apparent in the affinity of dopamine for the carrier system (Missale et al. 1984).

The data on dopamine uptake are reinforced by the observation that the Na^+-dependent ^{3}H-cocaine binding, reported to be directly linked to the control of dopamine uptake, is decreased in the striatum of lead-exposed rats (Table 1). In nucleus accumbens ^{3}H-cocaine binding is only Na^+-independent suggesting a different regulatory mechanism of the uptake system in comparison with striatum. In both areas the Na^+-independent binding is unaffected by lead poisoning (Missale et al. 1984). The changes in dopamine turnover are dose dependent and reversible. In fact the effect on dopamine turnover are attenuated in striatum and nucleus accumbens by a less severe lead intoxication (0.04 g/liter). Dopamine turnover in striatum and nucleus accumbens of exposed animals returns to control values 30 days after the last assumption of lead (Memo et al. 1981). A useful approach to explore and to unmask the lead-induced alterations in central dopaminergic transmission has been the challenge of exposed animals with dopaminergic agonists and antagonists. In accord with clinical studies where benzamides such as tiapride are used to treat hyperkinetic disorders, sulpiride is able to antagonize more efficently than haloperidol the hyperkinetic behaviour induced by lead intoxication; this observation has a neurochemical correlation with binding data indicating that dopamine receptors labeled by sulpiride but not by spiroperidol are affected by lead poisoning (Lucchi et al. 1981).

The use of indirect dopaminomimetics, such as amphetamine, induces an hyperkinetic behaviour which is less pronounced in lead poisoned animals (Memo et al. 1980a). The decreased ability of amphetamine to stimulate locomotor activity is not paralleled neurochemically by a reduced ability of the drug to decrease dopamine turnover (measured as DOPAC levels) in the striatum and nucleus accumbens of these animals. The explanation for this discrepancy may rely on the involvement of other neurotransmitter systems and brain regions in addition to those investigated in mediating the locomotor response to amphetamine (Govoni et al. 1980; Memo et al. 1980b).

TUBERO INFUNDIBULAR DOPAMINERGIC SYSTEM

Not only nigrostriatal and mesolimbic dopaminergic systems are targets for lead intoxication but also the tubero infundibular dopamine neurons, controlling prolactin release, seem to be particularly sensitive to this metal. A decrease in dopamine turnover at the hypothalamic level in lead-exposed rats appears to be paralleled by an increase in circulating prolactin (Govoni et al. 1978). In addition an impairment of dopamine receptors in the pituitary, as indicated by a decreased ^{3}H-sulpiride binding, suggests a selective sensitivity of these receptors to the toxic action of circulating lead (Govoni et al. 1984) (Table 2).

The observation in rodents of a lead-induced dysfunction of the hypothalamic dopaminergic system has prompted a clinical investigation. Plasma prolactin, Zinc protoporphyrin (Zpp), and blood lead (PbB) were measured in the blood of occupationally exposed workers. Subjects were workers of pewter factories regularly controlled by the local Occupational Health Unit (USSL 41, Brescia, Italy). Although serum prolactin is in the normal range (1 to 10 ng/ml) in all subjects, dividing the population sample in subgroups having blood lead and zinc protoporphyrin below and above normal safe levels (40 μg/dl each), a picture emerges in which lead intoxication is accompanied by a significant rise in serum prolactin concentration (Fig. 1) (Fernicola et al. 1984).

TABLE 2

LEAD INDUCES CHANGES IN TUBERO INFUNDIBULAR DOPAMINERGIC TRANSMISSION

Parameter measured	Hypothalamus	Pituitary	Serum
Dopamine	no change	n.d.	---
DOPAC	decrease	n.d.	---
Dopamine receptor (^{3}H-Sulpiride)	small increase	decrease	---
Prl	----	n.d.	increase

n.d. = not determined.

We may tentatively correlate the rise in prolactin to an impairment of the dopaminergic system without relevant clinical symptoms. Prolactin may therefore represent a biological marker for central effects of lead at threshold levels of exposure.

CALCIUM METABOLISM

Part of the neurotoxic effects of lead have been linked to the ability of this ion to interact with other positively charged physiological ions (Silbergeld, 1982) or their carriers (Hexum, 1974). Neurotoxic effects of lead are seen at concentrations of this ion in tissues well below the level of toxicity of other neurotoxic metals such as manganese, copper, aluminum, cadmium and mercury. Particular attention has been given to the interaction of lead and calcium. Lead added in vitro to striatal synaptosomes is able to promote the influx of ^{45}Ca into the terminals (Silbergeld, 1977).

We observed that lead poisoning induces an increase in ^{3}H-nitrendipine (a specific probe for calcium channel) binding to striatal membranes (Rius et al. 1984). The treatment affects the number of binding sites. However, when the membranes are washed with chelating agents, the binding of lead-exposed rats returns to control values, indicating that the increase is due to the presence of lead in the membranes prepared from treated rats (Fig. 2).

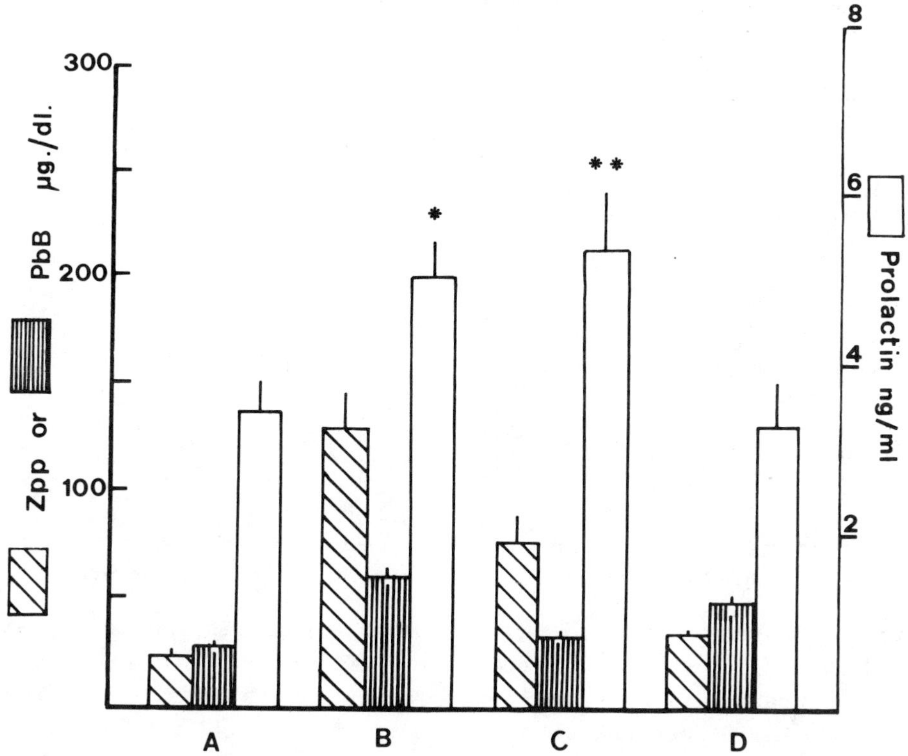

Fig. 1 Zinc protoporphyrin, lead and prolactin in blood of occupationally exposed workers. Group A: Zpp and PbB < 40 µg/dl, N = 22. Mean age 33±2.3; Group B: Zpp and PbB > 40 µg/dl, N = 33. Mean age 35±0.2; Group C: PbB < and Zpp > 40 µg/dl, N = 13. Mean age 37±3.6; Group D: PbB > and Zpp < 40 µg/dl, N = 8. Mean age 39±4.6.
Values represent means ± S.E.M.
*P < 0.01, **P < 0.02 respect to group A, Dunnet t-test.

Very interestingly preliminary data indicate that this effect is area-specific. In fact no changes in ^{3}H-nitrendipine binding are observed in hippocampus in spite of the fact that this brain area accumulates lead (Collins et al. 1984). In addition, the in vitro exposure to micromolar concentration of lead stimulates the binding of nitrendipine in a area-specific fashion. In fact lead stimulates nitrendipine binding maximally in striatum being more powerful than calcium on a molar basis, while in hippocampus almost no stimulation in binding occurs and intermediate values are observed using cortical membranes (manuscript in preparation). This regional selective sensitivity of ^{3}H-nitrendipine binding to lead is in line with previous observations indicating that this metal has different and specific effects on brain neurotransmitters according to the nucleus studied.

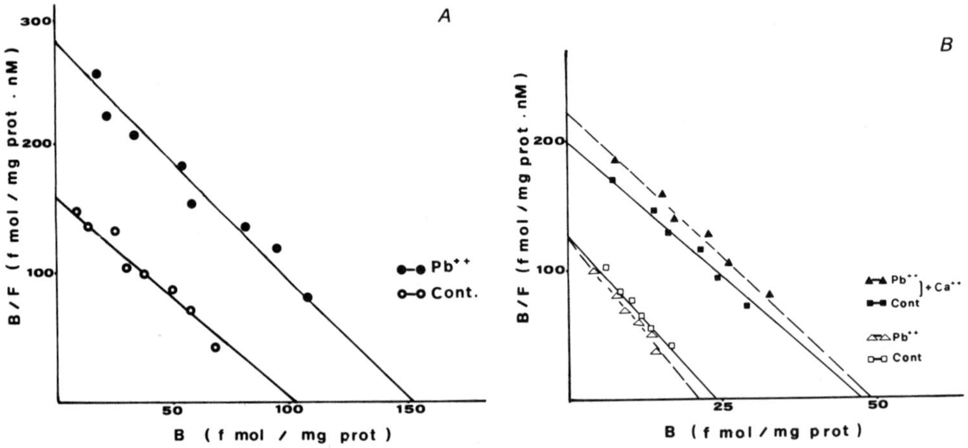

Fig. 2 Scatchard analysis of ^{3}H-nitrendipine binding to striatal membranes from control and lead intoxicated rats. Scatchard analysis was performed using at least 6 different ^{3}H-NDP concentrations ranging from 0.05 to 1.5 nM for Tris washed membranes (A) and from 0.05 to 0.5 nM for Tris EDTA-EGTA washed membranes (B) according to Gould et al. 1982.
EGTA-EDTA treated membranes were assayed either in absence or presence of 300 μM Ca^{++}.

Actually, it may be hypothesized that the differential sensitivity to lead of dihydropyridine binding sites, which are presumably linked to the regulation of calcium channels, may represent one of the fundamental mechanisms mediating the selective neurotoxicity of lead. An action of lead on transmitter release by interference with the processes governing the presynaptic concentration of ionized calcium has been suggested also by electrophysiological experiments on neuromuscular junctions (Cooper and Manalis, 1983). These electrophysiologic data show that lead first inhibits evoked release (as indicated by a reduced endplate potential (EPP)) and then stimulates the rate of spontaneous release (as indicated by an increase in the frequency of miniature endplate potentials (MEPPs)).

The effect of lead has been explained by hypothesizing that the metal blocks Ca^{++} channel on or near the external surface of the presynaptic membrane, thus reducing the EPP, and then enters the intracellular component where it enhances free Ca^{++} concentrations by altering the Ca^{++} sequestration by mitochondria and other intracellular organelles, thus causing the increased MEEP frequency. However, direct experiments with brain mitochondria (Silbergeld and Adler, 1978) indicate that lead stimulates rather than inhibits the binding of $^{45}Ca^{++}$ to them. Moreover experiments on brain cortex synaptosomes indicate that ruthenium red reverses lead-enhanced calcium uptake by synaptosomes (Silbergeld and Adler 1978). In addition experiments on synaptosomal ghosts, confirm that lead does not stimulate calcium uptake in synaptosomes void of mitochondria (Silbergeld, 1984a).

Silbergeld suggests that the effect of lead on spontaneous release in peripheral nerves might be mediated only at the extracellular side, possibly involving the Na-Ca exchange processes, or that free lead in cytosol may act like calcium to promote spontaneous release (Silbergeld, 1984a).

The interaction with mitochondrial calcium and calcium availability for neurotransmitter release, may not be the solely mechanisms by which lead alters neurotransmitter function and release. For example Missale et al. (1984) did not find alterations in DA release in striatum and in nucleus accumbens of in vivo lead-exposed rats, although DA-uptake processes were respectively decreased and increased in these two brain areas.

On the other hand, other authors found that in vivo lead treatment or in vivo lead addition increases DA release from nerve terminals (Silbergeld, 1977; Silbergeld and Adler, 1978).

In spite of these inconsistences, there is agreement that mitochondria are key structures in the basic action of lead.

On the other hand, recent data indicate that lead-calcium may interact also at the calmodulin level. In fact, lead may activate calmodulin-sensitive processes, both in peripheral models (erythrocytes; Goldstein and Ar, 1983) and in brain (Chao et al. 1984). All this evidence points to the interaction lead-calcium as a key event possibly underlying some of the neurotoxic actions of this heavy metal.

CONCLUDING REMARKS

The molecular mechanisms of lead toxicity are not fully elucidated; however the basic and clinical data on lead as a neurotoxin are relatively abundant and strongly indicate the necessity to reduce exposure to this toxin. Although it is not yet possible to integrate the cellular mechanism with the complex lead-induced behavioral dysfunctions, the literature data are consistent in indicating that dopaminergic transmission, gabaergic transmission and calcium ion homeostasis in CNS are deeply affected by this metal. The study of Pb neurotoxicity has in fact fostered the notion that metals may act as specific neurotoxins through complex molecular mechanism, rather than acting as non-specific protein denaturating agents. On this line, the problem of metal toxicity becomes even more complex in terms of interactions with mechanisms of normal brain functioning with drug treatments, health status and other environmental factors and metals (Shukla and Singhal, 1984).

Clinically these new concepts have promoted a greater attention to the search for methods of detecting early symptoms and biological markers of lead toxicity both in exposed workers in their families and in the general population as withnessed by the studies reported also in the introductory section of this paper (Needleman, 1983; Winneke et al. 1983; Winneke and Kraemer, 1984; Grandjean et al. 1978; Arnvig et al. 1980; Hanninen et al. 1979; Rice et al. 1978).

In addition, there is concern about the possible teratogenic effects; Needleman has in fact recently shown (Needleman, 1984) the existence of a correlation between umbilical blood lead concentrations and minor birth defects. On this line, Silbergeld has recently stressed the importance to progress in the study of the behavioural teratology of lead as a toxin able to reach the fetus in utero and to exert toxic effects on reproduction (Silbergeld, 1984b). In fact maternal fetal hormonal patterns are important in supporting normal brain development. On the other hand, relatively few studies are available on the neuroendocrine effects of lead as well as of other heavy metals. This may actually represent a fruitful field of investigation in the search for precocious biological markers of toxicity allowing an efficacious prevention.

ACKNOWLEDGEMENTS: This study was supported by contract CNR

830297656 of the Consiglio Nazionale delle Ricerche of Italy.

REFERENCES

Arnvig, E., Grandjean, P., and Beckman, J., 1980, Neurotoxic effects of heavy lead exposure determined with psychological tests, Toxicol. Lett., 5:399.

Bondy, S.C., and Agrawal, A.K., 1980, The inhibition of cerebral high affinity receptor sites by lead and mercury compounds Arch. Toxicol., 46:249.

Burchfiel, J., Duffy, F., Bartels, P.H., and Needleman, H.L., 1980, The combined discriminating power of quantitative electroencephalography and neuropsychologic measures in evaluating central nervous system effects of lead at low levels, In: "Low lead exposure", (H.L. Needleman, ed.), pp. 75, Raven Press, New York.

Bushnell, P.J., and Bowman, R.E., 1979, Effects of chronic lead ingestion on social development in infant rhesus monkeys, Neurobehav. Toxicol., 1:207.

Chao, S.H., Suzuki Y., Zysk, J.R., and Cheung, W.Y., 1984, Activation of calmodulin by various metal cations as a function of ionic radius, Molecular Pharmacol., 26:75.

Collins, M.F., Whittle, E., and Singhal, R.L., 1984, The effects of low-level lead exposure in developing rats: changes in circadian locomotor activity and hippocampal noradrenaline turnover, Can. J. Physiol. Pharmacol., 62:430.

Cooper, G.P., and Manalis, R.S., 1983, Influence of heavy metals on synaptic transmission: a review, Neurotoxicology, 4:69.

Dubas, T.C., and Hrdina, P.D., 1978, Behavioral and neurochemical consequences of neonatal exposure to lead in rats, J. Environ. Path. Toxic., 2:473.

Elwood, P.C., Gallacher, J.E.J., Phillips, K.M., Davies, B.E., and Toothill, C., 1984, Greater contribution to blood lead from water than from air, Nature, 310:138.

Fernicola, C., Coniglio, L., Govoni, S., and Trabucchi, M., 1984, Andamento delle concentrazioni plasmatiche di prolattina in un gruppo di lavoratori professionalmente esposti a piombo inorganico, 47° Congresso della Società Italiana di Medicina del Lavoro e Igiene Industriale, pp. 937.

Fjerdingstad, E.J., Danscher, G., and Fjerdingstad, E., 1974, Hippocampus: selective concentration of lead in the normal rat brain, Brain Res., 80:350.

Fox, D.A., 1979, Physiological and neurobehavioral alterations during development in lead exposed rats, Neurobehav. Toxicol., 1:193.

Goldstein, G.W., and Ar, D., 1983, Lead activates calmodulin sensitive processes, Life Sci., 33:1001.

Golter, M., Michaelson, I.A., 1975, Growth, behavior and brain catecholamines in lead exposed neonatal rats: a reappraisal, Science, 187:359.

Gould, R.J., Murphy, K.M.M., Snyder, S.H., 1982, ^{3}H-Nitrendipine labeled calcium channels discriminate inorganic calcium agonists and antagonists, Proc. Natl. Acad. Sci., U.S.A., 79:3656.

Govoni, S., Montefusco, O., Spano, P.F., and Trabucchi, M., 1978, Effect of chronic lead treatment on brain dopamine synthesis and serum prolactin release in the rat, Toxicol. Lett. 2:333.

Govoni, S., Memo, M., Spano, P.F., and Trabucchi, M., 1979, Chronic lead treatment differentially affects dopamine synthesis in various rat brain areas, Toxicology, 12:343.

Govoni, S., Memo, M., Lucchi, L., Spano, P.F., and Trabucchi, M., 1980, Brain neurotransmitter system and chronic lead intoxication, Pharmacol. Res. Commun., 12:447.

Govoni, S., Lucchi, L., Battaini, F., Spano, P.F., and Trabucchi, M., 1984, Chronic lead treatment affects dopaminergic control of prolactin secretion in rat pituitary, Toxicol. Lett., 20:237.

Grant, L.D., Howard, J.L., Alexander, S., Krigman, M.R., 1975, Low level lead exposure: behavioral effects, Environ. Health Perspect., 10:267.

Grandjean, P., Arnvig, E., and Beckman, J., 1978, Physiological dysfunctions in lead-exposed workers, Scand. J. Work. Environ. and Health, 4:295.

Gray, L.E., Reiter, L.W., 1977, Lead-induced developmental and behavioral changes in the mouse, Toxicol. Appl. Pharmacol. 41:140.

Hanninen, H., Mantere, P., Hernberg, S., Seppalainen, A.M., and Kock, B., 1980, Subjective symptoms in low-level exposure to lead, Neurotoxicology, 1:333.

Hexum, T.D., 1974, Studies on the reaction catalyzed by transport (Na, K) adenosine triphosphatase, I, Biochem. Pharmacol., 23:3441.

Lucchi, L., Memo, M., Airaghi, M.L., Spano, P.F., and Trabucchi, M., 1981, Chronic lead treatment induces in rat a specific and differential effect on dopamine receptors in different brain areas, Brain Res., 213:397.

Mahaffey, K.R., Annest, J.L., Roberts, J., and Murphy, R.S., 1982, National estimates of blood lead levels: US 1976-1980; association with selected demographic and socioeconomic factors, New Engl. J. Med., 307:575.

Maker, H.S., Lehrer, G.M., Silides, D.M., 1975, The effect of lead on mouse brain development, Environ. Res., 10:76.

Mc Carren, M., and Eccles, C.V., 1983, Neonatal lead exposure in rats: I. Effects on activity and brain metals, Neurobehav. Toxicol. and Teratol., 5:527.

Memo, M., Lucchi, L., Spano, P.F., and Trabucchi, M., 1980a, Lack of correlation between the neurochemical and behavioral effects induced by d-amphetamine in chronically lead-treated rats, Neuropharmacology, 19:795.

Memo, M., Lucchi, L., Spano, P.F., and Trabucchi, M., 1980b, Effect of lead treatment on GABAergic receptor function in rat brain, Toxicol. Lett., 6:427.

Memo, M., Lucchi, L., Spano, P.F., and Trabucchi, M., 1981, Dose--dependent and reversible effects of lead on rat dopaminergic system, Life Sci., 28:795.

Missale, C., Battaini, F., Govoni, S., Castelletti, L., Spano, P.F., and Trabucchi, M., 1984, Chronic lead exposure differentially affects dopamine transport in rat striatum, and nucleus accumbens, Toxicology, 33:81.

Modak, A.T., Weintraub, S.T., Stavinoha, W.B., 1975, Effect of chronic ingestion of lead on the central cholinergic system in rat brain regions, Toxicol. Appl. Pharmacol., 34:340.

Needleman, H.L., 1983, Lead at low dose and the behavior of children, Neurotoxicology, 4,3:121.

Needleman, H.L., Rabinowitz, M., Leviton, A., Linn, S., Schoenbaum S., 1984, The relationship between prenatal exposure to lead and congenital anomalies, JAMA, 251,22:2956.

Pijnenburg, A.J.J., and Van Rossum, J.M., 1973, Stimulation of locomotor activity following injection of dopamine into the nucleus accumbens, J. Pharm. Pharmacol., 25:1003.

Rice, C., Fischbein, A., Lilig, R., Sarkozi, L., Kon, S., and Selikoff, I.J., 1978, Lead contamination in the homes of employees of secondary lead smelters, Environ. Res., 15:375.

Rius, R.A., Lucchi, L., Govoni, S., and Trabucchi, M., 1984, In vivo chronic lead exposure alters ^{3}H-Nitrendipine binding in rat striatum, Brain Res., 322:180.

Shukla, G.S., and Singhal, R.L., 1984, The present status of biological effects of toxic metals in the environment: lead, cadmium, and manganese, Can. J. Physiol. Pharmacol., 62: 1015.

Silbergeld, E.K., Goldberg, A.M., 1973, A lead-induced behavioral disorder, Life Sci., 13:1275.

Silbergeld, E.K., and Goldberg, A.M., 1975, Pharmacological and neurochemical investigations of lead-induced hyperactivity Neuropharmacol., 14:431.

Silbergeld, E.K., 1977, Interactions of lead and calcium on the synaptosomal uptake of dopamine and choline, Life Sci., 20:309.

Silbergeld, E.K., and Adler, H.S., 1978, Subcellular mechanisms of lead neurotoxicity, Brain Res., 148:451.

Silbergeld, E.K., 1982, Neurochemical and ionic mechanisms of lead neurotoxicity, In "Mechanisms of actions of neurotoxic substances", (K.N. Prasad and A. Vernadakis, eds.), pp. 1, Raven Press, New York.

Silbergeld, E.K., 1984a, Mitochondrial mechanisms of lead neurotoxicity, In "Cellular and molecular basis of neurotoxicity of environmental agents", (Narahashi, ed.), in press, Raven Press, New York.

Silbergeld, E.K., 1984b, Behavioral teratology of lead, Neurobehavioral Teratology, 19:433.

Sobotka, T.J., Cook, M.P., 1974, Postnatal lead acetate exposure in rats: possible relationship to minimal brain dysfunction, Amer. J. Ment. Defic., 79:5.

Spano, P.F., Memo, M., Stefanini, E., Fresia, P., and Trabucchi, M., 1980, Detection of multiple receptors for dopamine, In "Receptors for neurotransmitters and peptide hormones", (G. Pepeu, M.J. Kuhar and S.J. Enna, eds.), pp. 243, Raven Press, New York.

Winder, C., Garter, L.L., and Lewis, P.D., 1983, The morphological effects of lead on the developing central nervous system, Neuropathology and Appl. Neurobiology, 9:87.

Winder, C., and Kitchen, I., 1984, Lead neurotoxicity: a review of the biochemical, neurochemical and drug induced behavioral evidence, Progress in Neurobiology, 22:59.

Winneke, G., Brockhaus, A., and Baltissen, R., 1977, Neurobehavioral and systemic effects of longterm blood lead-elevation in rats, Arch. Toxicol., 37:247.

Winneke, G., Lilienthal, H., and Werner, W., 1982, Task dependent neurobehavioral effects of lead in rats, New Toxicol. for Old Arch. Toxicol., 5:84.

Winneke, G., Kraemer, U., Brockhaus, A., Ewers, U., Kujanek, G., Lechner, H., and Janke, W., 1983, Neuropsychological studies in children with elevated tooth-lead concentrations, Int. Arch. Occup. Environ. Health, 51:231.

Winneke, G., Kraemer, U., 1984, Neuropsychological effects of lead in children: interactions with social background variables, Neuropsychobiology, 11:195.

Zenick, H., Goldsmith, M., 1981, Drug discrimination learning in lead-exposed rats, Science, 212:569.

EXPERIMENTAL MODELS and ASSESSMENT of NEUROTOXIC MECHANISMS

CRITERIA AND STRATEGIES FOR NEUROBEHAVIORAL ASSESSMENT

Stata Norton

Pharmacology, Toxicology and Therapeutics
University of Kansas College of Health Sciences
Kansas City, Kansas

INTRODUCTION

Neurobehavioral evaluation of damage to the nervous system requires different strategies depending on several factors. As in any toxicological experiment, the purpose of the evaluation needs to be clearly identified since the result can be varied markedly depending on the intent of the experiment. For example, selection of species, strain, sex, and age of the test animal may well affect the result. Doses and duration of exposure must be fixed. However, in some instances, the aim may be to look for a range of effects without a prior identification of a specific test protocol or end point. When the point of the experiment is so broad that the aim is to identify any type of damage, the difficulties of selecting strategies are clearly magnified. For example, in the study of a potential carcinogen an experiment may be set up which is intended to detect an increase in carcinogenesis in a species over a lifetime exposure to a potential carcinogen. This is not possible in neurobehavior. Such an experiment cannot be carried out, that is, to attempt to detect any change in behavior over a lifetime exposure to a potential neurotoxicant.

Some criteria must be established for any experiment intended to evaluate neurobehavioral damage. Four are listed below.

1. Exposure Considerations

Dose, duration and route of exposure depend on the nature of the experiment. Nevertheless a good strategy is to attempt to develop dose-response data, using at least three doses of the toxic agent. Sometimes dose-response is not possible, either because a qualitatively different response is obtained over a reasonable range of doses or because technical difficulties of administration set narrow limits.

2. Practical Considerations

Various factors such as cost, performance time, and interpretability of results in terms of purpose must be considered. If the aim is to screen large numbers of chemicals for possible neurotoxicity, a strategy is chosen which is different from an aim to evaluate chemicals for production of one effect, such as delayed neurotoxicity.

3. Reversible/Irreversible Effects

The time frame of the experiment relative to exposure must be established. Different strategies are required for effects predicted to occur during the period of exposure than for effects which are irreversible or which last well beyond the exposure.

4. Selection of Target Area

Where possible, decision of expected peripheral or central nervous system effects should be made. In addition, sensory versus motor systems may be selected as targets of interest. Alternatively, the interest may be only in effects on memory, learning and other so-called higher nervous system functions.

The strategies discussed below will be concerned with the third and fourth criteria just listed. The first and second considerations are outside the scope of this discussion.

STRATEGIES FOR NEUROBEHAVIORAL DAMAGE

Perhaps it is well to start with a definition of those nervous system functions which are included here. "Neurobehavioral toxicity" is interpreted to mean any significant alteration in motor function resulting from acute or chronic damage to any part of the nervous system. Motor output or behavior of any animal may be modified by damage to sensory or motor systems and also by damage to integrative systems or "higher centers". Thus, damage to the 8th cranial nerve can be detected by testing the non-conditional "startle response" (a motor response) or by use of conditional motor responses to tones. In both types of test, it is a motor movement that is recorded. Tests of learning, memory and various other complex responses are equally dependent on movement of the animal in performing the tests. Without movement of the animal as an end point, neurotoxicity must be evaluated biochemically, physiologically or morphologically. Only in the case of human neurotoxicity is there the luxury of evaluating symptoms or subjective findings of the test organism.

Perhaps the first rule for selecting a neurobehavioral test for study of a chemical is to use a test which is known to detect other compounds which have the predicted type of damage. There are three important characteristics of a good test: specificity, reproducibility and validity. In this context specificity has two components. One is that a test may detect a wide range of types of nervous system damage (low specificity), the second is that a test may be highly specific for a type of damage. The first component implies that there are some generalized behavioral responses to various types of nervous system damage and there is evidence that this is true. As an example of a generalized test, if the intent is to test a chemical for ability to cause a distal axonopathy, a behavioral test for hind limb motor weakness will be chosen, based on information from effects of agents known to cause distal axonopathies. Reproducibility is measured by the variability between animals and between experiments. It is determined by the effect of uncontrolled or unknown variables in the test procedure and it determines the number of replicates to be employed. Low reproducibility may effectively exclude some tests from general use until more is known about the variables which need to be controlled. The validity of a test for behavioral toxicology is determined by the degree to which the results parallel affects on morphological, biochemical or physiological parameters in the same animals or species or parallels of the different parameters between species. It is rare for the above information on a test method to be other than fragmentary. It is often possible to ask if the risk of false positive or false negative results is known. That is, have enough types of chemicals been evaluated so that one can estimate the probability of interpreting an inactive compound as active (false positive) or an active compound as inactive (false negative)?

A second rule is to set up sequential test protocols in order to improve predictability and interpretation of results. Using the example of a test for delayed neurotoxicity with distal axonopathy, it would not be sufficiently accurate to assume damage to motor nerve fibers in the hind limb was present based solely on observation of progressive hind limb weakness beginning about 10 days after a single exposure to a chemical. Although these findings taken alone would be compatible with the interpretation that the chemical caused a distal axonopathy, there are other possible interpretations, including general debility from as remote a site as liver damage. The strategy is obvious in such a case. Other information, such as progression of signs and food consumption, is considered. Morphological verification of axonal involvement is a critical step. More than that, morphological examination of the entire central nervous system may be required if a new type of chemical is involved. Biochemical and physiological measurements can be added for selected parameters.

The general protocol for sequential analysis of an unknown agent for which the behavioral action can be predicted is shown in Fig. 1.

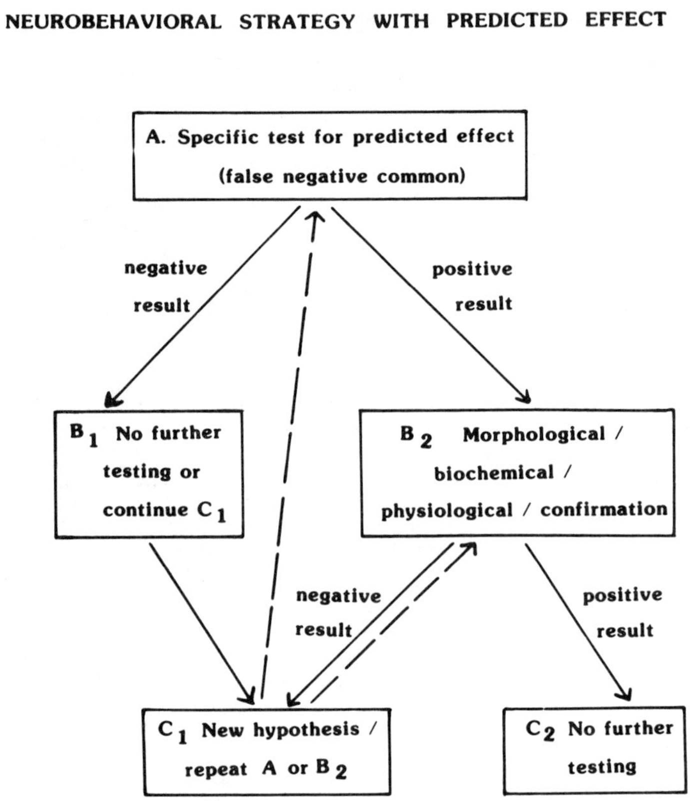

Fig. 1. Strategy for a toxic agent with a predicted effect.

As an example of the tests employed in the design in Fig. 1, test A for a chemical predicted to cause a distal axonopathy could be gait analysis. A positive result, showing ataxia and altered gait, would be confirmed by morphological examination of peripheral nerve (Test B). When the target area is not predicted, the strategy is more complicated. The first aim to select a test with a low specificity. If the test does give positive results from damage to many areas of the nervous system, then it is also likely to generate false positive results, through effects on other systems. Given this propensity for false positives in the first test, a second behavioral test needs to be added following a positive result in the first test. The second test should have greater specificity and be selected to identify a possible target area, depending on the first results. An example of this procedure is the observation that exposure of rat fetuses to ionizing radiation causes postnatal hyperactivity and this indication of brain damage can be refined by gait analysis, suggesting at least one focus of damage in the motor system (Mullenix et al., 1975).

A general protocol for sequential analysis of an unknown agent for which no specific action on the nervous system is predicted is shown in Fig. 2.

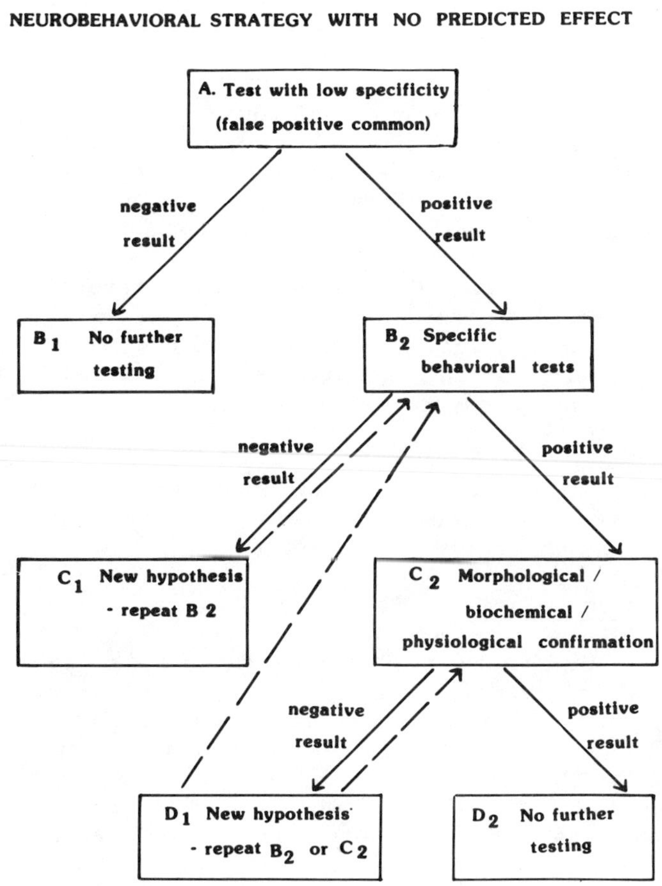

Fig. 2. Strategy for a toxic agent without a predicted specific target.

In the protocol in Fig. 2, steps B and C can be repeated using as many different tests as desired until all appropriate hypotheses have been examined.

TYPES OF NERVOUS SYSTEM DAMAGE

An example of the procedure in Fig. 2 would be analysis of possible neurotoxic effect of a new chemical with no known CNS toxicity. Test A could be a test for altered locomotor activity, either hyper- or hypoactivity, measuring circadian activity for 24 or 48 hours. A positive result would be followed by another test for activity (e.g. test B = exploratory activity) or a test for learning/memory (e.g. test B = spatial maze or passive avoidance conditioning) or for sensory deficit (e.g. test B = auditory startle). In each case, positive results with test B would be followed by appropriate morphological examination of the CNS (Test C).

1. Reversible Damage

In many types of exposure to toxic agents, the effect is acute and reversible, so that the nervous system is affected during the presence of the chemical but recovers upon removal of the toxic agent. This situation is comparable to the action of drugs on the nervous system, with rare exceptions.

When damage is predicted to be readily reversible, and the intent is to detect acute effects of a chemical, behavioral effects may occur at doses which do not produce detectable morphological, biochemical or physiological changes. Part of the reason for this is the brief nature of the changes and the difficulty of making invasive measurements during a changing level of toxic agent. By definition a reversible agent leaves no trace of its passage after a final time. An important characteristic of behavioral tests in this situation is that they may be the most sensitive of the different categories of measurement.

2. Irreversible Damage

When the damage to the nervous system is predicted to be irreversible, or reversible only in part through limited capacity for regeneration or compensation, the criterion of time is added to the strategy. For example, a high dose of an agent causing a delayed neuropathy characterized as a distal axonopathy, may result in death of an animal through inability to walk and therefore inability to eat. However, lower doses, as is known from human exposure, may result in survival with varying degrees of recovery of hind limb function requiring a period of a year or more for final outcome. Even in the presence of complete recovery of function in a given behavioral test it may be possible to detect morphological damage by examination of the nerve or muscle if the organism has compensated for the damage to the nervous system. Therefore, in the case of irreversible damage, the strategy may include morphological tests in the presence of negative behavioral tests when the time-frame would allow compensation to occur.

CATEGORIES OF BEHAVIORAL TESTS

Behaviors can be conveniently categorized in 7 groups: motor, sensory, integrated sensorimotor, emotional, cognitive, reproductive and immature behaviors (Table 1). These categories are based on types of functional data available from different tests and are not intended to encompass all aspects of laboratory animal behavior. In the following discussion only some tests in each category will be listed. It is to be understood that many behavioral tests have been devised which monitor one or more of the 7 categories of behavior. Many tests suitable for evaluation of behavior have been excluded here because they are not in common use in toxicology, because they duplicate information obtained by other tests described or because they evaluate behaviors not in one of the 7 categories. No brief overview, such as this one, can do justice to the rich resources of research methods for evaluation of behavior. The focus here is on tests which are currently being used to evaluate the effects of toxic agents on the nervous system. Examples of use of the tests in behavioral toxicology are given.

1. Tests of Motor Function

Damage to the peripheral or spinal motor nerves can be monitored by several tests. The end is weakness which usually is greater in the hind legs than fore legs.

Gait alteration and ataxia can be detected by recording footprints (Mullenix et al., 1975; Comer and Norton, 1984).

Negotiation of a narrow pathway has been devised as a measure of motor development (Altman and Sudarshan, 1975) and can be used to measure motor weakness.

Hind foot splay on dropping from a short distance has been reported to measure motor neuropathy (Edwards and Parker, 1977).

Rotarod performance in which the animal, usually a rodent, maintains balance on a rotating rod has a long history of use. The effect of a chemical causing distal axonopathy is readily determined (Kaplan and Murphy, 1972). There is a major component of habituation or learning in this test.

Table 1. Categories of Tests for Neurobehavioral Assessment

	Example
1. Motor functions	
a. Gait	(Mullenix et al. 1975)
b. Hind foot splay	(Edwards and Parker 1977)
c. Rotarod	(Kaplan and Murphy 1972)
d. Balancing rods	(Altman and Sudarshan 1975)
2. Sensory functions	
a. Startle response	(Wecker and Ison 1984)
b. Tremor	(Gerhart et al. 1983)
c. Auditory discrimination	(Stebbins and Rudy 1978)
d. Visual discrimination	(Evans 1978)
e. Odor discrimination	(Wood 1978)
f. Vibration sensitivity	(Maurissen et al. 1983)
3. Sensorimotor integration	
a. Conditioned active avoidance	(Rodier et al. 1979)
b. Conditioned passive avoidance	(Sandstead et al. 1977)
c. Circadian activity	(Reiter et al. 1975)
d. Locomotor activity	(Norton et al. 1976)
4. Emotional alterations	
a. Exploratory	
Open field	(Walsh and Cummins 1976)
Closed corridor	(Reiter et al. 1980)
b. Aggressive behavior	(Archer 1973)
5. Cognitive behavior (Learning/memory)	
a. Spatial maze	(Olton et al. 1979)
b. Operant fixed interval/fixed ratio	(Wenger et al. 1984)
c. Goal box	(Miller 1984)
6. Reproductive behavior	
a. Male mating behavior	(Zenick 1984)
b. Female estrus behavior	(Erskine 1983)
7. Preweaning behavior	
a. Surface righting	(Vorhees et al. 1979; Comer and Norton 1982)
b. Negative geotaxis	(Vorhees et al. 1979; Comer and Norton 1982)
c. Reflex suspension	(Vorhees et al. 1979; Comer and Norton 1982)
d. Auditory startle	(Vorhees et al. 1979; Comer and Norton 1982)

All of these tests for motor function will detect motor rigidities involving spinal or higher centers as well as weakness. Also, sensory damage can affect all of these tests since all complex motor performance involves sensory information from muscles and joints as well as sensory cranial nerves.

2. Tests of Sensory Damage

The startle response is a test for auditory or visual damage which has been refined to a high degree of sophistication (Fechter and Young, 1983; Wecker and Ison, 1984). The combination of two sensory modalities allows information about sensory processing as well as detection of direct damage to the sensory pathway.

Tremor may involve damage to the peripheral sensory nervous system as well as spinal pathways and a method for recording tremor has been utilized in toxicology (Gerhart et al., 1983).

Conditioned discriminations in which an animal learns to discriminate tones (Stebbins and Rudy, 1978), shapes or light intensities (Evans, 1978) or odors (Wood, 1978) have been used to detect specific types of sensory damage. Vibration sensitivity has been reported as a measure of damage to Pacinian corpuscles and large sensory fibers (Maurissen et al., 1983).

3. Integrated Sensorimotor Tests

The tests listed above under the separate categories of motor and sensory cannot be completely specific for one or the other modality but a high degree of selectivity can be detected by careful consideration of methodology. Many times both sensory and motor systems are involved and higher centers which integrate the two systems may also be damaged. Additional information can be gained by adding one of the tests which requires complex integration and comparing results over a range of doses. Tests which measure damage to the same nervous system components should have parallel dose-response effects.

Conditioned avoidance, both passive (Rodier et al., 1979) and active (Sandstead et al., 1977) requires sensory function to detect to light or sound of the conditioning stimulus. Passive avoidance is less dependent on degree of motor function than active avoidance. When toxicity testing involves active avoidance, motor function may determine the response. An example of use of two tests is in the report from Kishi and co-workers (1978) showing that escape latency (motor response to shock) correlates well with conditional active avoidance in rats exposed to mercury vapor, suggesting that the main effect may be on motor function.

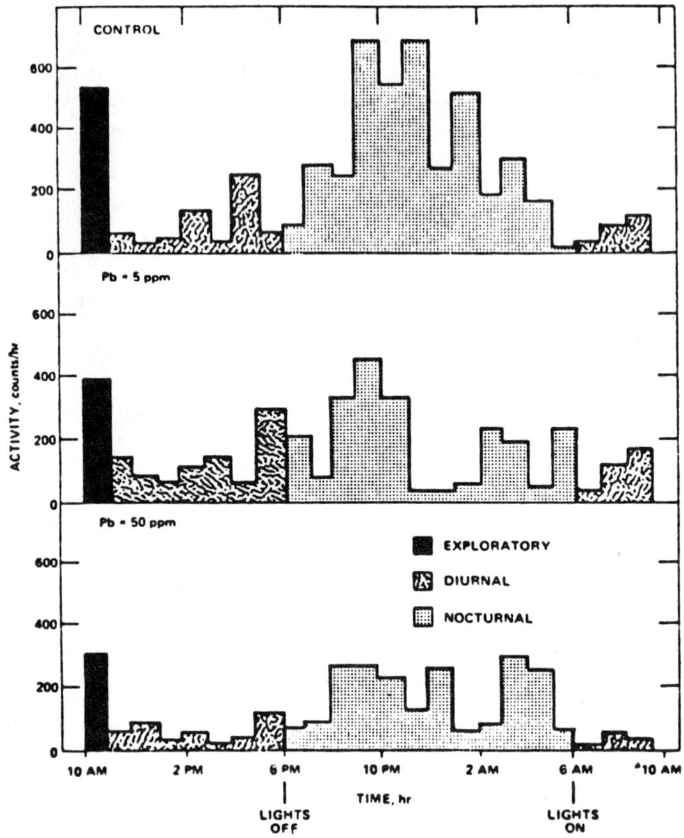

Fig. 3. Circadian activity of control and lead-treated animals in a residential maze. (Reprinted by permission, Reiter et al., 1975).

Locomotor activity tied to the diurnal cycle can be used to detect sensorimotor damage since response to the light/dark cycle requires detection of difference of illumination and motor activity during the cycle can be monitored by various devices (Norton et al., 1975; Wenger et al., 1984a).

In the rodent the circadian cycle is quite marked (Fig. 3). Rats carry on feeding-associated behaviors and other motor behaviors predominately during the dark portion of a day-night cycle. Some agents preferentially alter dark-associated activities (e.g. Reiter et al., 1975) while other toxic substances affect both the light and dark portion (e.g. Wenger et al., 1984a).

One common consequence of generalized damage to the central nervous system, such as the sequelae of encephalopathies, is hyperactivity. Even in the absence of a demonstrated encephalopathy, hyperactivity is a frequent result of localized brain damage (Norton, 1976). As a result, detection of central nervous system damage, when a specific target is not predicted, should include a test of spontaneous motor activity over at least a 24 hour period. When the spontaneous locomotor behavior of a rat is analyzed in detail, the "hyperactivity", which is usually recorded as increased movement past various spatial recording devices, shows a more complex structure (Norton et al., 1976). In the hyperactive rat all behavioral acts are performed for a shortened duration and the sequencing of acts is disrupted compared with controls. These observations led to the study of sequences of behavioral acts as a method which reliably detects low levels of generalized central nervous system damage, such as prenatal phenytoin exposure (Mullenix et al., 1983).

4. Emotional Alterations

There is no way that a subjective phenomenon such as emotion can be measured directly nor even defined in a meaningful way in animals. By analogy with subjective human experience, some animal behaviors have been given labels which imply emotions. As long as serious attempts are not made to equate these labels with human emotion, the labels can be accepted.

The argument that activity in an open space (open field behavior) has a component of "fear" or "anxiety" has been challenged in a careful analysis (Walsh and Cummins, 1976). Nevertheless the open field test is one of the most common tests. It is used to measure locomotion, usually of rats or mice, in a novel environment. Variability is high and the test conditions which affect open field behavior are not well defined. Exploration of spatially closed environment (i.e. corridors) has also been used (Reiter et al., 1980) and seems to be somewhat less variable.

"Aggression", defined as attacking another animal, has been used as a test of altered emotion (Archer, 1973).

None of the tests involving emotional behavior have received wide use in toxicology.

5. Cognitive Behavior

Effects of toxic agents on learning and memory are of considerable interest. Like terms for "emotion", learning and memory in non-human species may not be directly equatable to human learning and memory since the human condition can be communicated directly. Apart from possible differences in the mechanism by which the central nervous systems of different species of animals store and retrieve information, mechanisms of interpretation of stimuli can determine an animal's response to a task involving learning and memory. To take a trivial example, the honey bee can "learn" and "remember" where it has found a good source of flower nectar and then can communicate the location to other bees in the hive. Is this process mechanistically comparable to storage and retrieval in the human brain or are we looking at different processes to which we apply the same words? As an example in the mammalian brain, the cat has been considered psychologically unable to see color because it will not express a preference for the color of a food object in learning experiments. However, physiologists and anatomists detect all the apparatus for color vision. The failure of the cat to "learn" in this experiment may not be storage or retrieval of information about the color of objects but a lack of ability to link this information to feeding behavior.

In spite of these caveats, tests of learning and memory are plentiful. They measure the ability of an animal to modify its behavior on repeated exposure to a stimulus. Even here it should be considered that learning to respond to one type of stimulus may not be generalizable to all responses involving learning, even within the same species. For example, "learning to walk" could involve different fundamental processes than "learning to read".

Both operant and Pavlovian conditioning methods, and some test methods not using deliberate conditioning, involve learning. In tests not based on conditioning, such as repeated exposure to a novel environment, learning is often called habituation. Specific tests of learning and memory usually involve deliberate conditioning procedures. Passive and active avoidance methods, particularly the former, are often used. Various operant schedules, with simple or mixed fixed interval/fixed ratio schedules of reward or punishment have been tried. No specific set of schedules can be proposed, partly for the reasons given above and partly because the intent of different studies varies. Generally, complex operant schedules are used to detect lower levels of brain damage while tests which are more readily learned are used when damage is predicted to be more severe. Even this generalization, while intuitively probable, lacks rigorous proof. There is evidence that low rates of operant responding are more likely to be increased than high rates and, conversely, high rates are more easily decreased than low rates. Since low rates of responding are characteristic of many fixed interval schedules and high rates for fixed ratio schedules, the schedule may be chosen with this consideration.

A few recent conditioning studies will be mentioned as examples of current methodology. Miller (1984) studied learning and extinction in young rats following early postnatal exposure to triethyltin. There was a dose-related increase in errors in a radial arm maze in which accuracy depended on spatial recall. Spatial learning/recall in a radial maze has been related to hippocampal function (Olton et al., 1979). Miller also reported that triethyltin impaired rate of learning in a goal-box alley way but did not impair performance of the acquired task.

A study of the effect of lead on operant behavior in a fixed interval schedule showed marked individual differences in responding of lead-treated rats but a high level of behavioral variability also existed in the control rats (Cory-Slechta et al., 1983). Correlations between blood lead levels and response rates were also very variable. Because of the high variability of responding in this study, which was a replication of a previous study, it is uncertain that this schedule for operant behavior is a reliable test for brain damage. Comparisons with other tests are needed.

Wenger and co-workers (1984b) have recently compared the behavioral effects of trimethyltin exposure at three dose levels on circadian activity and a multiple fixed ratio-fixed interval schedule. The operant results in this study paralleled the effects on circadian activity and behavioral effects in both tests paralleled the light microscopic findings of loss of granule cells in the hippocampal fascia dentata. More studies of this type, which combines behavioral tests and morphological tests, are needed.

6. Reproductive Behavior

Reproductive behavior has received attention in toxicology because exposure to some chemicals has been shown to alter human fertility. Reproductive behavior, in the context of this discussion, includes mating and maternal behavior. Both fertility and reproductive outcome and associated behaviors are under hormonal control in rodents, which are the common test animals for studying reproductive behavior. The endocrine system may be directly affected by toxic exposure, secondarily altering behavior, or neuroendocrine control may be altered via effects on the hypothalamus.

Quantitative evaluation of male mating behavior has been defined (Beach, 1947; Lanier et al., 1979). An example of use of male mating behavior in toxicology is the recent report by Zenick and co-workers (1984) on carbon disulfide in the male rat. Female mating behavior and maternal behavior have received less attention in toxicology although much is known about the nature of this behavior. For a recent example see the report by Erskine (1983).

7. Preweaning Behavior

In some types of toxic exposure there is specific interest in early postnatal behavior. With some chemicals, fetal damage may be of greater concern than adult neurotoxicity since the developing brain involves several unique features which may increase sensitivity to toxic agents. It is well recognized that the development of offspring is delayed in thyroid deficiency and a number of toxic agents are recognized as potential goitrogens (Thomas and Bell, 1982). In addition, light body weight is a common finding in neonates of female rats exposed to toxic substances and the potential exists for delayed development via neuroendocrine toxicity.

Several early postnatal behaviors have been studied and knowledge is accumulating on their merits as measures of behavior. The most common tests are surface righting, negative geotaxis, reflex suspension and auditory startle (Vorhees et al., 1979; Comer and Norton, 1982). The usual measure is time of achieving a criterion for performance. In control albino rats, surface righting is rapidly accomplished by postnatal day 9; negative geotaxis or return from a head down to a head up position on a screen is performed readily by day 12; reflex suspension on a rod by forelimbs can be sustained for 30 seconds by day 15; and auditory startle to a sharp noise develops by 12 days of age. Acquisition of all of these responses is delayed by thyroid deficiency (Comer and Norton, 1982).

CONCLUSIONS

This brief survey of behavioral tests has been intended to indicate the range of behaviors which are commonly examined in neurotoxicology. In order to have a truly logical strategy for detection of neurotoxicity, much more precise information is needed regarding the correlation of structure and function. We do not understand the function of most of the structures that receive the sensory information and translate it into motor output utilizing information stored in the multiply-wired systems of the brain. At best we can achieve some simple generalizations, realizing that these will alter with better understanding.

One type of information which can be obtained is on the reproducibility of the tests both within and between different laboratories and between different strains or species of laboratory animals. This is important in selection of tests in the strategies in Fig. 1 and Fig. 2. Reproducibility can be measured by the precision of results with standard compounds which produce positive effects in the test.

A second important kind of information which is urgently needed is validity testing. A range of standard neurotoxicants with known effects needs to be examined in each of the tests. This will give information on the kinds of agents which each test detects and allow estimation of false positives and false negatives in each test. For example, locomotor behavior throughout the diurnal cycle has been studied for a variety of toxic agents, drugs and stereotaxic brain lesions. The test appears to detect a wide range of types of brain damage, usually in the form of hyperactivity. Comparable findings of hyperactivity in humans have been related to brain damage, particularly in children. To draw the parallel between a test in laboratory animals and humans is the last link required to complete the validity of a behavioral test. Unfortunately, extrapolation of results from animals to man is the most difficult and least understood aspect.

In summary, application of the strategies proposed here for evaluation of neurotoxicants is more a goal than accomplished procedure. We need more information on many of the tests already in use and this can be obtained. In addition we need a greater understanding of the relationship of brain structure to function. With the continued study of neurotoxicants we can achieve the first goal and the information so obtained may help us to achieve the second goal.

REFERENCES

Altman, J. and Sudarshan, K. Postnatal development of locomotion in the laboratory rat. Anim. Behav. 23: 896-920.

Archer, J. Tests for emotionality in rats and mice. A review. Anim. Behav. 21: 205-235, 1973.

Beach, F. A. A review of physiological and psychological studies of sexual behavior in mammals. Physiol. Rev. 27: 240-307, 1947.

Comer, C. P. and Norton, S. Effects of perinatal methimazole exposure on a developmental test battery for neurobehavioral toxicity in rats. Toxicol. Appl. Pharmacol. 22: 133-141, 1982.

Comer, C. P. and Norton, S. Behavioral consequences of perinatal hypothyroidism in postnatal and adult rats. Pharmacol. Biochem. Behav. 22: in press, 1985.

Cory-Slechta, D. A., Weiss, B. and Cox, C. Delayed behavioral toxicity of lead with increasing exposure concentration. Toxicol. Appl. Pharmacol. 71: 342-352, 1983.

Edwards, P. M. and Parker, V. H. A simple, sensitive and objective method for early assessment of acrylamide neuropathy in rats. Toxicol. Appl. Pharmacol. 40: 589-591, 1977.

Erskine, M. S. Effects of an anti-androgen and 5 α-reductase inhibitors on estrus duration in the cycling female rat. Physiol. Behav. 30: 519-524, 1983.

Evans, H. L. Behavioral assessment of visual toxicity. Environ. Health Perspec. 26: 53-57, 1978.

Fechter, L. D. and Young, J. S. Discrimination of auditory from nonauditory toxicity by reflex modulation audiometry: effects of triethyltin. Toxicol. Appl. Pharmacol. 70: 216-227, 1983.

Gerhart, J. M., Hong, J.-S. and Tilson, H. A. Studies on the possible sites of chlordecone-induced tremor in rats. Toxicol. Appl. Pharmacol. 70: 382-389, 1983.

Kaplan, M. and Murphy, S. D. Effect of acrylamide on rotarod performance and sciatic nerve β-glucuronidase of rats. Toxicol. Appl. Pharmacol. 22: 259-268, 1972.

Kishi, R., Hashimoto, K., Shimizu, S. and Kobayashi, M. Behavioral changes and mercury concentrations in tissues of rats exposed to mercury vapor. Toxicol. Appl. Pharmacol. 46: 555-566, 1978.

Lanier, D. L., Estep, D. Q. and Dewsbury, D. A. Role of prolonged copulatory behavior in facilitating reproductive success in a competitive mating situation in laboratory rats. J. Comp. Physiol. Psychol. 93: 781-792, 1979.

Maurissen, J. P. J., Weiss, B. and Davis, H. T. Somatosensory thresholds in monkeys exposed to acrylamide. Toxicol. Appl. Pharmacol. 71: 266-279, 1983.

Miller, D. B. Pre- and postweaning indices of neurotoxicity in rats: effects of triethyltin (TET). Toxicol. Appl. Pharmacol. 72: 557-565, 1984.

Mullenix, P., Norton, S. and Culver, B. Locomotor damage in rats after X-irradiation in utero. Exp. Neurol. 48: 310-324, 1975.

Mullenix, P., Tassinari, M. S. and Keith, D. A. Behavioral outcome after prenatal exposure to phenytoin in rats. Teratology 27: 149-157, 1983.

Norton, S. Hyperactive behavior of rats after lesions of the globus pallidus. Brain Res. Bull. 1: 193-202, 1976.

Norton, S., Mullenix, P. and Culver, B. Comparison of the structure of hyperactive behavior after brain damage from X-irradiation, carbon monoxide and pallidal lesions. Brain Res. 116: 49-67, 1976.

Olton, D. S., Becker, J. T. and Handelmann, G. E. Hippocampus, space and memory. Behav. Brain Sci. 2: 313-365, 1979.

Reiter, L. W., Anderson, G. E., Laskey, G. W., and Cahill, D. F. Developmental and behavioral changes in the rat during chronic exposure to lead. Environ. Health Perspect. 12: 119-123, 1975.

Reiter, L., Kidd, K., Heavner, G. and Ruppert, P. Behavioral toxicity to acute and subacute exposure to triethyltin in the rat. Neurotoxicology 2: 97-112, 1980.

Rodier, P. M., Reynolds, S. S. and Roberts, W. N. Behavioral consequence of interference with CNS development in the early fetal period. Teratology 19: 327-336, 1979.

Sandstead, H. H., Fosmire, G. J., Halas, E. S., Jacob, R. A., Strobel, D. A. and Marks, E. O. Zinc deficiency: effects on brain and behavior of rats and rhesus monkey. Teratology 16: 229-234, 1977.

Stebbins, W. C. and Rudy, M. C. Behavioral ototoxicity. Environ. Health Perspec. 26: 43-51, 1978.

Thomas, J. A. and Bell, J. U. Endocrine toxicology. In, Principles and Methods of Toxicology. Ed. A. W. Hayes, Raven Press, N.Y., 1982, pp. 487-507.

Vorhees, C. V., Butcher, R. E., Brunner, R. L. and Sobotka, T. J. A developmental test battery for neurobehavioral toxicity in rats: a preliminary analysis using monosodium glutamate, calcium carrageenan, and hydroxyurea. Toxicol. Appl. Pharmacol. 50: 267-282, 1979.

Walsh, R. N. and Cummins, R. H. The open-field test: a critical review. Psychol. Bull. 83: 482-504, 1976.

Wecker, J. R. and Ison, J. R. Acute exposure to methyl or ethyl alcohol alters auditory function in the rat. Toxicol. Appl. Pharamcol. 74: 258-266, 1984.

Wenger, G. R., McMillan, D. E. and Chang, L. W. Behavioral effect of trimethyltin in two strains of mice. I. Spontaneous motor activity. Toxicol. Appl. Pharmacol. 73: 78-88, 1984a.

Wenger, G. R., McMillan, D. E. and Cheng, L. W. Behavioral effects of trimethyltin in two strains of mice. II. Multiple fixed ratio, fixed interval. Toxicol. Appl. Pharmacol. 73: 89-96, 1984b.

Wood, R. W. Stimulus properties of inhaled substances. Environ. Health Perspec. 26: 69-76, 1978.

Zenick, H., Blackburn, K., Hope, E. and Baldwin, D. An evaluation of the copulatory, endocrinologic, and spermatotoxic effects of carbon disulfide in the rat. Toxicol. Appl. Pharmacol. 73: 275-283, 1984.

THE ROLE OF NEUROCHEMISTRY IN BEHAVIOURAL TERATOLOGY AND TOXICOLOGY

Vincenzo Cuomo and Giorgio Racagni*

Institute of Pharmacology, University of Bari
Institute of Pharmacology and Pharmacognosy, University of Milan*, Italy

INTRODUCTION

Prenatal exposure to various drugs and environmental chemicals can cause abnormal embryonic or fetal development which results in alterations of structural and/or functional nature. Teratology, until the early 1970s, was concerned almost exclusively with the production of gross structural malformations with little focus on functional manifestations (Hutchings, 1978). In these last years, a newer aspect of teratology,focused on function instead of structure is achieving prominence. Postnatal functional abnormalities elicited by prenatal exposures may range from changes expressed as metabolic alterations to defects revealed mainly as behavioural deficits, hence the term "behavioural teratology" (Evans and Weiss, 1978). In this regard, it has been shown that a toxic effect may be detected by subtle behavioural changes before any of the classical symptoms of poisoning appear, and that there are substances which act as pure behavioural teratogens (Vorhees, 1979; Alder, 1983). Our recent findings and those of other authors have demonstrated that results of behavioural teratology and toxicology tests can fruitfully be compared to neurochemical data from the same animals. In this regard, neurochemical correlates of a behavioural dysfunction can help pinpoint neuronal systems involved in the behavioural change.

On the basis of these findings, when speaking of behavioural teratology, one should expect also a correlated neurochemical change, so that the term "biochemical teratology" would also be justified.

In the present paper, examples of correlations between neurochemical and behavioural changes produced by developmental (prenatal and early postnatal) exposure to environmental chemicals (methylmercury) and to psychotropic drugs (neuroleptics, antidepressants, antianxiety agents) are reported.

BEHAVIOURAL AND NEUROCHEMICAL CHANGES IN OFFSPRING OF RATS EXPOSED TO ENVIRONMENTAL CHEMICALS DURING GESTATION

Methylmercury

It has been clearly shown that methylmercury may induce subtle behavioural abnormalities at dose levels below those associated with overt symptoms of neurotoxicity. The study of the interactions of methylmercury with neurochemical systems of the developing brain, however, has not been explored extensively. In this regard, Bartolome et al. (1982) recently showed in rats that postnatal methylmercury exposure produced both acute and long-lasting effects on maturation of central catecholamine neurotransmitter systems, an effect that may be transmitter specific. Since studies of the effects of prenatal methylmercury exposure on the development of the catecholaminergic system as well as on behavioural models which are linked to catecholaminergic mechanisms are lacking, the purpose of our recent experiments (Cuomo et al., 1984) was to investigate the behavioural responsiveness to a dopaminergic agent (apomorphine) and to a noradrenergic agent (clonidine) in young and adult offspring of rats given methylmercury during gestation. Additionally, 3H-spiroperidol binding to striatal membranes and 3H-clonidine binding to cortical membranes of rats prenatally exposed to methylmercury were determined. The results of this study show a significant correlation between the behavioural changes and the alterations in the development of the central catecholaminergic system caused by prenatal administration of this heavy metal. In particular, 22-day-old pups exposed to methylmercury displayed an increased behavioural sensitivity to apomorphine as well as a significant increase in the number of 3H-spiroperidol binding-sites in striatal membranes.

Therefore, the abnormal behavioural response to apomorphine could be due to the production of dopamine receptor supersensitivity elicited by methylmercury. The results of studies of the noradrenergic system show that neither the effects of a challenge dose of clonidine on locomotor activity (clonidine-induced inhibition of rat locomotor activity may be considered a possible functional response to the activation of $alpha_2$-adrenoreceptors) nor the affinity and the density of 3H-clonidine binding-sites were modified significantly in offspring of rats exposed to methylmercury during gestation.

Thus,these findings demonstrate that the prenatal exposure to this heavy metal induces alterations in striatal dopamine receptor sensitivity of offspring whereas it does not affect the development of presynaptic $alpha_2$-adrenoreceptors which seem to be an important mechanism by which the activity of noradrenergic neurons is regulated (Langer, 1977; Racagni et al., 1982).

BEHAVIOURAL AND NEUROCHEMICAL CHANGES IN OFFSPRING OF RATS EXPOSED TO PSYCHOTROPIC DRUGS DURING GESTATION

Neuroleptics

Our recent findings (Cuomo et al., 1985) have shown that prolonged prenatal administration of haloperidol significantly influences in adult rats the behavioural responsiveness to a dopamine receptor agonist, like apomorphine. In particular, the intensity of stereotyped behaviour elicited by apomorphine in haloperidol pretreated animals was markedly attenuated with respect to controls. Parallely, the decrement in locomotion caused by apomorphine in adult animals exposed to haloperidol during prenatal life was significantly less intense than in vehicle-pretreated rats. These data, indicating a behavioural subsensitivity of the dopaminergic system of haloperidol exposed rats to pharmacological stimulation, are in agreement with those of Rosengarten and Friedhoff (1979) who showed a significant decrease in 3H-spiroperidol binding in the striatum of rats born to mothers treated with haloperidol during gestation.This decrease was still apparent at day 60 of postnatal life when we made behavioural measurements. Conversely, the prolonged administration of haloperidol during the first weeks of postnatal life, which seem to be vulnerable periods for the functional maturation of the central dopaminergic system in the rat (White and Tapp, 1977), produces an opposite response pattern. In particular, the intensity of apomorphine-induced stereotyped behaviour was significantly greater in 60-day-old haloperidol-pretreated animals than in controls and this was accompanied by a more marked reduction of locomotor activity in haloperidol-pretreated than in vehicle-pretreated rats (Cuomo et al., 1981). Furthermore, a significant increase in 3H-spiroperidol binding to caudate tissue was observed in rats if haloperidol was administered to their mothers postpartum during nursing (Rosengarten and Friedhoff, 1979). Even though increased central dopaminergic receptor sensitivity to apomorphine after prolonged haloperidol treatment in adult rats is well documented, there is no evidence (Cuomo et al., 1983) that alterations in behavioural sensitivity to this dopaminergic agonist persist up to 40 days after the last administration of the neuroleptic agent.

Therefore, these findings further confirm that the compensatory mechanisms occurring in response to chronic treatment with dopamine receptor blocking agents during development are markedly different from those occurring in response to their prolonged administration during adulthood.

Antidepressants

Clinical studies indicate that neurological alterations have occurred in neonates of women treated during pregnancy with "typical antidepressants", such as tricyclic agents (Webster,1973; Musa and Smith,1979).These clinical reports have been paralleled by recent experimental findings showing that prenatal administration of tricyclic antidepressants (imipramine, amitriptyline) in rats can lead profound neurobehavioural and neurochemical changes in offspring of exposed dams. In particular, Jason et al. (1981) found that in imipramine pretreated pups eye opening occurred significantly earlier, development of the surface righting reflex was delayed and development of negative geotaxis was altered. Hypothalamic levels of noradrenaline and adrenaline were unchanged in imipramine exposed pups at 7, 14 and 30 days of age, but dopamine levels, unaffected at 7 and 14 days, were significantly lower than controls at 30 days. Moreover, the number of cortical beta adrenergic receptors, measured by 3H-dihydroalprenolol binding, was significantly decreased by 18.7% at 14 days and 9.1% at 30 days; affinity for binding was increased at 30 days of age. Furthermore, Bigl et al. (1982) have demonstrated that the administration of amitriptyline to pregnant rats markedly reduced locomotor activity in 8-and 21-day-old offspring. Parallel neurochemical data show that amitriptyline affected serotonin metabolism during the early stages of postnatal development.The concentration of serotonin was significantly reduced in the 1-day-old rat brain, while that of 5-HIAA was increased in the 8-day-old brain. The serotonin concentration of the brain from the amitriptyline-treated adult was also reduced in comparison to the saline-treated controls. Of the other neurotransmitters studied, the only changes which occurred were in the concentration of noradrenaline (which rose in the 15-day-old group) and in GABA which increased in the 21-day-old group.

Finally, a comparative evaluation (Cuomo et al., 1984a) of the effects induced by prenatal exposure to a typical antidepressant (desipramine) and to two atypical antidepressants (viloxazine and mianserin), at dose levels which do not influence reproductive success or neonatal mortality, shows that physical signs,such as pinna detachment (unfolding of external ear) and eye opening, were not modified by prenatal exposure to any of the antidepressants tested. However, at 23 days of age, rats pretreated with desipramine, mianserin and viloxazine (only in males) showed higher levels of locomotor activity with respect to control group. At 60 days of age, locomotor activity levels in desipramine-exposed animals were still higher than in saline-pretreated rats. The comparison of these data with our recent findings (Racagni et al., 1982; Cuomo et al., 1983a) indicates that the locomotion of rats subjected to prolonged treatment with desipramine, viloxazine and mianserin during adulthood was not modified with respect to control animals.

Thus, this study further suggests that the behavioural consequences of prolonged treatment with some psychotropic agents are critically dependent upon the period of their administration. Furthermore, desipramine, viloxazine and mianserin could be included in the class of chemical agents which cause behavioural changes in offspring of treated animals at subteratogenic doses.

Antianxiety drugs

Prolonged exposure to the antianxiety agent diazepam during gestation can produce persistent behavioural abnormalities in offspring (Kellog et al., 1980). Similar treatment of pregnant rats with diazepam did not influence either the density or affinity of benzodiazepine binding sites in brain regions (cortex, striatum, cerebellum) of offspring during postnatal development (Massotti et al.,1980). However,these authors suggest that daily administration of diazepam during pregnancy may result in an alteration in the mechanism of coupling between GABA and benzodiazepine receptor. The results of Watanabe et al. (1983), indicating that chronic diazepam treatment during pregnancy retards the development of central opiate receptors, could be due to a similar mechanism. It is of interest to compare the behavioural and neurochemical changes produced by prenatal and early postnatal exposure to benzodiazepines, respectively. In this regard, Coen et al. (1983) showed that the administration of a benzodiazepine derivative (chlordiazepoxide) to lactating mothers in their drinking water caused a notable deficit in the acquisition of the conditioned avoidance response in 60-day-old offspring. Moreover, 3H-flunitrazepam binding-sites in cerebral cortex and hippocampus were decreased by the treatment whereas no change was detected in cerebellum. On the other hand, 3H-muscimol binding-sites increased in hippocampus with no changes in cerebral cortex and cerebellum. According to the different regional distribution of benzodiazepine type 1 and type 2 receptors, these authors suggest that type 2 receptors are selectively affected by the treatment, and that the GABAergic receptor system is also permanently altered by administration of chlordiazepoxide during early postnatal life.

Finally, it has been demonstrated (Kellog et al., 1984) that while restraint stress increased the utilization of NE by hypothalamic NE neurons (over basal values) in control animals, stress decreased the NE utilization in animals prenatally exposed to diazepam. Additionally, prenatal exposure to diazepam attenuated the stress-induced increase in plasma corticosterone and altered the stress-induced increase in prolactin. All effects of prenatal exposure were prevented if the pregnant dams were administered a specific benzodiazepine antagonist concurrently with diazepam. On the basis of these results, Kellog et al. (1984) suggest that diazepam interacts during development with the same neuronal substrates which mediate stress-related responses in adults.

ACKNOWLEDGEMENTS

This paper was partially supported by a grant of Italian Ministry of Education

REFERENCES

Alder, S., 1983, Behavioural Teratology, in :"Application of Behavioural Pharmacology in Toxicology", G. Zbinden, V. Cuomo, G. Racagni, B. Weiss, eds., Raven Press, N.Y..

Bartolome, J., Trepanier, P., Chait, E. A., Seidler, F.J., Deskin, R., and Slotkin, T.A., 1982, Neonatal methylmercury poisoning in the rat: effects on development of central catecholamine neurotransmitter system, Toxicol. Apppl. Pharmacol., 65: 92.

Bigl, V., Dalitz, E., Kunert, E., Biesold, D., and Leonard, B. E., 1982, The effect of d-amphetamine and amitriptyline administered to pregnant rats on the locomotor activity and neurotransmitters of the offspring, Psychopharmacology ,77:371

Coen, E., Abbracchio, M. P., Balduini, W., Cagiano, R., Cuomo, V., Lombardelli,G., Peruzzi,G., Ragusa, M.C., and Cattabeni,F., 1983, Early postnatal chlordiazepoxide administration: permanent behavioural effects in the mature rat and possible involvement of the GABA-benzodiazepine system, Psychopharmacology , 81: 261.

Cuomo, V., Cagiano, R., Coen, E., Mocchetti, I., Cattabeni, F., and Racagni, G., 1981, Enduring behavioural and biochemical effects in the adult rat after prologed postnatal administration of haloperidol, Psychopharmacology , 74: 166.

Cuomo, V., Cagiano, R., Brunello,N., Fumagalli,R., and Racagni,G., 1983a, Behavioural changes after acute and chronic administration of typical and atypical antidepressants in rats: interactions with reserpine, Neurosci. Lett. , 40: 315.

Cuomo, V., Cagiano, R., Mocchetti,I., Coen, E., Cattabeni,F., and Racagni, G.,1983, Biochemical and behavioural effects after early postnatal administration of neuroleptics in rats, in: "Application of Behavioural Pharmacology in Toxicology", G. Zbinden,V. Cuomo,G. Racagni,B. Weiss,eds., Raven Press,N.Y.

Cuomo, V., Ambrosi, L., Annau, Z., Cagiano, R., Brunello, N., and Racagni, G., 1984, Behavioural and neurochemical changes in offspring of rats exposed to methylmercury during gestation Neurobehav. Toxicol. Teratol. , 6: 249.

Cuomo, V., Cortese, I., Cagiano, R., Renna, G., and Racagni, G., 1984a, Behavioural changes in rats after prenatal administration of typical and atypical antidepressants, Arch. Toxicol. , 7: 504.

Cuomo, V., Cagiano, R., Renna, G., Serinelli, A., Brunello, N.,and Racagni,G., 1985, Comparative evaluation of the behavioural consequences of prenatal and early postnatal exposure to haloperidol in rats, Neurobehav. Toxicol. Teratol. ,7: 489.

Evans, H.L., and Weiss, B., 1978, Behavioural Toxicology, in : "Contemporary Research in Behavioural Pharmacology", D.E. Blackman, O.J. Sanger, eds., Plenum Press, N.Y.

Hutchings, D.E., 1978, Behavioural teratology: embriopathic and behavioural effects of drugs during pregnancy, in :"Studies of the development of behaviour and the nervous system: Early influences", G. Gottlieb, ed., Academic Press, N.Y.

Jason, K.M., Cooper, T.B., and Friedman, E., 1981, Prenatal exposure to imipramine alters early behavioural development and beta adrenergic receptors in rats, J. Pharmacol. Exp. Ther. 217: 461.

Kellog, C., Tervo, D., Ison, J.R., and Parisi, T., 1980, Prenatal exposure to diazepam alters behavioural development in rats Science , 207: 205.

Kellog, C., Ison, J.R., Simmons, R.D., and Miller,M.K., 1984, Prenatal diazepam exposure in rats: long-lasting functional changes in the offspring, in : "Clinical Neuropharmacology" G. Racagni, R. Paoletti, P. Kielholz,eds., Raven Press,N.Y.

Langer, S.Z., 1977, Presynaptic receptors and their role in the regulation of transmitter release, Brit. J. Pharmacol. , 60: 481.

Massotti, M., Alleva, F.R., Balazs, T., and Guidotti, A., 1980, GABA and benzodiazepine receptors in the offspring of dams receiving diazepam: ontogenetic studies, Neuropharmacology 19: 951.

Musa, A. and Smith, C., 1979, Neonatal effects of maternal chlorimipramine therapy, Ach. Dis. Child. , 54: 405.

Racagni, G., Mocchetti, I., Renna, G., and Cuomo, V.,1982, In vivo studies on central noradrenergic synaptic mechanisms after acute and chronic antidepressant drug treatment:biochemical and behavioural comparison, J. Pharmacol. Exp. Ther., 223: 227.

Rosengarten, H., and Friedhoff, A.J., 1979, Enduring changes in dopamine receptor cells of pups from drug administration to pregnant and nursing rats, Science, 203: 1133.

Vorhees, C.V., Brunner, R.L. and Butcher, R.E., 1979, Psychotropic drugs as behavioural teratogens, Science, 205: 1220.

Watanabe, Y., Shibuya, T., Salafsky, B., and Hill, H.F., 1983, Prenatal and postnatal exposure to diazepam: effects on opioid receptor binding in rat brain cortex, Eur. J. Pharmacol., 96: 141.

Webster, P., 1973, Withdrawal symptoms in neonates associated with maternal antidepressant therapy, Lancet, 2: 318.

White, B.C., and Tapp, W.N., 1977, Unilateral catecholamine depletion of the corpus striatum and amphetamine induced turning: an ontogenetic study, Psychopharmacology, 53: 211.

RECEPTOR BINDING TECHNIQUES IN NEUROTOXICOLOGY

Lucio G. Costa[1], Marina Marinovich[2] and Corrado L. Galli[2]

[1]Department of Environmental Health, University of Washington, Seattle, Washington, (USA) and [2]Laboratory of Toxicology, Institute of Pharmacology and Pharmacognosy University of Milano, Milano (Italy)

This chapter is intended to be an overview on receptor binding techniques and their application to the study of the neurotoxicity of chemicals. Although the theoretical basis of radioligand binding assays, the experimental methodologies and the basic processes of interpretation of binding data will be briefly considered, the reader is referred to other publications for more detailed theoretical and practical reviews (Peck and Kelner, 1983; Yamamura et al., 1978; Titeler, 1981; Williams and Lefkowitz, 1978). A few reviews on the use of radioligand techniques in neurotoxicology have also been recently published (Bondy, 1979; 1982; DeHaven and Mailman, 1983).

Introduction

Transmission of messages between cells in the nervous system involves the release of a chemical neurotransmitter from one cell and its subsequent recognition by a second cell. Specific enzymes synthetize the neurotransmitter from one or more precursors. The neurotransmitter is usually stored in vescicles in the presynaptic ending and released in the synaptic cleft upon arrival of a stimulus. After their interaction with the second cell, neurotransmitters are rapidly inactivated by enzymatic degradation or by an uptake mechanism into the neuron that released them or into glial cells. The specific protein on the postsynaptic cell to which the neurotransmitter binds is known as the receptor (Cooper et al. 1982). The concept of receptor goes back to 1905, when John Langley introduced the idea of a specific "receptive substance" in the myoneural junction, as the site of action for nicotine and curare: ".....So we may suppose that in all cells two constituents at least are to be distinguished, a chief substance, which is concerned with the chief function of the cell as contraction and secretion, and receptive substances which are acted upon by chemical bodies and in certain cases by nervous stimuli. The receptive substance affects or is capable of affecting the metabolism of the chief substance....." (Langley, 1905). For many years scientists have been investigating the properties of neurotransmitter receptors by means of electrophysiological, behavioral and pharmacological methods. However, biochemical studies of neurotransmitter receptors have mostly occurred during the past ten years. In particular, the availability of radiolabeled ligands and the development of rapid filtration techniques have been the key to the success in measuring small amounts of drug and neurotransmitter receptors in the brain. Since the word receptor is now used with different meanings by many scientists, a definition of this term is needed. As recently discussed by Laduron (1984), a receptor involves three processes: (1) binding of the agonist to the recognition site (or acceptor); (2) generation of a transmission signal; and (3) a physiological response. All three steps need to be present in order to apply the term "receptor" to this system (Laduron, 1984). Furthermore, specific criteria need to be fulfilled for a binding site to be called receptor. These include drug displacement, correlation between drug affinity _in vitro_ and pharmacological potency _in vivo_, regional distribution or tissue specificity, subcellular distribution, stereospecificity, saturability, reversibility and high affinity (Laduron, 1984). The term receptor, however, is also used, in a more narrow sense, to indicate the specific protein that recognizes and binds the neurotransmitter (Snyder, 1984). This chapter will deal mostly with receptors as recognition sites, as these are the sites identified with radioligand binding techniques. Most of these sites have met the criteria outlined before.

Apart from studies by Paton and Rang (1965) on the uptake of radioactive atropine by intestinal muscle and studies by several investigators on the binding of [^{125}I]-alpha-bungarotoxin to acetylcholine nicotinic receptors in the electric organs of eels (Changeaux et al. 1970; Raftery et al. 1971), the first receptor type to be identified in the mammalian brain was the opiate receptor (Pert and Snyder, 1973; Terenius, 1973; Simon et al., 1973). It is noteworthy that this occurred before the endogenous ligands were discovered; the same happened, a few years later, with the benzodiazepine receptors (Braestrup and Squires, 1977). The historical development of radioligand binding methods for the principal neurotransmitters is summarized in Table 1.

In addition to the receptor sites included in Table 1, other receptor types and subtypes should be briefly mentioned. Nicotinic cholinergic receptors have been identified in the brain (Morley et al., 1983a). Muscarinic receptors have now been proposed to exist in two subtypes, M_1 and M_2, the first concentrated in sympathetic ganglia, hippocampus corpus striatum and cerebral cortex, the latter preponderant in ileum cerebellum and heart and regulated by GTP (Hirschowitz et al., 1984). Adrenergic receptors, once subdivided into alpha and beta, are now divided into alpha $_1$, alpha $_2$, beta $_1$, and beta $_2$, (Snyder, 1984). Selective ligands for each subtype have been developed and each adrenergic receptor subtype appears to act through different mechanisms (Exton, 1982; Leclerc et al., 1981). As many as four or five subtypes of dopamine receptors have been proposed (Seeman, 1980). However, only the D_1-receptor, linked to adylate cyclase and the D_2-receptor, appear to have physiological significance (Leff and Creese, 1983). Receptors for 5-hydroxytryptamine (Peroutka and Snyder, 1979) and adenosine (Burnstock, 1981) have also been divided into two subclasses. Recently, a novel, bicuculline-insensitive, GABA receptor has been labeled with [^{3}H]

Table 1

Development of receptor binding techniques

Year	Receptor	Reference
1973	Opiate	Pert and Snyder, 1973 Terenius, 1973 Simon et al., 1973
1973	Glycine	Young and Snyder, 1973
1974	Muscarinic	Yamamura and Snyder, 1974 Burgen et al., 1974
1975	GABA	Enna and Snyder, 1975
1975	Serotonin	Bennett and Snyder, 1975
1975	Dopamine	Creese et al., 1975 Seeman et al., 1975
1975	Beta-adrenergic	Alexander et al., 1975 Bylund and Snyder, 1976
1976	Alpha-adrenergic	Williams and Lefkowitz, 1976 Greenberg et al., 1976
1977	Benzodiazepine	Braestrup and Squires, 1977
1980	Adenosine	Wu et al., 1980 Bruns et al., 1980

Baclofen (Hill and Bowery, 1981). At least five subclasses of opiate receptors (μ, δ, σ, κ and ε) have been identified (Martin, 1984). Subclasses have also been proposed. For example, within the receptor type, selective for morphine, there is a μ_1 subtype which is selectively inhibited by naloxonazine and is implicated in analgesia but not in respiratory depression (Goodman and Pasternak, 1984).

Moreover, during the last few years receptor sites on brain membranes for numerous neuropeptides have been labeled, such as subtance P, cholecystokinin, vasoactive intestinal polypeptide, calcitonin, neurotensin, angiotensin II and tyrotropin releasing hormone (see Snyder, 1980; Iversen, 1983, for reviews).

SOME THEORETICAL ASPECTS OF BINDING ASSAYS

1. Law of mass action and saturation binding assays

The simplest mechanistic assumption that can be made about the interaction of a radioactive ligand, L, with a receptor, R, is that a simple molecule of L reacts, in a reversible manner, with a single receptor molecule, R, to form a complex, RL:

$$L + R \underset{K-1}{\overset{K1}{\rightleftarrows}} RL \tag{1}$$

At equilibrium

$$\frac{(R)\ (L)}{(RL)} = Kd \tag{2}$$

where Kd is the equilibrium dissociation constant of the complex, (L) and (R) the concentrations of free ligand and free receptor, respectively, and (RL) the concentration of ligand bound to the receptor. The total concentration of receptors, R_t is then equal to (R) + (RL).
Equation 2 becomes:

$$\frac{(Rt-RL)\ (L)}{RL} = Kd \tag{3}$$

Which can be rearranged to:

$$\frac{(RL)}{(Rt)} = \frac{1}{(1+Kd/L)} = \frac{(L)}{Kd + (L)} \tag{4}$$

where the ratio (RL)/(Rt) is the fraction of total receptors occupied by the radioactive ligand, that is, the fractional occupancy. The concentration of L can be varied from very high to extremely low concentrations. At concentrations of L that are so high to make the ratio Kd/L approach zero, the fractional occupancy approaches 1, i.e. the receptors have become fully occupied or saturated by the radioactive ligand (Titeler, 1981). If the concentrations of L are very low, the ratio Kd/L is >>1, and the fractional occupancy approaches zero. When Kd = (L), the ratio (RL)/(Rt) = 1/2, that is, fractional occupancy is 50%. Hence, the concentration of L required for half-maximal occupancy of the receptor is equal to Kd. Equation

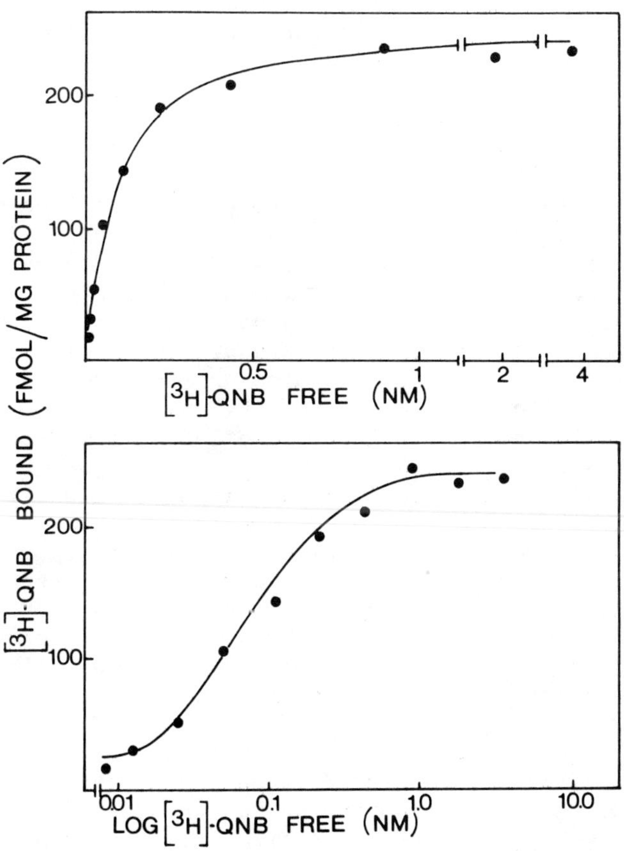

Figure 1. Saturation binding of [^{3}H]-QNB to homogenates from rat submandibular glands. The amount of [^{3}H]-QNB specifically bound is plotted against the concentration of free [^{3}H]-QNB. The lower graph is plotted on semilogarithmic paper. Data from Costa and Murphy (unpublished).

(4) can be rearranged to give:

$$(RL) = \frac{(Rt)\ (L)}{Kd + (L)} \tag{5}$$

Equation (5) is used in binding studies to derive the dissociation constant K_d and the number of binding sites Rt. The radioligand is added over a range of concentrations to a fixed concentration of receptors. The level of binding approached asymptomatically at high ligand concentrations is Rt and the concentration of free ligand that elicits a level of binding equal to (Rt)/2 represents the Kd (Williams and Lefkowitz, 1978). If the Log (L) is plotted against (RL), the plot is a symmetrical sigmoidal curve (Klotz, 1982; Figure 1). These considerations apply only to a situation in which the reaction is a simple bimolecular reaction (Equation(1)) and the measurements are made at equilibrium. Equation (3) can be rearranged to give the equation derived by Scatchard (1949):

$$\frac{(RL)}{L} = [(Rt) - (RL)]\ Kd^{-1} \tag{6}$$

Thus, if the ratio of (RL)/(L) (also expressed as B(bound)/F(free)), is plotted versus the concentration of bound ligand, (RL) or B, one gets a straight line with a slope of -1/Kd and intercept with the abscissa of (Rt) or B_{max} (Figure 2). The advantage of the Scatchard transformation of saturation binding data is that the data are linearized, which is particularly valuable in binding systems that have a high level of non-specific binding (Williams and Lefkowitz, 1978). Use of the correct value for (L) (i.e. F, free ligand concentration) is very important. If only a small fraction of L is bound, then the concentration of total L can be used to approximate the concentration of free L. This condition is usually met when the total binding site concentration is considerably lower than the K_d of the ligand. However, in certain cases estimation of free ligand concentration needs to be carefully considered (Siiteri, 1984). The dissociation constant K_d can also be measured by experimentally determining the two kinetic constants k_1 and k_{-1} of equation (1) (Williams and Lefkowitz, 1978; Titeler 1981), and the K_d values determined by each method should be in agreement.

Scatchard plots are often non-linear but can present convexities and concavities. A curved Scatchard plot can be due to coopera tive interactions among receptors or to the ligand binding to two or more sites with different affinities. However, a non-linear Scatchard plot should not be taken *a priori* as evidence of cooperativity or multiple binding sites. It only indicates that the data do not fit a simple two-state model in which ligand and receptor exist at equilibrium as bound or free. Methodological artifacts which can lead to non linear Scatchard plots are: (1) Use of non-equilibrium conditions; (2) instability of ligand or receptor; (3)

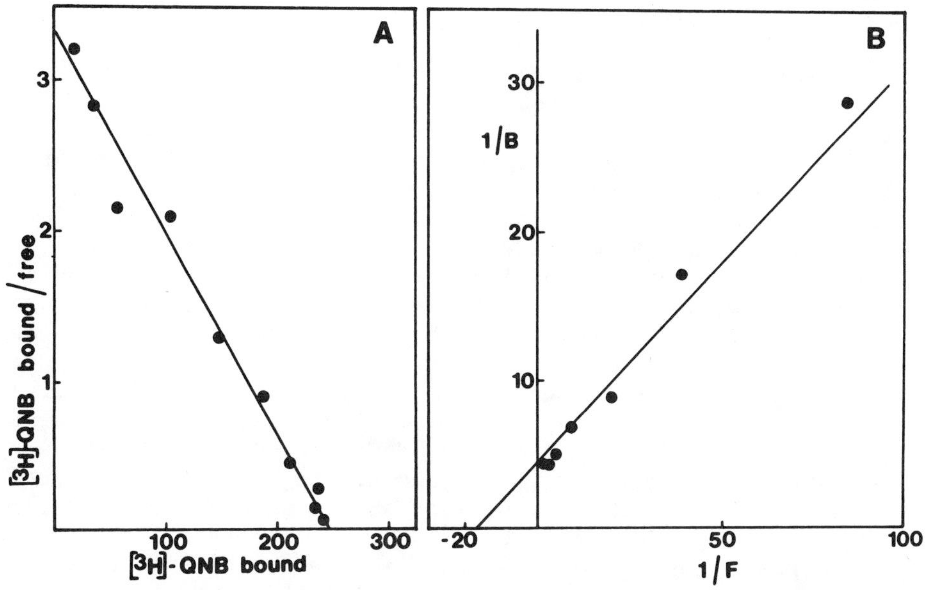

Figure 2. Scatchard plot (panel A) and double reciprocal plot (panel B) of specific [^{3}H]-QNB binding to rat submandibular glands. Data points are the same as in Figure 1. Three data points are not reported in panel B for reasons of graphical clarity. Data from Costa and Murphy (unpublished).

dilution of radioactivity with endogenous ligand; (4) high concentrations of ligand or receptor (Peck and Kelner, 1983; Munson, 1983). Many methods have been published to interpret curved Scatchard plot by graphical (Rosenthal, 1967; Pennock, 1973) or computer analysis (Munson and Rodbard, 1980) and many articles have warned about misinterpretation of Scatchard plots (Norby et al., 1980; Chamness and McGuire, 1975; Ketelslegers et al., 1984). Furthermore, the theoretical validity of the use of the Scatchard plot has been recently the object of discussion (Klotz, 1982; 1983; Munson and Rodbard, 1983).

Besides the Scatchard plot, many other methods can be used to analyze a rectangular hyperbola. These include the Hill plot (Hill, 1910), the Lineweaver-Burke plot (Lineweaver and Burke, 1934), the direct-linear plot (Eisenthal and Cornish-Bowden, 1974) and the Woolf plot (Keightley and Cressie, 1980). The use of these methods, their advantages and pitfalls are summarized by Zivin and Wand (1982).

2. Competition binding studies

Inhibition of the binding of a radioactive ligand to its receptor by an unlabeled compound may occur by competitive or non-competitive interactions. A mutually exclusive binding of both labeled and unlabeled ligand to the receptor is the mechanism of competitive inhibition, while the inhibition is non-competitive when the unlabeled ligand inactivates (reversibly or irreversibly) the ligand-binding capacity of the receptor (Peck and Kelner, 1983). If the inhibition is competitive, increasing concentrations of inhibitor will increase the value of the K_d of the ligand (i.e. decrease its affinity) without changing the number of binding sites. In case of non-competitive inhibition, the number of binding sites increases or decreases by varying the concentration of inhibitor. Therefore, the inhibition of the binding of a radioligand is not indicative of a competitive mechanism. Saturation binding studies and Scatchard or double-reciprocal analyses of ligand binding data in the presence of various concentrations of inhibitor should be used to establish the exact nature of this inhibition. This is simply the application to the receptor binding assay of the same concept that enzymologists have been using when analyzing enzyme inhibition data.

Displacement data are usually analyzed by calculating the IC_{50} value of the inhibitor, that is, the concentration of unlabeled compound which produces 50% inhibition of the binding of the radioactive ligand. The IC_{50} value can be then converted, by the equation of Cheng and Prusoff (1983) to the inhibition constant, Ki

$$Ki = \frac{IC_{50}}{1 + \frac{[L]}{K_d}} \tag{7}$$

where [L] is the concentration of ligand used in the displacement curve and the K_d is derived from separate saturation experiments. For this relationship, the ligand concentration should be kept below its K_d value, and caution should be used in selecting the concentrations of unlabeled ligand (excessive levels of competing ligand could result in displacement of secondary non specific sites and the artifactual production of multiple binding sites; Peck and Kelner, 1983). This equation is valid only if the law of mass action is followed, that is, if competition curves produce a Hill coefficient not different from one. Hill coefficients (Hill, 1910) can be calculated for displacement curves as they are for saturation curves. The Hill equation, adapted for competition experiments is (Titeler, 1981):

$$\log \frac{(\%\ \text{inhibition})}{(100-\%\ \text{inhibition})} = n_H \cdot \log (I) \tag{8}$$

A plot of the first term of the equation versus log (I) (concentration of the nonradioactive competing drug) will yield the Hill coefficient, n_H. A Hill coefficient greater than 1 indicates positive cooperativity, a Hill coefficient less than 1 indicates negative cooperativity or multiple sites, while a Hill coefficient of 1 indicates independent binding of the drug to sites with a single affinity.

3. Determination of nonspecific binding

Specific binding sites, such as receptors, exist in small finite numbers in tissues and therefore can be saturated with drug molecules. However, every ligand also binds to non-specific sites, usually other tissue components, such as lipids, proteins, or to the filters or the tubes. The number of nonspecific sites is usually very large compared to the number of specific binding sites and increases linearly over the concentration range of the radioactive drug used. Thus, nonspecific binding is usually nonsaturable and of low affinity. The difference in specific and nonspecific sites allows the experimenter to differentiate the two types of interactions of radioactive drugs with membrane. Practically, an unlabeled compound that is pharmacologically and/or chemically similar to the radioligand is used to determine nonspecific binding. This unlabeled drug is usually incubated in large excess (100 to 1000 fold more than the radioligand) with the tissue and the radioligand. The excess cold drug, with an affinity for the receptor site similar or higher than the radioligand, will reduce its binding to the receptor and only minimally affect its binding to the nonspecific sites. If too high concentrations of cold displacer are used, this can displace the radioligand from its nonspecific sites and generate artifactual multiple binding sites. Important to consider are the properties of the radioactive drug, particularly its affinity for the receptor. If the affinity is very high (K_d $<10^{-9}$), then very low concentrations of the drug can be used and this tends to minimize the nonspecific binding. Nonspecific binding to filters can be decreased by pretreating them with certain solutions (e.g. poly-L-lysine) prior to filtration.

METHODOLOGICAL ASPECTS OF RECEPTOR BINDING ASSAYS

The methods used to measure binding of radioactive ligands are technically simple and rapid. However, many parameters can influence the outcome of a binding assay. These include the tissue preparation, the ionic composition and strength of the buffer, the length and temperature of the incubation, the volume of incubation and the procedure used to separate the bound from the free ligand. In establishing a new binding procedure all these parameters have to be carefully experimentally evaluated so that optimal conditions are achieved. When utilizing established methodologies they have to be taken into account, since also small procedural variations might lead to changes in the results of binding experiments.

1. Tissue Preparation

Tissues can be processed for binding studies in a variety of ways. Normally, the tissue is homogenized in the appropriate buffer and then washed several times by centrifugation. Various procedures can be used to obtain fractions particularly enriched in synaptosomal membranes or to obtain highly enriched subcellular fractions (Mailman and Morell, 1982). The tissue can be used fresh or stored frozen for various times until assayed. Some receptor binding sites are not affected by either procedure (e.g. [^{3}H]-QNB), while others (e.g. [^{3}H] GABA, [^{3}H]-serotonin) are. The method used to sacrifice the experimental animal appears to have no effect on receptor binding (Uphouse et al. 1981). For certain binding assays (e.g. GABA, benzodiazepine) additional washings of tissue are required to remove endogenous ligands. Preincubation of homogenates at 37°C prior to the binding assay is used to accelerate the rate of metabolic degradation for endogenous substances such as neuropeptides. Careful preparation and washing of the tissue to be used for binding assay is especially important if an *in vivo* treatment had taken place in order to remove any residual chemical which might interfere with the assay.

2. Radioactive ligand

A large number of radioligands for binding studies are available from commercial sources. Most ligands are either tritiated or iodinated. Tritiated ligands offer the advantages of a long radioactive half-life and no significant alteration of the chemical structure of the ligand because of the presence of the isotope. The radioligand should have a high specific radioactivity to allow detection of small concentrations of neurotransmitter receptors, as well as a high affinity for the receptor site, which will allow the use of low concentrations of radioligand, reducing the likelihood of nonspecific binding. Substitution of an aromatic halide (Br or I) with tritium gas ($^3H_2$) or hydrogenation of an unsaturated double bond are two popular methods of synthesis of tritiated ligands. Iodination (with ^{131}I or ^{125}I) can provide a radioactive molecule with very high specific activity. However, iodinated ligands have the disadvantage of a short radioactive half-life, require more precautions in handling and iodination can cause potential alterations in biological activity.

A radioligand should be chemically stable under the assay conditions employed and its chemical purity should be checked routinely, particularly after a long period of storage.

3. Separation of bound from free ligand

The radioligand is incubated with the tissue until equilibrium is reached, that is, until the rate of association and dissociation are equal. The time of incubation, dependent upon the temperature, can range from less than a minute to several hours. Temperatures normally used range from 4°C to 37°C. After equilibrium is reached, the radioligand bound to the receptors has to be separated from the unbound ligand. This can be accomplished by filtration or centrifugation, although other methodologies such as equilibrium dialysis or gel filtration have also been used (Yamamura et al. 1978; Williams and Lefkowitz, 1978).

Filtration techniques are unsurpassed for speed and efficiency. The incubation mixture is rapidly filtered under vacuum suction through a 2.4 cm filter (for example, Whatman GF/C). If a small volume is used for the incubation, the sample can be diluted with buffer before filtration. The filters are washed rapidly with cold buffer to remove nonspecifically trapped ligand. The radioactivity retained on the filter (representing the ligand bound to the receptors) is then quantified by liquid scintillation spectroscopy. Some radioligands bind to the filters and in certain cases the binding is displaceable by an unlabeled ligand. Hence, an appropriate filter should be chosen or the filters should be treated with chemicals able to reduce this displaceable binding to non-receptor sites. A second problem with the use of filtration is represented by the possible loss of protein which may pass through the filters. Depending upon the amount of protein in the incubation, different types of filters can be selected. Protein determination can also be done in the filtrate to assay any loss.

Centrifugation is usually preferred when ligands with lower affinities, or rapid dissociation rates are being used or when binding to filters cannot be reduced. At the end of the incubation period the samples are rapidly centrifuged and the resulting pellet either dissolved with a tissue solubilizer, or, when a microfuge is being used, the tip of the microfuge is cut and directly counted. The major disadvantage of the centifugation method is that higher levels of unbound radioligand remain trapped in the pellet, thus increasing nonspecific binding. Careful and rapid washing of the pellet with buffer or saline will help remove unbound radioligand.

USE OF RADIOLIGAND BINDING TECHNIQUES IN NEUROTOXICOLOGY

As discussed by DeHaven and Mailman (1983), there are two main applications of receptor binding assays to neurotoxicology. One can determine if a neurotoxicant interacts with a receptor directly or if it alters other components of the nervous system which in turn lead to changes in receptor binding.

To establish if a toxicant can interact with a receptor directly (either as an agonist or an antagonist), displacement assays are usually performed in vitro. As mentioned in the previous section, simple inhibition of the binding of a radioligand does not imply that the compound tested interacts directly with the receptor recognition site. When this is the case, as with many pharmacological agents, the test compound competitively displaces the radioligand and when saturation curves are performed, this results in a decrease in the affinity of the latter. The in vitro displacement assay will not determine if the unlabeled compound activates the receptor or acts as an antagonist. A biochemical assay of receptor function in vitro is necessary for this determination. For example, if a compound inhibits the binding of [^{3}H]-dihydroalprenolol to beta-adrenergic receptors, one should determine whether it stimulates adenylcyclase or antagonizes its stimulation by a beta-adrenergic agonist. In some cases, a preliminary differentiation between agonists and antagonists can be done with regard to opiate receptors, and it is possible to determine if a compound acts as an agonist or an antagonist by measuring its potency in displacing the radioligand in the absence and in the presence of sodium ions. The inhibitory potency of opiate agonists on the stereospecific binding of [^{3}H]-dihydromorphine is not affected by sodium ions, whereas that of pure antagonists is greatly enhanced (Chau-Pham et al. 1978).

Neurotoxicants often inhibit the binding of a radioligand by interacting with certain chemical groups on the receptor macromolecule. A typical example is that of mercurial compounds, described in the next section, which interact with sulfhydryl groups. Furthermore, the binding of radioligands can be affected by perturbation of the membrane environment surrounding the receptor. For example, phospholipids can alter opiate and muscarinic receptor binding (Abood et al. 1977; Aronstam et al., 1977). Nonspecific membrane interactions have been described for the food color Erythrosin B (Mailman et al, 1980; DeHaven and Mailman, 1983). In another study, Ciofalo (1981) looked at the ability of a series of lipid-soluble, membrane stabilizing compounds in inhibiting the binding of [^{3}H]-WB 4101 to alpha$_1$-adenoreceptors in beef cortical membranes. With few exceptions, their potency in inhibiting [^{3}H]-WB 4101 binding correlated with the membrane/buffer partition of the drug, each of which was pharmacologically devoid of alpha-adrenergic activity. This further indicates that specific receptor function can be modified by perturbation of the lipid environment of the receptor macromolecule. Moreover, various perturbers can alter different neuroreceptors to a different extent, probably depending on the lipid microenvironment for critical conformation of the receptor, which varies with the macromolecule (Ciofalo, 1980; 1981).

Alterations in receptor binding can also occur following in vivo exposure to a neurotoxicant. If a compound affects one or more components of neurotransmission (synthesis, release, degradation or uptake of neurotransmitters) changes in receptor binding could occur. Similar receptor binding alterations could occur if a chemical and/or a metabolite directly interact with the receptor as an agonist or an antagonist. The density of neurotransmitter receptors can vary depending on the availability of the neurotransmitter. There is often an inverse relation between the intersynaptic level of a ligand and the density of the corresponding receptors on the cell membranes (Damstra and Bondy, 1982). Thus, the density of neurotransmitter receptors can increase (up-regulation) or decrease (down-regulation). Such mechanisms of synaptic modulation and of regulation of neuronal sensitivity have been extensively reviewed (see for example Daly et al., 1980; Shain and Carpenter, 1981). Receptor modification after treatment with various drugs can be responsible for the development of tolerance or supersensitivity (Creese and Sibley, 1980; Friedhoff and Miller, 1982; Schwartz et al. 1983). For example, chronic treatment with neuroleptics causes a supersensitivity of dopamine receptors, whereas chronic treatment with the beta-adrenergic agonist isoproterenol induces a decrease in the density of beta-adrenergic receptors (Creese and Sibley, 1980). The effect of chronic exposure to cholinesterase inhibitors, either insecticides or drugs, on muscarinic receptors (described in the next section), is a good example of receptor down-regulation caused by a chemical not interacting directly with the receptor. Compounds such as disulfoton (Costa et al. 1982a) or neostigmine (Costa et al. 1981a) cause inhibition of acetylcholinesterase and a consequent accumulation of acetylcholine at the receptor site. Stimulation of muscarinic receptors by endogenous acetylcholine is believed to be responsible for their down-regulation. The same phenomenon is observed both *in vivo* and *in vitro* if muscarinic receptors are directly stimulated with a cholinergic agonist such as carbachol or oxotremorine (Marks et al., 1981; Siman and Klein, 1979).

A neurotoxicant can also affect other cellular components (e.g. membrane, intermediate metabolism, DNA) and cause cell death. A loss of neurons in a certain brain area will be detected as a loss of receptor binding. When that particular area contains various receptor types, decrease in the binding of more than one neurotransmitter receptor would be found. A neuropathological examination of the affected area is helpful in determining whether the loss of receptor binding is solely secondary to neuronal degeneration.

EXAMPLES OF NEUROTOXICITY STUDIES UTILIZING RECEPTOR BINDING TECHNIQUES

Receptor binding techniques have not been widely used in neurotoxicology, as compared to neuropharmacology. However, many studies have been published in the last five years describing the effects of various neurotoxicants on neurotransmitter receptors after *in vivo* administration, as well as *in vitro* binding interactions. This section will review most of these studies trying to emphasize those in which an alteration of receptor binding could be correlated with physiological or pharmacological alterations, or those in which receptor binding assays helped in identifying a possible mechanism of action of a neurotoxicant.

1. Pesticides

Many studies on receptor binding alterations have involved pesticides, in particular insecticides such as organophosphates and pyrethroids, and these will be discussed in more detail. The primary mechanism of action of organophosphorus insecticides is inhibition of acetylcholinesterase (Murphy, 1980). Several investigators had noted that a tolerance to their toxic effects could be induced in mammals (Barnes and Denz, 1951; Rider et al., 1952; reviewed by Costa et al., 1982b). That is, animals repeatedly exposed to sublethal doses of an insecticide initially show signs of poisoning typical of acetylcholinesterase inhibitors, but the signs of poisoning diminish or disappear with continued dosing. Bombinski and DuBois (1958) noted that brain acetylcholinesterase was highly inhibited in animals that had been made tolerant to repeated injections of the insecticide disulfoton (0,0-diethyl-S-[2-(ethylthio) ethyl] phosphorodithioate), and that acetylcholine levels in the brain of tolerant animals were elevated. Thus, these earlier studies suggested that this phenomenon permitted animals to tolerate higher concentrations of endogenous acetylcholine at neuroeffector sites. This concept was supported by the studies of Brodeur and DuBois (1964) who found that rats made tolerant to disulfoton were also resistant to the direct acting cholinergic agonist carbachol. They were the first to suggest that the tolerance to disulfoton might be the result of development of refractoriness of the cholinergic receptors to the acetylcholine that accumulates with prolonged acetylcholinesterase inhibition. Studies by McPhillips (McPhillips and Dar, 1967; McPhillips, 1969) also suggested that the decreased sensitivity of isolated organs taken from rats made tolerant to disulfoton was due to a change in the responsiveness of the cholinergic receptor system. This hypothesis was later reproposed (Russell et al. 1975) and could be tested experimentally by the use of radioligand binding techniques. The specific cholinergic muscarinic antagonist [^{3}H]-quininuclidinyl benzilate (^{3}H-QNB) was used to label muscarinic receptors in various tissues (Yamamura and Snyder, 1974). Mice and rats were repeatedly treated with disulfoton, until the initial signs of toxicity decreased and then disappeared. At this time the animals were considered tolerant to the toxicity of disulfoton. Receptor binding assays were performed in various brain areas and in some peripheral tissues (Costa et al. 1981b; 1982a; 1984; Costa and Murphy, 1982; Schwab et al. 1981; 1983). The results are summarized in Table 2. Saturation binding studies showed that the decreased binding of [^{3}H]-QNB was due to a reduced density of muscarinic receptors while their affinity for the ligand was unchanged. In mice with a reduced number of brain muscarinic receptors, the hypothermic and antinociceptive effects of the muscarinic agonist oxotremorine were significantly decreased (Costa et al. 1982 a). Thus, the decreased density of muscarinic receptors in mice made tolerant to disulfoton was correlated with a subsensitivity to two centrally mediated (Ringdahl and Jenden, 1983) effects of oxotremorine. Chronic administration of disulfoton also decreased the density of muscarinic receptors in the ileum (Costa et al., 1981b; Schwab et al., 1983) and in the pancreas (Costa et al., 1984; Table 2). The alteration of muscarinic receptors in the ileum was paralleled by an increase in the EC_{50} value for the contractile effect of oxotremorine, i.e. the tissue was resistant to the action of oxotremorine *in vitro* (Schwab et al., 1983). Similarly, pancre-

Table 2

$[^3H]$ QNB binding in various tissues from disulfoton-tolerant animals[a]

Tissue	Mice	Rats
	$[^3H]$ QNB binding (% of control)[b]	
Forebrain	59	56
Hindbrain	73	85
Cortex	68	76
Cerebellum	84	78
Striatum	60	52
Hippocampus	79	62
Medulla-pons	-	67
Ileum	36	66
Heart	-	81*
Atria	-	98*
Submandibular gland	-	72
Pancreas	-	59

[a] Data adapted from: Schwab et al, 1981; 1983; Schwab, 1981; Costa et al. 1981b; 1984; Costa and Murphy, 1982; and unpublished results.

[b] Percent changes of Bmax values. No changes in affinity constant were found.

* Not significantly different from control.

ata removed from rats treated with disulfoton were more resistant than control to the stimulation of amylase release induced by carbachol in vitro (Costa et al. 1984). Similar alterations of muscarinic receptors in the brain and the ileum were found after chronic treatment with other organophosphates, such as paraoxon (Smit et al., 1980a), DFP (Ehlert et al., 1980; Yamada et al., 1983; Sivam et al., 1983) and Tetram (Gazit et al., 1979). Time-course studies showed that here is a good correlation between the development of tolerance and the decrease in muscarinic receptor binding (Costa et al., 1981b; Ehlert et al., 1980).

Although other hypotheses on the mechanism of tolerance to organophosphates need to be further investigated (Russell et al., 1983; Costa et al., 1982b), there is an overall good correlation between the subsensitivity of various tissues from organophosphate tolerant animals and alterations of cholinergic muscarinic receptors. Results obtained in the heart, however, seem to contradict this hypothesis. Rats made tolerant to disulfoton were more resistant than controls to the effect of carbachol on heart rate in vivo (McPhillips and Dar, 1967; Schwab et al., 1983) as well as to the negative chronotropic effect of oxotremorine in an isolated atrial preparation (Perrine and McPhillips, 1970; Schwab et al. 1983). However, binding of muscarinic antagonists and agonists was not altered in cardiac tissue from these animals (Schwab et al., 1983; Smit et al. 1980b; Yamada et al., 1983). This suggests that, in addition to receptor loss, other mechanisms distal to the ligand recognition sites or removed from the receptor complex may contribute to the subsensitivity of tissues to muscarinic cholinergic agonists.

Chronic exposure to organophosphates has also been shown to alter cholinergic nicotinic receptors in rat brain. This has been observed in DFP-treated rats, using [^{3}H]-acetylcholine as a ligand (Schwartz and Kellar, 1983) as well as in disulfoton-treated rats, using [^{3}H]-nicotine to label brain nicotinic receptors (Costa and Murphy, 1983).

There is some evidence that the nicotinic cholinergic receptors present in the brain differ from that in the neuromuscular junction or in the electric organ of Torpedo (Morley et al. 1983a;b). Some organophosphates can interact directly with the "peripheral" nicotinic receptor. Eldefrawi et al., (1982) reported that monocrotophos, (0,0-dimethyl-0-(2-methyl-carbamoyl-1 methylvinyl) phosphate), its 2,2-dimethyl analog dicrotophos, azinphos-methyl (0,0-dimethyl-S[4-oxo-1,2,3-benzotriazin-3(4H)-yl methyl] phosphorodithioate) and dichlorvos (2,2-dichlorovinyl dimethyl phosphate) at a concentration of 10^{-4}M, were able to inhibit the binding of 10^{-6}M [^{3}H]-acetylcholine to the nicotinic receptor of Torpedo electric organ membranes. The affinity for the cholinergic receptor was much less than that for acetylcholinesterase and the binding was completely reversible. These data do not indicate whether these organophosphates (and some carbamates such as aminocarb, aldicarb and carbaryl) activate or inhibit the receptor. It is known, however, that the carbamate neostigmine is able to cause skeletal muscle contraction after complete inactivation of acetylcholinesterase by DFP (Riker, 1953), suggesting that it acts as an agonist of the nicotinic receptor. Interestingly, the same organophosphates which displaced [^{3}H]-acetylcholine from nicotinic receptors in Torpedo were ineffective in inhibiting the binding of [^{3}H] nicotine to cholinergic nicotinic receptors in rat brain membranes (Costa, unpublished observations).

Certain bicyclic organophosphorus compounds are highly toxic to mammals, their intraperitoneal LD_{50} in mice being as low as 0.2 mg/kg (Bellet and Casida, 1973). The toxic signs produced by these compounds do not resemble the characteristic manifestations of poisoning by anticholinesterase agents, that is, there is no indication of parasympathetic stimulation. Even after high doses causing convulsive seizures and death within five minutes, brain acetylcholinesterase activity is not inhibited (Bellet and Casida, 1973). Further studies confirmed that bicyclic phosphates are very weak phosphorylators of acetylcholinesterase and alpha-chymotrypsin (Ozoe et al., 1982). Since bicyclic phosphates can be formed during the thermal decomposition of polyurethane foams containing reactive phosphates as fire retardants (Petajan et al. 1975), it was important to identify their mechanism of action. Electrophysiological studies showed that these compounds can act as GABA antagonists (Bowery et al. 1976) and biochemical experiments indicated that they increase cyclic GMP content in the cerebellum (Mattsson et al. 1977). By using receptor binding techniques it was possible to determine that bicyclic phosphates do not interact with the GABA receptor site but are able to inhibit the binding of [^{3}H]-dihydropicrotoxinin to its recognition site on the GABA-ionophore receptor complex (Ticku and Olsen, 1979).

Another insecticide, 2-isothiocyanatoethyltrimethylammonium iodide, which is a potent inhibitor of choline acetyltransferase but has no effect on cholinesterase activity, interacts directly with the nicotinic acetylcholine receptor in insects. This insecticide inhibited the binding of [^{125}I]-alpha-bungarotoxin in extracts of flies (Drosophila melanogaster) and cockroach (Periplaneta Americana) with IC_{50} values of 10^{-6} - 10^{-5}M (Gepner et al. 1978). Since these are physiologically relevant concentrations, the investigators suggested that, like nicotine, 2-isothiocyanatoethyltrimethylammonium iodide, exerts its insecticidal action by interacting with the alpha-bungarotoxin-sensitive acetylcholine receptors (Gepner et al. 1978). They also suggested that the alpha-bungarotoxin binding assay in Drosophila and/or Periplaneta could provide a rapid way to screen potential insecticides for action on a cholinergic receptor.

Chlordimeform and other related formamidine compounds are a rather new class of pesticides, which find use as insecticides and acaricides (Hollingworth and Lund, 1982). A number of mechanisms have been proposed for their action including inhibition of monoaminooxidase (Aziz and Knowles, 1973), inhibition of prostaglandin biosynthesis (Yim et al. 1978), uncoupling of mitochondrial phosphorylation (Abo-Khatwa and Hollingworth, 1973), local anesthetic activity (Chinn et al. 1977) and inhibition of neurotransmitter uptake (Johnson and Knowles, 1981). Some of these effects might not be involved in the toxicity of chlordimeform (see for example Hollingworth et al. 1979). Recent studies have shown that chlordimeform is a potent agonist at the octopamine receptor (Evans, 1982) and stimulates the octopamine-sensitive adenyl cyclase in invertebrates (Murdock and Hollingworth, 1980). There is no strong evidence of octopamine receptors in the vertebrate nervous system, however, the pharmacological profile of invertebrate octopamine receptors is very similar to that of vertebrate alpha-adrenergic receptors, in particular the $alpha_2$ subtype (Evans, 1982). Pupillary and cardiac responses to chlordimeform and Amitraz in rats were found to be mediated by $alpha_2$-adrenoceptors (Hsu and Kakuk, 1984). In vitro receptor binding confirmed and extended these observations (Table 3). Chlordimeform inhibited the binding of $[^3H]$ clonidine to $alpha_2$-adrenoceptors, while it was a much weaker inhibitor of $alpha_1$-, and beta-adrenoceptor binding and was totally ineffective toward GABA and benzodiazepine binding sites. (Table 3).

Table 3

Effect of Chlordimeform on neurotransmitter receptor binding in mouse brain *in vitro*[a]

$[^3H]$ Ligand	Receptor type	IC_{50} ($x10^{-6}M$)
Clonidine	$alpha_2$-adrenergic	11.8
WB-4101	$alpha_1$-adrenergic	166
Dihydroalprenolol	beta-adrenergic	851
Muscimol	GABAA	>1000
Diazepam	Benzodiazepine	>1000

[a] Data from L. G. Costa, previously unpublished

Chlordecone (Kepone^R) is another pesticide which affects the nervous system. Kepone is active in a variety of biochemical systems. It inhibits neurotransmitter uptake (Ho et al. 1981), Na^+,K^+-and Mg^{++}-ATPases (Desaiah, 1981) and mitochondrial oxidative phosphorylation (End et al. 1981). One study (Seth et al. 1981a) examined its effects on neurotransmitter receptor binding when administered to both developing and adult rats. Offspring of rats, which were exposed to 6 ppm chlordecone from 60 days prior to mating through day 12 post-partum, were sacrificed at 30 days of age. Binding of [^{3}H]-spiperone to striatal membranes was increased by 27% in male, but not female, offspring of chlordecone-exposed dams. Adult rats exposed to 30 ppm chlordecone in the diet for 90 days had decreased binding of [^{3}H]-spiperone in the striatum and of [^{3}H]-QNB and [^{3}H]-muscimol in the cerebellum. However, striata and cerebella had an increased protein content compared to control, indicating that the receptor binding alterations were due to an effect of chlordecone on protein synthesis (Seth et al., 1981a).

Recent studies have investigated the effects of pyrethroid insecticides on neurotransmitter receptors. Pyrethroids had no effect on the binding of [^{3}H]-acetylcholine to its binding sites on the nicotine receptor/channel complex of Torpedo electric organ membranes, however, they inhibited the binding of [^{3}H]-perhydrohistrionicotoxin ([^{3}H]H_{12}-HTX) to the channel site (Abbassy et al., 1983). The correlation between the potencies in inhibiting [^{3}H]-H_{12}-HTXg binding and the toxicity of nine pyrethroids to house flies, mosquitoes and cockroaches was, however, very poor (Abbassy et al. 1983). On the other hand, studies with 37 pyrethroids revealed an absolute correlation between mouse intracerebroventricular toxicity and in vitro inhibition of the binding of [^{35}S]-t-butylcyclophosphorothioate (^{35}S-TBPS), a new ligand for the picrotoxinin binding site on the GABA/ionophore receptor complex (Lawrence and Casida, 1983). Pyrethroids have no effect on [^{3}H]-muscimol binding in vitro (Cremer et al. 1980; Costa, unpublished observation), while another study showed that three pyrethroid insecticides (decamethrin and cis-and trans-permethrin) inhibited the binding of [^{3}H] kainic acid to mouse forebrain homogenates in vitro (Staatz et al., 1982). Their potency in vitro correlated with their intracerebroventricular toxicity in mice.

The mechanism of action of certain chlorinated hydrocarbon insecticides such as lindane, toxaphene and dieldrin had never been clarified. However, it was recently shown that a series of chlorinated insecticides of these three classes are potent competitive inhibitors (IC_{50}s = 10^{-6}M - 10^{-8}M) of the binding of [^{35}S] - TBPS to rat brain membranes (Lawrence and Casida, 1984). The mammalian toxicity of these compounds was closely related to their potency for inhibition of TBPS binding. A modified receptor assay incorporating liver microsomes and NADPH was developed to compensate in part for oxidative detoxication and bioactivation (Lawrence and Casida,

1984). It was found, for example that the potency of aldrin and heptachlor increases two to three-fold in the presence of this system suggesting that they undergo metabolic activation. This well designed and executed study indicates the TBPS-picrotoxinin binding site on the GABA/ionophore receptor complex as the site of action of certain chlorinated insecticides. On the other hand, other compounds such as DDT, mirex or kepone had no effect on [^{35}S]-TBPS binding (Lawrence and Casida, 1984).

The studies summarized above indicate that neurotransmitter receptor binding assays have brought an important contribution to the understanding of the mechanism of action of several pesticides. Chronic exposure to cholinesterase inhibitors such as the organophosphorus insecticides has been shown to cause decreases in the density of cholinergic receptor in a variety of tissues. These findings offer an explanation, at least partial, of the phenomenon of tolerance to organophosphate toxicity and to the observed subsensitivity to cholinergic agonists. Furthermore, they are a stimulus for further research to determine the potential deleterious effects of such alterations and their reversibility, and also offer an <u>in vivo</u> model to study the down-regulation of muscarinic receptors. <u>In vitro</u> studies suggested that some organophosphates could interact directly with the nicotinic receptor in the neuromuscular junction, an observation which is worth further investigation.

<u>In vitro</u> binding studies have also helped to clarify the possible site of action of compounds such as the bicyclic phosphates, some chlorinated hydrocarbon insecticides and the pyrethroids. Since this latter class of compounds seems to interact with various targets, more studies on their effects on neurotransmitter receptors are warranted. Finally, the studies with Kepone offer an example of the caution that must be exerted before reaching any conclusion on the effect of a neurotoxic chemical on receptor binding.

2. Metals and Organometals

Lead is probably the most studied of all metals and its behavioral and neurochemical effects have been recently reviewed (Silbergeld, 1982; Winder and Kitchen, 1984). Several studies have dealt with the effects of lead on neurotransmitter receptor binding, both <u>in vitro</u> and after <u>in vivo</u> administration. Inorganic lead (as lead nitrate) was found to inhibit the the binding of [^{3}H]-QNB to muscarinic receptors in rat brain membrane preparations (Aronstam and Eldefrawi, 1979). However, Bondy and Agrawal, (1980) reported that lead acetate caused only a 20% inhibition of [^{3}H]-QNB binding to rat brain cortical membranes, while yet another study (Costa and Fox, 1983) indicated a lack of effect of lead acetate (up to 10^{-4} M) on [^{3}H]-QNB binding in rat visual cortex, <u>in vitro.</u> Interestingly, an organic form of lead, tri-n-butyl lead acetate, was a much more potent inhibitor of [^{3}H]-QNB binding than inorganic lead (Bondy and Agrawal, 1980).

Alterations of muscarinic receptors were also found after developmental exposure to lead acetate (Costa and Fox, 1983). Neonatal rats were exposed to lead from parturition to weaning (0 to 21 days postnatal) via the milk of dams who consumed a 0.2% lead acetate solution. Blood concentrations of lead rose to 65 g/dl at 21 days of age, but declined to 7 g/dl at 90 days of age when neurochemical and psychophysical tests were conducted. A regional analysis of [^{3}H]-QNB binding in brain of lead exposed rats indicated a specific decrease in the density of muscarinic binding sites in the visual cortex (Costa and Fox, 1983), but not in other brain areas. This alteration appears to correlate with the observed supersensitivity to the effect of scopolamine on visual discrimination behavior (Fox et al., 1982) and with deficits observed in visual evoked cortical potential studies (Fox et al. 1979). However, the molecular mechanism of these receptor binding alterations has not been determined.

Some studies have examined the effects of lead on GABA and dopamine receptors. Memo and his colleagues (Memo et al., 1980) exposed rats to lead acetate from birth to six weeks of age and found that binding of [^{3}H] GABA was significantly decreased in the striatum and increased in the cerebellum. In both cases the change was due to an alteration in the number of GABA receptors. Silbergeld et al. (1980), after a similar lead treatment, confirmed the increase of GABA binding in the cerebellum, but did not find any alteration in the striatum. Lead had no effect in vitro on the binding of [^{3}H] GABA (Silbergeld et al. 1980) or [^{3}H] Muscimol (Bondy and Agrawal, 1980; Costa and Fox, unpublished observation). Using the same developmental exposure model described earlier (Costa and Fox, 1983), decreases of [^{3}H] muscimol binding were found in the hippocampus and the visual cortex (Fox and Costa, 1984). Lead tri-n-butyl acetate but not lead acetate inhibited the binding of [^{3}H]-spiperone to striatal membranes in vitro (Bondy and Agrawal, 1980). An investigation on dopamine receptors was made in rats exposed to 2.5 mg/ml lead acetate from birth to 4-6 weeks of age. Initially no effects on striatal dopamine receptors were found, as measured by binding of [^{3}H]-spiperone (Govoni et al., 1979). However, a subsequent study by the same investigators (Lucchi et al., 1981) using [^{3}H]-sulpiride (a ligand specific for D_2 dopamine receptors), revealed an increased density of binding sites in striata from lead-exposed rats. A lack of alteration of striatal [^{3}H]-spiperone binding after in vivo lead exposure was also reported by DeHaven et al., (1984).

The effects of mercury and methylmercury on neurotransmitter receptor binding have also been studied by several investigators. Both compounds inhibit the binding of [^{3}H]-QNB to muscarinic receptors in vitro (Bondy and Agrawal, 1980; Von Burg et al. 1980;

Eldefrawi et al., 1977; Abd-Elfattah and Shamoo, 1981; Aronstam and Eldefrawi, 1979) and mercury chloride was found to be 100-350 times more potent than methylmercury. This suggests that the effect on muscarinic receptors is due to an interaction of mercury with sulfhydryl residues, as inorganic mercury inhibits sulfhydryl enzymes to a greater extent than do organic mercurials (Waku and Nakazawa, 1979).

The inhibition by methylmercury of [^{3}H]-acetylcholine binding to cholinergic receptors of the electric organ of *Torpedo ocellata* (Eldefrawi et al., 1977) might also be ascribed to an interaction with sulfhydryl groups. In fact, the purified nicotinic receptor from *Torpedo* has been shown to contain two -SH groups per binding site (Shamoo et al., 1976).

Two studies by Corda and her colleagues (Corda et al., 1981; Concas et al., 1983) examined the effects of acute and chronic treatment with methylmercury on benzodiazepine receptors. Both treatments were found to increase the total number of binding sites for [^{3}H]-diazepam in various brain areas (cortex, striatum, retina) and particularly the cerebellum. Methylmercury failed to alter [^{3}H]-spiperone and [^{3}H] GABA binding in the same areas. Organic mercurials, such as parahydroxymercurybenzoate and mersalyl, have been reported to inhibit binding to beta$_1$-adrenoceptors in renal cortical membranes, the effect being due to their interaction with sulfhydryl groups (Moustafa et al. 1984).

A recent study (Cuomo et al., 1983) examined the effect of a single injection of methylmercury (8 mg/kg *per os*) to pregnant rats on neurotransmitter receptors of the offspring. Binding of [^{3}H]-spiperone was significantly increased in the striatum of 22 day-old rats from exposed mothers. This alteration was correlated with an increased sensitivity to the effects of apomorphine on locomotor activity. On the other hand, the locomotor response to clonidine, as well as alpha$_2$-adrenoceptor binding were unchanged.

Trimethyltin (TMT) is an organometal which causes a characteristic neurotoxic syndrome (Dyer et al. 1982; Wenger et al. 1982) and neuronal degeneration of the limbic system (Bouldin et al. 1981; Brown et al. 1979; Chang et al. 1982). A few studies have examined its effects on receptor binding. TMT does not inhibit the binding of [^{3}H]-QNB, [3H]-GABA and [^{3}H]-clonidine, *in vitro* (Costa et al., 1982; Doctor et al., 1982; Costa, unpublished observations). No alterations of [^{3}H]-QNB binding were found in mouse forebrain up to 14 h after *in vivo* administration of 4.26 mg/kg TMT (Costa et al., 1982), nor in [^{3}H]-QNB, [^{3}H]-Muscimol and [^{3}H]-Spiperone binding in mouse striatum following four 2.13 mg/kg injections of TMT, one week apart (Costa, Doctor and Murphy, unpublished results). After the same chronic treatment with TMT, however, there was an increased density of alpha$_2$-adrenoceptors in the cerebral cortex (Costa and

Murphy, unpublished results). Administration of 7.0 mg/kg TMT to rats had no effect on [^{3}H]-Spiperone binding in the striatum measured seven days after injection (DeHaven, et al. 1982). On the other hand, Summer and Hirsch (1982) found decreases in [^{3}H]-binding in the hippocampus, amygdala and frontal cortex of rats and mice, starting from four days after TMT administration. Ali et al. (1983) reported changes in [^{3}H]-Spiperone binding (increase at 7 and 14 days after 3.0 mg/kg TMT and in [^{3}H]-QNB binding (decrease at 2 and 7 days after TMT) in mouse brain. A recent study (Loullis et al. 1983) showed a 21% decrease of muscarinic receptors in the hippocampus of rats, two weeks following administration of 3.5 mg/kg TMT. This decrease is probably due to the loss of pyramidal cells observed in the hippocampus. Apart from this last study, interpretation of these receptor binding data is somewhat difficult, and their relationship with the mechanisms of TMT neurotoxicity not readily apparent. It would seem, however, that TMT toxicity is due to mechanisms other than receptor changes. Another organotin compound, triethyltin, was found to be inactive toward alpha-adrenergic and GABA receptors in vitro (Fox, 1982).

Manganese, cadmium and vanadium have also been studied with regard to their interactions with neurotransmitter receptors. Repeated treatment of rats with manganese chloride (10 or 15 mg/kg/day for 2 weeks) caused an increase of [^{3}H]-spiperone binding to striatal membranes while cerebellar GABA, frontal cortical serotonin and striatal muscarinic binding were depressed (Seth et al. 1981b). These findings were confirmed in another study (Gerhart and Tilson, 1982) in which striatal [^{3}H]-spiperone binding was increased and hippocampal [^{3}H]-muscimol binding was decreased following administration of 10, 20, or 40 mg manganese/ml of drinking water. This increase in dopaminergic receptors did not correlate, however, with an alteration in the responsiveness to apomorphine (Gerhart and Tilson, 1982).

The effect of manganese on muscarinic receptors was investigated by Donaldson and LaBella (1984). Incubation of rat brain tissue in the presence of catecholamine autooxidation products catalyzed by manganese led to a dose-dependent decrease in high affinity binding of [^{3}H]-QNB. Such an effect might be due to free radicals or cytotoxic quinones arising from the manganese-catalyzed autooxidation of dopamine. In contrast, administration of manganese to neonatal rats for two weeks resulted in an increase of [^{3}H]-QNB binding in the striatum which correlated with an inhibition of lipid peroxidation. The authors suggest that the effects of manganese on receptor binding might be due to its dual ability to act as a prooxidant or powerful antioxidant (Donaldson and LaBella, 1984).

Cadmium (1 mM in the drinking water for 8 days) decreased muscarinic receptor binding by 50% in the striatum of rats and to a lesser degree in the hippocampus (Hedlund et al. 1979). Vanadium, as orthovanadate (VO_4^{3-}), was reported to inhibit [^{3}H]-QNB binding *in vitro* by about 40% at a concentration of 1 mM (Danielsson et al. 1983).

The results of receptor binding studies with metals and organometals are not always easy to interpret in relation to their mechanism of neurotoxicity, in particular because of the variety of biochemical processes which are affected by this class of compounds. Some of their effects are due to the interaction with chemical groups on the receptor macromolecules, as in the case of mercury compounds. Decreases in receptor binding might be also due to loss of neurons as suggested by some results obtained with trimethyltin. Other interactions of metals with neurotransmitter receptors need to be further investigated before any conclusion or hypothesis on their significance can be formulated. Of a certain interest are the long term alterations in receptor binding found following developmental exposure to metals, in particular lead, since it is known that young individuals are particularly susceptible to their neurotoxicity.

3. Miscellaneous compounds

Oximes, such as 2-PAM, which serve as potent reactivators of acetylcholinesterase, are commonly used in organophosphate poisoning. These compounds are, however, ineffective in protecting against soman (O-pinacolyl methyl-phosphonofluoridate) toxicity. A new series of bispyridinium oximes, commonly called H-oximes (deJong and Wolring, 1981) have been shown to be potent antidotes against poisoning by soman (Oldiges and Krügal, 1981). Their reactivating potency for soman-inhibited acetylcholinesterase is stronger than that of classical antidotes, but not strong enough to explain exclusively the antidotal effect. Indeed, it was shown that these oximes interact with the muscarinic cholinergic receptors. They inhibited the binding of the specific muscarinic antagonist [^{3}H]-N-methyl-4-piperidyl benzilate to mouse brain homogenates and antagonized acetylcholine-induced contraction of the guinea-pig ileum with similar potencies (Amitai et al. 1980). These results, later confirmed and expanded (Kuhnen-Clausen et al. 1983), suggest that some bispyridinium compounds may exert their therapeutic action by blocking muscarinic receptors. This example also indicates that the use of a receptor binding technique in combination with a methodology measuring a physiological response (in this case the isolated ileum preparation) is useful in elucidating the site of action of novel compounds and their pharmacological effect.

The vinyl monomer acrylamide is known for its effect on peripheral nerves (central-peripheral distal axonopathy). However, several investigators have noted that it produces effects in the central nervous system (Tilson, 1981). Several studies have been recently published on the effects of acrylamide on dopamine receptors. Agrawal and Bondy (Agrawal et al., 1981a,b; Bondy et al.,

1981) found an increased B max for [^{3}H]-spiperone in the striatum of rats 24 h after a single dose of 100 mg/kg or after 10 mg/kg/day for 10 days. Unilateral lesions with kainic acid suggested that the effect of acrylamide on striatal post-synaptic receptors was post-synaptic in nature (Hong et al., 1982). An attempt was made to correlate the alteration in [^{3}H] spiperone binding to an alteration in the response to apomorphine (Agrawal et al. 1981b). However, a decrease in motor activity after apomorphine was observed in acrylamide-treated rats, instead of an increase in the sensitivity to this dopaminergic agonist (as expected because of the increase in [^{3}H]-spiperone binding).

Chronic exposure of rats to toluene by inhalation (0.7% in air) caused a decrease in the density of [^{3}H]-5-hydroxytriptamine ([^{3}H]-5HT) binding in the whole brain (Yamawaki et al. 1982). The hippocampus and the medulla oblongata-pons were the two brain regions showing the highest decrease in [^{3}H]-5HT binding. The biochemical data, however, did not parallel behavioral observations (Yamawaki et al. 1982). In another study (Celani et al., 1983), subacute treatment of rats with toluene (3000 ppm, 6 h/day for three days) caused a decrease in the affinity of striatal dopaminergic receptors and of cortical serotonin binding sites, without any change in their number. Other neurotransmitter receptors were not investigated, so that it is difficult to establish the specificity of such alterations (nonspecific membrane effects are, in fact, probable with solvents such as toluene).

Exposure to chemicals during pre- and/or early post-natal stages of development is of particular concern since it can cause abnormalities in the development of brain function and eventually lead to long-term irreversible alterations. The effects of such exposures on neurotransmitter receptors have been investigated for a variety of compounds. Examples of long term alterations following developmental exposure to lead, methylmercury or kepone have been described above. Many other compounds, such as caffeine, nicotine, or ethanol and various drugs have been shown to alter neurotransmitter receptor binding following prenatal or postnatal exposure, and the results obtained with some of these are summarized in Table 4. These biochemical investigations are an important corollary to behavioral and electrophysiological studies aimed at defining the potential neurobehavioral teratogenicity of chemicals.

4. Other uses of receptor binding assays

One of the applications of receptor binding techniques is the radioreceptor assay (Enna, 1978) which allows the quantitative determination of hormones, neurotransmitters and drugs in body fluids and tissues. ACTH and GABA were the first hormone and neurotransmitter to be assayed by radioreceptor assay (Lefkowitz, 1970; Enna and Snyder, 1976). Radioreceptor assays for a variety of

Table 4

Receptor binding alterations following pre-natal exposure to drugs

Prenatal Exposure	Receptor	Tissue	Increase/ Decrease	Reference
Diphenylhydantoin	Benzodiazepine	Cortex	Decrease	1
Nicotine	Cholinergic nicotinic	Cortex	Increase	2
Chlordiazepoxide	GABA	Whole brain	Increase	8
Haloperidol	Opiate	Striatum	Decrease	3
	Dopamine	Striatum	Increase	3
	Dopamine	Striatum	Increase	6
Ethanol	Dopamine	Striatum	Decrease	4
Streptomycin*	Dopamine	Striatum	Increase	5
	Serotonin	Cortex	Increase	5
Caffeine	Adenosine	Cerebellum Brain Stem	Increase	7
Monosodium Glutamate*	Benzodiazepine	Retina	Decrease	9
	Opiate	Thalamus	Decrease	10

(1) Gallager and Mallorga, 1980; (2) Sershen et al., 1982; (3) Edley, 1983; (4) Lucchi et al., 1983; (S) Seth et al., 1982; (6) Rosengarten and Friedhoff, 1979; (7) Marangos et al., 1984; (8) Peruzzi et al., 1983; (9) Regan et al., 1981; (10) Young et al. 1983.

* Postnatal

drugs have been since developed and clinical determination of drug levels probably represent the main use of this technique. The principle of radioreceptor assay procedures is based on the fact that the amount of radioligand bound to its receptor is quantitatively reduced by the amount of unlabeled ligand present (Enna,

1978). Thus, an unknown quantity of the competing drug or hormone can be calculated by determining the percentage inhibition of radioligand binding and comparing this with the inhibition produced by known quantities of the compound in question in a parallel, standard curve (Barnett and Nahorski, 1983)

One of the limitations of radioreceptor assays is their specificity, since any substance having some affinity for the neurotransmitter receptor site will displace the radioactive ligand. Thus, precautions should be taken to ensure that the only substance in the sample that will interfere with ligand binding is the substance being analyzed (Enna, 1978). An application of radioreceptor assay for toxicological purposes has been attempted with the benzodiazepines (Aaltonen and Scheinin, 1982). Benzodiazepine levels were measured in the serum of 21 patients with acute benzodiazepine overdosage. The radioreceptor assay was simple and rapid (no extraction of the samples was required), specific and reproducible. Concentrations measured by radioreceptor assay showed a good correlation with those obtained by gas-liquid chromatography. This also indicates that eventual metabolites of the benzodiazepine (which would not be differentiated from the parent compounds in the radioreceptor assay) possess very low benzodiazepine-like pharmacological activity (Klotz et al., 1980).

Radioligand binding techniques can also be used to label sites other than neurotransmitter or drug receptors. For example, [^{3}H]-ouabain binds to the catalytic site of the Na^+,K^+-ATPase (Akera et al., 1970). Inhibition of ouabain binding by various compounds correlates with their ability to inhibit Na^+K^+-ATPase activity measured by hydrolysis of ATP and inhibition of [^{3}H]ouabain binding might be used to screen compounds for their effect on Na^+, K^+-ATPase. Kepone (Desaiah et al., 1980), organotins (Prasada Rao et al., 1984; Costa, unpublished results) and erythrosin B (Silbergeld, 1981) have been shown to inhibit [^{3}H]-ouabain binding as well as Na^+, K^+-ATPase. However, the study with erythrosin B has been criticized (Mailman et al., 1980), since the effect of erythrosin B appears to be due to non-specific interactions with brain membranes.

[^{3}H]-Imipramine and [^{3}H]-desimipramine appear to bind to the uptake sites for serotonin and norepinephrine, respectively (Paul et al., 1981; Rehavi et al., 1982). However, the correspondence of their binding sites with the uptake sites has been recently challenged. [^{3}H] Nipecotic acid, [^{3}H]-mazindol and [^{3}H]-hemicholinium-3 have been used to label the uptake sites for GABA dopamine and choline, respectively. Thus, these binding assays might be used to investigate the effects of neurotoxicants on neurotransmitter uptake. Various toxins which bind to specific sites on ion channels are also of interest. For example, [^{3}H]-tetrodotoxin and [^{3}H] saxitoxin bind to the sodium channel (Catterall, 1980) while [^{3}H]-perhydrohistrionicotoxin ([^{3}H]H_{12}-HTX) binds to the nicotinic receptor/channel complex (Aronstam et al. 1981). As described before, various pyrethroid insecticides are able to inhibit [^{3}H]-H$_{12}$-HTX binding in the presence of carbachol (Abbassy et al. 1983). Radiolabeled compounds such as nitrendipine, which binds to the calcium channel have also been developed (Ehlert et al. 1982). Thus, progress in the field of radioligands for various sites will offer new tools to the biochemical neurotoxicologist for testing possible sites of action of neurotoxic chemicals.

CONCLUSIONS

The studies summarized here illustrate some applications of receptor binding assays to neurotoxicology. Although the available literature is still limited, it appears that the use these techniques has already provided important contributions to the study of neurotoxic chemicals. With the development of new, more specific radioligands and the characterization of more receptor types or subtypes, new tools are offered to the neurotoxicologist to investigate the effect of chemicals on neurotransmission. A judicious use of these techniques is warranted to make the results thus obtained useful and meaningful. In particular, nonspecific effects of the neurotoxicant which may alter the binding experiment, should be considered. Furthermore, studies on receptor binding sites should be run in parallel with experiments aimed at testing the functional status of the receptors. That is, there should be a correlation between a change in receptor binding and alterations in physiologi cal or pharmacological responses, measured by biochemical, behavioral or electrophysiological tests. It is also useful to investigate other components of neurotransmission (uptake, synthesis, release, degradation) to obtain a more complete picture of the effects of a neurotoxicant. Moreover, morphological examination of brain tissue where the receptor binding changes are found, are useful to determine if neuronal death had occurred. Thus, receptor binding techniques have been, and will be, an important addition to the methodologies available to the neurotoxicologist; however, only the cooperation of various scientific disciplines, each with its different technical approaches, will permit a successful advancement toward the understanding of the mechanism of action of neurotoxicants.

ACKNOWLEDGMENTS

The experimental studies by the first author cited herein were supported in part by NIEHS grant ES-03424 awarded to Sheldon D. Murphy (Seattle, WA). The authors thank Dr. S. D. Murphy for advice and support and Mrs. Ruth Larsen for typing this manuscript.

REFERENCES

Aaltonen, L. and Scheinin, M. Application of radioreceptor assay of benzodiazepines for Toxicology. Acta Pharmacol. Toxicol. 50: 206-212 (1982).

Abbassy, M.A.,Eldefrawi, M.E. and Eldefrawi, A.T. Pyrethroid Action on the Nicotinic Acetylcholine Receptor/Channel. Pesticide Biochem. Physiol. 19: 299-308 (1983).

Abd-Elfattah, A.S.A. and Shamoo,A.E. Regeneration of a Functionally Active Rat Brain Muscarinic Receptor By D-Penicillamine After Inhibition with Methylmercury and Mercuric Chloride. Mol. Pharmacol. 20: 492-497 (1981).

Abood, L.G., Saleti, N., MacNeil, M., Bloom, L. and Abood, M.E. Enhancement of opiate binding by various molecular forms of phosphatidylserine and inhibition by other unsaturated lipids. Biochem. Biophys. Acta 468: 51-62 (1977).

Abo-Khatwa, N. and Hollingworth, R.M. Chlordimeform: uncoupling activity against rat liver mitochondria. Pest. Biochem. Physiol. 3: 358-369 (1973).

Agrawal, A.K., Squibb, R.E. and Bondy, S.C. The effects of acrylamide treatment upon the dopamine receptor. Toxic. Appl. Pharmacol. 58: 84-99 (1981a).

Agrawal, A.K., Seth, P.K., Squibb, R.E., Tilson, H.A., Uphouse, L.L. and Bondy, S.C. Neurotransmitter receptors in brain regions of acrylamide-treated rats. I: Effects of a single exposure to acrylamide. Pharmacol. Biochem. Behav. 14: 527-531 (1981b).

Akera, T., Larsen, F.S. and Brody, T.M. Correlation of cardiac sodium - and potassium - activated adenosine triphosphatase activity with ouabain-induced inotropic stimulation. J. Pharmacol. Exp. Ther. 173: 145-151 (1970).

Alexander, R.W., Williams, L.T. and Lefkowitz, R.J. Identification of cardiac beta-adrenergic receptors by (-) [^{3}H] alprenolol binding. Proc. Natl. Acad. Sci. USA 72: 1564-1568 (1975).

Ali, S.F., Cranmer, J.M., Goad, P.T., Sukker. W., Harbison, R.D. and Cranmer, M.F. Trimethyltin induced changes of neurotransmitter levels and brain receptor binding in the mouse. Neurotoxicology 4(1): 29-36 (1983).

Amitai, G., Kloog, Y., Balderman, D. and Sokolovsky, M. The interaction of bis-pyridinium oximes with mouse brain muscarinic receptors. Biochem. Pharmacol. 29: 483-488 (1980).

Aronstam, R.S. and Eldefrawi, M.E. Transition and Heavy Metal Inhibition of Ligand Binding to Muscarinic Acetylcholine Receptors from Rat Brain. Toxicol. Appl. Pharmacol. 48: 489-496 (1979).

Aronstam, R.S., Abood, L.G. and Baumgold, J. Role of phospholipids in muscarinic binding by neural membranes. Biochem. Pharmacol. 26: 1689-1695 (1977).

Aronstam, R.S., Eldefrawi, A.T., Pessah, I.N., Daly, J.W., Albuquerque, E.X. and Eldefrawi, M.E. Regulation of [^{3}H] perhydrohistrionicotoxin binding to Torpedo electroplax by effectors of the acetylcholine receptor. J. Biol. Chem. 256: 2843-2850 (1981).

Aziz, S.A. and Knowles, C.O. Inhibition of Monoamine Oxidase by the Pesticide Chlordimeform and related compounds. Nature 242: 417-418 (1973).

Barnes, I.M. and Denz, F.A. The chronic toxicity of p-Nitrophenyl diethyl thiophosphate (E.605). J. Hyg. 49: 430-441 (1951).

Barnett, D.B. and Nahorski, S.R. Drug assays in plasma by radioreceptor techniques. Trends Pharmacol. Sci. 4: 407-409 (1983).

Bellett, E.M. and Casida, J.E. Bicyclic phosphorous esters: high toxicity without cholinesterase inhibition. Science 182: 1135-1136 (1973).

Bennett, J.P. and Snyder, S.H. Stereospecific binding of D-Lysergic acid diethylamide (LSD) to brain membranes: relationship to serotonin receptors. Brain Res. 94: 523-544 (1975).

Bombinski, T.S. and Dubois, K.P. Toxicity and mechanism of action of di-syston. AMA Arch. Ind. Health 17: 192-199 (1958).

Bondy, S.C. Rapid Screening of Neurotoxic agents by in vivo and in vitro means. In "Effects of Foods and Drugs on the Development and Function of the Nervous System: Methods for Predicting Toxicity", Proceeding of the Fifth FDA Science Symposium, 1979, pp. 133-143.

Bondy, S.C. Neurotransmitter Binding Interaction as a Screen for Neurotoxicity. In: "Mechanisms of action of neurotoxic substances", (K.N. Prasad and A. Vernadakis, Eds.), Raven Press, NY, 1982, pp. 25-50.

Bondy, S.C. and Agrawal, A.K. The Inhibition of Cerebral High Affinity Receptor Sites by Lead and Mercury Compounds. Arch. Toxicol. 46: 249-256 (1980).

Bondy, S.C., Tilson, H.A. and Agrawal, A.K. Neurotransmitter receptors in brain regions of acrylamide-treated rats. II: Effects of extended exposure to acrylamide. Pharmacol. Biochem. Behav. 14: 533-537 (1981).

Bouldin. T.W., Goines, N.D., Bagnell, C.R. and Krigman, M.R. Pathogenesis of trimethyltin neuronal toxicity: Ultrastructural and Cytochemical Observations. Am. J. Pathol. 104: 237-249 (1981).

Bowery, N.G., Collins, J.F. and Hill, R.G. Bicyclic Phosphorus esters that are potent convulsants and GABA antagonists. Nature 261: 601-603 (1976).

Braestrup, C. and Squires, R.F. Specific Benzodiazepine receptors in rat brain characterized by high-affinity [^{3}H] diazepam binding. Proc. Natl. Acad. Sci. USA 74: 3805-3809 (1977).

Brodeur, J. and Du Bois, K.P. Studies on the mechanism of acquired tolerance by rats to O,O-diethyl S-2 (ethylthio) ethyl phosphorodithioate (DiSyston). Arch. Int. Pharmacodyn. 149: 560-570 (1964).

Brown, A.W., Aldridge, W.N., Street, B.W. and Verschoyle, R.D. The behavioral and neuropathologic sequelae of intoxication by trimethyltin compounds in the rat. Am. J. Pathol. 97: 59-82 (1979).

Bruns, R.F., Daly, J.W. and Snyder, S.H. Adenosine receptors in brain membranes: binding of N^6-cyclohexyl [^{3}H] adenosine and 1,3-diethyl-8-[^{3}H] phenylxanthine. Proc. Natl. Acad. Sci. USA 9: 5547-5551 (1980).

Burgen, A.S.V., Hiley, C.R. and Young, J.M. The binding of [^{3}H]-propylbenzylcholine mustard by longitudinal muscle strips from guinea-pig small intestine. Br. J. Pharmacol. 50: 145-151 (1974).

Burnstock, G. (Ed.) Purinergic Receptors. Chapman & Hall, London, (1981).

Bylund, D.B. and Snyder, S.H. Beta adrenergic receptor binding in membrane preparations from mammalian brain. Mol. Pharmacol. 12: 568-580 (1976).

Catterall, W.A. Neurotoxins that act on voltage-sensitive sodium channels in excitable membranes. Ann. Rev. Pharmacol. Toxicol. 20: 15-43 (1980).

Celani, M.F.,Fuxe, K., Agnati, L.F., Andersson, K., Hansson, T., Gustafsson, J.A., Battistini, N. and Eneroth, P. Effects of subacute treatment with toluene on central monoamine receptors in the rat. Reduced affinity in [^{3}H] 5-hydroxytryptamine binding sites and in [^{3}H] spiperone binding sites linked to dopamine receptors. Toxicol. Lett. 17: 275-281 (1983).

Chamness, G.C. and McGuire, W.L. Scatchard Plots: Common Errors in Correction and Interpretation. Steroids. 26(4): 538-542 (1975).

Chang, L.W., Tiemeyer, T.M., Wenger, G.R., and McMillan, D.E. Neuropathology of mouse hippocampus in acute trimethyltin intoxication. Neurobehav. Toxicol. Teratol. 4: 149-156 (1982).

Changeaux, J.P., Kasai, M., Huchet, M. and Meunier, J.C. Neurobiologic moleculaire - Extraction a partir du tissu electrique de-gymnote d'une proteine dresentant plusieurs proprietes caracteristiques du recepteur physiologique del' acetylcholine. C.R. Acad. Sci. Paris 270: 2864-2867 (1970).

Chau-Pham, T.T., King, G. and Dewey, W.L. Sodium-induced alterations of opiate effects on the binding of [^{3}H]-dihydromorphine to mouse brain homogenates. Life Sci. 23: 1293-1300 (1978).

Cheng, Y.C. and Prusoff, W.H. Relationship between the Inhibitor Constant (KI) and the concentration of Inhibitor which causes 50 percent inhibition (I_{50}) of an enzymatic reaction. Biochem. Pharmacol. 22: 3099-3108 (1973).

Chinn, C., Lund, A.E. and Yim, G.K.W. Central actions of lidocaine and a pesticide: chlordimeform. Neuropharmacol. 16: 867-872 (1977).

Ciofalo, F. Effect of some antiarrhythmics on [^{3}H] clonidine binding to alpha$_2$-adrenergic receptors. Eur. J. Pharmacol. 65: 309-312 (1980).

Ciofalo, F. Effects of some membrane perturbers on alpha$_1$-adrenergic receptor binding. Neurosci. Lett. 21: 313-318 (1981).

Concas, A., Corda, M.G., Salis, M., Mulas, M.L., Milia, A., Corongiu, F.P. and Biggio, G. Biochemical Changes in the Rat Cerebellar Cortex Elicited by Chronic Treatment with Methyl Mercury. Toxicol. Lett. 18: 27-33 (1983).

Cooper, J.R., Bloom, R.E. and Roth, R.H. The Biochemical Basis of Neuropharmacology. Oxford University Press, NY, 1982.

Corda, M.G., Concas, A., Rossetti, Z., Guarneri, P., Corongiu, F.P. and Biggio, G. Methyl mercury enhances [^{3}H] diazepam binding in different areas of the rat brain. Brain Res. 229: 264-269 (1981).

Costa, L.G. and Murphy, S.D. Passive avoidance retention in mice tolerant to the organophosphorus insecticide disulfoton. Toxicol. Appl. Pharmacol. 65: 451-458 (1982).

Costa, L.G. and Fox, D.A. A selective decrease of cholinergic muscarinic receptors in the visual cortex of adult rats following developmental lead exposure. Brain Research 276: 259-266 (1983).

Costa, L.G. and Murphy, S.D. [^{3}H] nicotine binding in rat brain: alteration after chronic acetylcholinesterase inhibition. J. Pharmacol. Exp. Ther. 226: 392-397 (1983).

Costa, L.G., Schwab, B.W., Hand, H. and Murphy, S.D. Decreased muscarinic binding sites in small intestine from mice treated with neostigmine. Life Sci. 29: 1675-1682 (1981a).

Costa, L.G., Schwab, B.W., Hand, H. and Murphy, S.D. Reduced [^{3}H]-quinuclidinyl benzilate binding to muscarinic receptors in disulfoton-tolerant mice. Toxicol. Appl. Pharmacol. 60: 441-450 (1981b).

Costa, L.G., Schwab, B.W., and Murphy, S.D. Differential alterations of cholinergic muscarinic receptors during chronic and acute tolerance to organophosphorus insecticides. Biochem. Pharmacol. 31: 3407-3413 (1982a).

Costa, L.G., Schwab, B.W. and Murphy, S.D. Tolerance to anticholinesterase compounds in mammals. Toxicology 25: 79-97 (1982b).

Costa, L.G., Doctor, S.V. and Murphy, S.D. Antinociceptive and hypothermic effects of trimethyltin. Life Sci. 31: 1093-1102 (1982c).

Costa, L.G., Shao, M., Basker, K and Murphy, S.D. Chronic administration of an organophosphorus insecticide to rats alters cholinergic muscarinic receptors in the pancreas. Chem. Biol. Interactions 48: 261-269 (1984).

Creese, I., Burt, D.R. and Snyder, S.H. The dopamine receptor: Differential binding of d-LSD and related agents to agonist and antagonist states. Life Sci. 17: 1715-1720 (1975).

Creese, I. and Sibley, D.R. Receptor adaptations to centrally acting drugs. Ann. Rev. Pharmacol. Toxicol. 21: 357-391 (1980).

Cremer, J.E., Cunningham, V.J., Ray, D.E. and Sarna, G.S. Regional changes in brain glucose utilization in rats given a pyrethroid insecticide. Brain Research 194: 278-282 (1980).

Cuomo,V., Ambrosi, L., Cagiano, R., Brunello, N. and Racagni, G. Behavioral and neurochemical changes in offspring of rats exposed to methyl mercury during gestation. Soc. Neurosci. Abstr. 9: 1246 (1983).

Daly, J.W., Hoffer, B.J. and Dismukes, K. (Eds). Mechanisms of regulation of neuronal sensitivity. Neurosc. Res. Prog.Bull. 18: 323-456 (1980).

Damstra, T. and Bondy, S.C. Neurochemical approaches to the detection of neurotoxicity. In: "Nervous System Toxicology" (C.L. Mitchell, Ed.), Raven Press, NY, 1982, pp. 349-373.

Danielsson, E., Unden, A. and Bartfai, T. Orthovanadate induces loss of muscarinic cholinergic binding sites. Biochem. Biophys. Res. Comm. 110: 567-572 (1983).

DeHaven, D.L., Walsh,T.J. and Mailman, R.B. The effects of trimethyltin on dopaminergic and serotoninergic function of the central nervous system. Soc. Neurosci. Abstr. 8: 562 (1982).

DeHaven, D.L., Krigman,M.R., Gaynor, J.J. and Mailman, R.B. The effects of lead administration during development on lithium-induced polydipsia and dopaminergic function. Brain Res. 297: 297-304 (1984).

DeHaven, D.L. and Mailman, R.B. The use of radioligand binding techniques in neurotoxicology. In: "Reviews in Biochemical Toxicology", vol. 5 (E. Hodgson, J.R. Bend and R.M. Philpot, Eds.), Elsevier, NY, 1983, pp. 193-238.

DeJong, L.P.A. and Wolring, G.Z. Reactivating potency of oximes and their effect on aging. In: "Protection against highly toxic substances", 2nd Symposium, Prins Maurits Laboratory TNO, Rijswijk NL, 1981 pp. 319-326.

Desaiah, D. Interaction of chlordecone with biological membranes. J. Toxicol. Environ. Health 8: 719-730 (1981).

Desaiah, D., Gilliland, T., Ho, I.K. and Mehendale, H.M. Inhibition of mouse brain synaptosomal ATP-ases and ouabain binding by chlordecone. Toxicol. Lett. 6: 275-285 (1980).

Doctor, S.V., Costa, L.G., Kendall,D.A. and Murphy, S.D. Trimethyltin inhibits uptake of neurotransmitters into mouse forebrain synaptosomes. Toxicology 25: 213-221 (1982).

Donaldson, J. and LaBella, F.S. The effects of manganese on the cholinergic recetor _in vivo_ and _in vitro_ may be mediated through modulation of free radicals. Neurotoxicol. 5(1): 105-112 (1984).

Dyer, R.S., Walsh,T.J., Wonderlin, W.F. a nd Bercegeay, M. The trimethyltin syndrome in rats. Neurobehav. Toxicol. Teratol. 4: 127-133 (1982).

Edley, S.M. Effects of prenatal haloperidol on receptors in the developing rat striatum: opposite changes in naloxone and spiperone binding. Soc. Neurosci. Abstr. 9: 874 (1983).

Ehlert, F.J., Kokka, N. and Fairhurst, A.S., Altered [^{3}H] quinuclidinyl benzilate binding in the striatum of rats following chronic cholinesterase inhibition with diisopropylfluorophosphate. Mol. Pharmacol. 17: 24-30 (1980).

Ehlert, F.J., Roeske, W.R., Itoga, E. and Yamamura, H.I. The binding of [^{3}H] nitrendipine to receptors for calcium channel antagonists in the heart, cerebral cortex and ileum of rats. Life Sci. 30: 2191-2202 (1982).

Eisenthal, R. and Cornish-Bowden, A. The direct linear plot. A new graphical procedure for estimating enzyme kinetic parameters. Biochem. J. 139: 715-710 (1974).

Eldefrawi, A.T., Mansour, N.A. and Elderfrawi, M.E. Insecticides affecting acetylcholine receptor interactions. Pharmacol. Ther. 16: 45-65 (1982).

Eldefrawi, M.E., Manson, N.A. and Eldefrawi, A.T., Interactions of acetylcholine receptors with organic mercury. In: "Membrane Toxicity", (Miller, M.W. and Shamoo, A.E., Eds.) Plenum Press, NY, 1977, pp. 449-463.

End, D.W., Carchman, R.A. and Dewey, W.L. Neurochemical correlates of chlordecone neurotoxicity. J. Toxicol. Environ. Health 8: 707-718 (1981).

Enna, S.J. Radioreceptor assay techniques for neurotransmitters and drugs. In: "Neurotransmitter Receptor Binding", (H.I. Yamamura, S.J. Enna and M.J. Kuhar, Eds.), Raven Press, NY, 1978, pp. 127-139.

Enna, S.J. and Snyder, S.H. Properties of gamma-Aminobutyric acid (GABA) receptor binding in rat brain synaptic membrane fractions. Brain Res. 100: 81-97 (1975).

Enna, S.J. and Snyder, S.H. A simple, sensitive and specific radioreceptor assay for endogenous GABA in brain tissue. J. Neurochem. 26: 221-224 (1976).

Evans, P.D. Properties of modulatory octopamine receptors in the locust. In: "Neuropharmacology of insects", Ciba Foundation Symposium 88, Pitman, London, 1982. pp. 48-69.

Exton, J.H. Molecular Mechanisms involved in alpha-adrenergic responses. In: "More about receptors", (J.W. Lamble, Ed.), Elsevier North Holland, 1982, pp. 66-75.

Fox, D.A. Pharmacological and biochemical evaluation of triethyltin's anticonvulsant effects. Neurobehav. Toxicol. Teratol. 4: 273-278 (1982).

Fox, D.A. and Costa, L.G. Visual cortical and hippocampal loss of GABAergic receptors in lead exposed rats: electrophysiological and pharmacological correlates. Toxicologist 4(1): 114 (1984).

Fox, D.A., Lewkowski, J.P. and Cooper, G.P. Persistent visual cortex excitability alterations produced by neonatal lead exposure. Neurobehav. Toxicol. 1: 101-106 (1979).

Fox, D.A., Wright, A.A. and Costa, L.G. Visual acuity deficits following neonatal lead exposure: Cholinergic interactions. Neurobehav. Toxicol. Teratol. 4: 689-693 (1982).

Friedhoff, A.J. and Miller, J.C. Clinical implications of receptor sensitivity modification. Ann. Rev. Neurosci. 6: 121-148 (1982).

Gallager, D.W. and Mallorga, P. Diphenylhydantoin: Pre- and Postnatal administration alters diazepam binding in developing rat cerebral cortex. Science 208: 64-66 (1980).

Gazit, H., Silman, I. and Dudai, Y. Administration of an organophosphate causes a decrease in muscarinic receptor levels in rat brain. Brain Res. 174: 351-356 (1979).

Gerhart, J.M. and Tilson, H.A. Manganese Chloride Exposure Alter High Affinity Receptor Binding and Drug-Induced Activity in Male Rats. Toxicologist 2(1): 87 (1982).

Gepner, J.I., Hall, L.M. and Sattelle, D.B. Insect acetylcholine receptor as a site of insecticide action. Nature 276: 188-190 (1978).

Goodman, R.R. and Pasternak, G.W. Multiple opiate receptors. In: "Analgesics: Neurochemical, Behavioral and Clinical Perspectives", (M. Kuhar and G.W. Pasternak, Eds.), Raven Press, NY, 1984, pp. 69-96.

Govoni, S. Memo, M., Spano, P.F. and Trabucchi, M. Chronic lead treatment differentially effects dopamine synthesis in various rat brain areas. Toxicology 12: 343-349 (1979).

Greenberg, D.A., U'Prichard, D.C. and Snyder, S.H. Alpha-noradrenergic receptor binding in mammalian brain: differential labeling of agonist and antagonist states. Life Sci. 19: 69-76 (1976).

Hedlund, B., Gamarra, M. and Bartfai, T. Inhibition of striatal muscarinic receptor in vivo by cadmium. Brain Res. 168: 216-218 (1979).

Hill, A.W. The possible effects of the aggregation of the molecules of hemoglobin on its dissociation curves. J. Physiol. 40: IV (1910).

Hill, D.R. and Bowery, N.G. ^{3}H-Baclofen and ^{3}H-GABA bind to bicuculline-insensitive $GABA_B$ sites in rat brain. Nature, 290: 149-152 (1981).

Hirschowitz, B.I., Hammer, R., Giachetti, A., Keirns, J.J. and Levine, R.R., Eds. Subtypes of Muscarinic Receptors. Trends Pharmacol. Sci. suppl., Elsevier, 1984, pp. 103.

Ho, I.K., Fujimori, K., Huang, T.P. and Chang-Tusi, H. Neurochemical evaluation of chlordecone toxicity in the mouse. J. Toxicol. Environ. Health 8: 701-706 (1981).

Hollingworth, R.M., Leister, J. and Ghali, G. Mode of action of formamidine pesticides: an evaluation of monoamine oxidase as the target. Chem. Biol. Interactions 24: 35-49 (1979).

Hollingworth, R.M. and Lund, A.E. Biological and Neurotoxic Effects of Amidine Pesticides. In: "Insecticide mode of action", (R. O'Brien, Ed.) Academic Press, 1982, pp. 189-227.

Hong, I.S., Tilson, H.A., Agrawal, A.K., Karoum, F. and Bondy, S.C. Postsynaptic location of acrylamide-induced modulation of striatal ^{3}H-Spiroperidol binding. Neurotoxicol. 3: 108-112 (1982).

Hsu, W.H. and Kakuk, T.J. Effect of Amitraz and Chlordimeform on heart rate and pupil diameter in rats: mediated by alpha$_2$-adrenoreceptors. Toxicol. Appl. Pharmacol. 73: 411-415 (1984).

Iversen, L.L. Nonopioid neuropeptides in mammalian CNS. Ann. Rev. Pharmacol. Toxicol. 23: 1-27 (1983).

Johnson, T. and Knowles, C.O. Inhibition of Rat Platelet 5-Hydroxytryptamine Uptake by Chlordimeform. Toxicol. Lett. 9: 1-4 (1981).

Keightley, D.D. and Cressie, N.A.C. The Woolf plot is more reliable than the Scatchard plot in analysing data from hormone receptor assays. J. Steroid Biochem. 13: 1317-1323 (1980).

Ketelsleger, I.M., Pirens, G., Maghuin-Rogister, G., Hennen, G. and Freres, J.M. The choice of erroneous models of hormone receptor interactions: a consequence of illegitimate utilization of Scatchard graphs. Biochem. Pharmacol. 33: 707-710 (1984).

Klotz, I.M. Numbers of receptor sites from Scatchard graphs: facts and fantasies. Science 217: 1247-1249 (1982).

Klotz, I.M. Ligand-receptor interactions: what we can and cannot learn from binding measurements. Trends Pharmacol. Sci. 4: 253-255 (1983).

Klotz, U., Kangas, L. and Kanto, J. Clinical Pharmacology of Benzodiazepines. G. Fisher Verlag, Stuttgart, 1980.

Kuhnen-Clausen, D., Hagedorn, I., Gross, G., Bayer, H. and Hucho, F. Interactions of bisquaternary pyridine salts (H-oximes) with cholinergic receptors. Arch. Toxicol. 54: 171-179 (1983).

Laduron, P.M. Criteria for receptor sites in binding studies. Biochem. Pharmacol. 33: 833-839 (1984).

Langley, J.N. On the reaction of cells and of nerve endings to certain poisons. Chiefly as regards the reaction of striated muscle to nicotine and to curari. J. Physiol. 33: 374-413 (1905).

Lawrence, L.J. and Casida, J.E. Stereospecific action of pyrethroid insecticides on the gamma-aminobutyric acid receptor-ionophore complex. Science: 221: 1399-1401 (1983).

Lawrence, L.J. and Casida, J.E. Interactions of lindane, toxaphene and cyclodienes with brain-specific t-butylbicyclophosphorothionate receptor. Life Sci. 35:171-178 (1984).

Leclerc, G., Rovot, B., Velly, J. and Schwartz, J. Beta-adrenergic receptor subtypes. In: "Towards understanding receptors", (J.W. Lamble, Ed.), Elsevier North Holland, 1981, pp. 78-83.

Leff, S.E. and Creese, I. Dopamine receptors re-explained. Trends Pharmacol. Sci. 4: 463-467 (1983).

Lefkowitz, R., Roth, J. and Pastan, I. Radioreceptor assay of adrenocorticotropic hormone: new approach to assay of polypeptide hormones in plasma. Science 170: 633-635 (1970).

Lineweaver, H. and Burk, D. The determination of enzyme dissociation constants. J. Am. Chem. Soc. 56: 658-666 (1934).

Loullis, C.C., Dean, R.L., Benson, D.I., Lippa, A.S., Bartus R.T. and Coupet, J. Trimethyltin: behavioral, neurochemical and neuroanatomical effects. Soc. Neurosci. Abstr. 9: 420 (1983).

Lucchi, L., Memo, M. Airaghi, M.L., Spano, P.F. and Trabucchi, M. Chronic lead treatment induces in rat a specific and differential effect on dopamine receptors in different brain areas. Brain Res. 213: 397-404 (1981).

Lucchi, L. Covelli, V., Petkov, V.V., Spano, P. and Trabucchi, M. Effects of ethanol, given during pregnancy on the offspring dopaminergic system. Pharm. Biochem. Behav. 19: 567-570, (1983).

Mailman, R.B. and Morell, P. Neurotoxicants and membrane-associated functions. In: "Reviews in biochemical toxicology", vol. 4 (E. Hodgson, J.R. Bend and R.M. Philpot, Eds.), Elsevier, New York, 1982, pp. 213-255.

Mailman, R.B., Ferris, R.M., Tang, F.L.M., Vogel, R.A., Kilts, C.D., Lipton, M.A., Smith, D.A., Mueller, R.A. and Breese, G.R. Erythrosine (Red No. 3) and its nonspecific biochemical actions: what relation to behavioral changes? Science 207: 535-537 (1980).

Marangos, P.J., Boulenger, J.P. and Patel, J. Effects of chronic caffeine on brain adenosine receptor: regional and ontogenetic studies. Life Sci. 34: 899-907 (1984).

Marks, M.J., Artman, L.D., Patinkin, D.M. and Collins, A.C. Cholinergic adaptations to chronic oxotremorine infusion. J. Pharmacol. Exp. Ther. 218: 337-343 (1981).

Martin, W.R. Pharmacology of opioids. Pharmacol. Rev. 35: 283-323 (1984).

Mattsson, H., Brandt, K. and Heilbronn, E. Bicyclic phosphorus esters increase the cyclic GMP level in rat cerebellum. Nature 268: 52-53 (1977).

McPhillips, J.J. Altered sensitivity to drugs following repeated injections of a cholinesterase inhibitor to rats. Toxicol. Appl. Pharmacol. 14: 67-73 (1969).

McPhillips, J.J. and Dar, M.S. Resistance to the effect of carbachol on the cardiovascular system and on the isolated ileum of rats after subacute administration of an organophosphorus cholinesterase inhibitor. J. Pharmacol. Exp. Ther. 156: 507-513 (1967).

Memo, M., Lucchi, L., Spano, P.F. and Trabucchi, M. Effects of chronic lead treatment on GABAergic receptor function in rat brain. Toxicol Lett. 6: 427-432 (1980).

Morley, B.J., Farley, G.R. and Javel, E. Nicotinic acetylcholine receptors in mammalian brain. Trends Pharmacol. Sci. 4: 225-227 (1983a).

Morley, B.J., Dwyer, D.S., Strang-Brown, P.F., Bradley, R.J. and Kemp, G.E. Evidence that certain peripheral anti-acetylcholine receptor antibodies do not interact with brain BuTX binding sites. Brain Res. 262: 109-116 (1983b).

Moustafa, E., Snavely, M.D. and Insel, P.A. Selective inhibition by organic mercurials of binding to the beta population of rat renal cortical beta-adrenergic receptors. Biochem. Pharmacol. 33: 1148-1151 (1984).

Munson, P.J. Experimental artifacts and the analysis of ligand binding data: results of a computer simulation. J. Recept. Res. 3(1&2): 249-259 (1983).

Munson, P.J. and Rodbard, D. LIGAND: a versatile computerized approach for characterization of ligand binding systems. Anal. Biochem. 107: 220-239 (1980).

Munson, P.J. and Rodbard, D. Number of receptor sites from Scatchard and Klotz graphs: a constructive critique. Science 220: 979-981 (1983).

Murdock, L.L. and Hollingworth, R.M. Octopamine-like actions of formamidines in the firefly light organ. In: "Insect Neurobiology and Insecticide Action (Neurotox '79)", Soc. Chem. Ind., London, pp. 415-422.

Murphy, S.D. Pesticides. In: Toxicology: The basic science of poisons, (J. Doull, C.D. Kiaassen and M.O. Amdur, Eds.), MacMillan, N.Y., 1980, pp. 357-408.

Norby, J.G., Ottolenghi, P. and Jensen, J. Scatchard Plot: Common misinterpretation of binding experiments. Anal. Biochem. 102: 318-320 (1980).

Oldiges, H. and Krugel, M. Tierexperimentelle Untersuchungen mit potentiellen Antidoten zur Therapic einer Alkylphosphatvergiftung. In: "Protection against highly toxic substances", 2nd Symposium, Prins Maurits Laboratory TNO, Riijswijk NL, (1981), pp. 319-326.

Ozoe, Y. Mochida, K. and Eto, M. Reaction of toxic bicyclic phosphates with acetylcholinesterase and alpha-chimotrypsin. Agric. Biol. Chem. 46: 2527-2531 (1982).

Paton, W.D.M. and Rang, H.P. The uptake of atropine and related drugs by intestinal smooth muscle of the guinea-pig in relation to acetylcholine receptors. Proc. R. Soc. London Ser. B 163: 1-44 (1965).

Paul, S.M., Rehavi, M., Rice, K.C., Ittah, Y. and Skolnick, P. Does high affinity [^{3}H] imipramine binding label serotonin reuptake sites in brain and platelet? Life Sci. 28: 2753-2760 (1981).

Peck, E.J., Jr. and Kelner, K.L. Receptor Measurement. In: "Handbook of Neurochemistry", vol. II (A. Lajtha, Ed.) Plenum Press, NY, 1983, pp. 53-75.

Pennock, B.E. A calculator for finding binding parameter from Scatchard plot. Anal. Brochem. 56: 306-309 (1973).

Peroutka, S.J. and Snyder, S.H. Multiple serotonin receptors: differential binding of [^{3}H] 5-hydroxytryptamine, [^{3}H] lysergic acid diethylamide and [^{3}H] spiroperidol. Mol. Pharmacol. 16: 687-699 (1979).

Perrine, S.E. and McPhillips, J.J. Specific subsensitivity of the rat atrium to cholinergic drugs. J. Pharmacol. Exp. Ther. 175: 496-502 (1970).

Pert, C.B. and Snyder, S.H. Opiate receptor: demonstration in nervous tissue. Science 179: 1011-1014 (1973).

Peruzzi, G., Abbracchio, M.P., Cagiano, R. Coen, E., Cuomo, V., Galli, C.L., Lombardelli, G., Marinovich, M. and Cattabeni, F. Enduring behavioral and biochemical effects of perinatal treatment with caffeine and chlordiazepoxide. In: "Application of Behavioral Pharmacology in Toxicology" (G. Zbinden, V. Cuomo, G. Racagmi and B. Weiss, Eds.), Raven Press, NY, 1983, pp. 217-236.

Petajan, J.H., Vorhees, K.J., Packam, S.C., Baldwin, R.C., Einhorn, I.N., Grunnet, M.L., Dinger, B.G. and Birky, M.N. Extreme toxicity from combustion products of a fire-retarded polyurethane foam. Science 187: 742-744 (1975).

Prasada Rao, K.S., Chetty, C.S., Trottman,C.H. and Desaiah, D. Inhibition of rat brain synaptosomal ATPases by Plictran. Toxicologist 4(1): 55 (1984).

Raftery, M.A., Schmidt, J., Clark, D.G. and Wolcott, R.G. Demonstration of a specific alpha-bungarotoxin binding component in elecrophorus electricus electroplex membranes. Biochem. Biophys. Res. Commun. 45: 1622-1629 (1971).

Regan, J.W., Roeske, W.R., Ruth, W.H., Deshmukh, P. and Yamamura, H.I. Reductions in retinal gamma-aminobutyric acid (GABA) content and in [^{3}H]-flunitrazepam binding after postnatal monosodium glutamate injections in rats. J. Pharm. Exp. Ther. 218: 791-796 (1981).

Rehavi, M., Skolnick, P., Brownstein, M.J. and Paul, S.M. High-affinity binding of [^{3}H] desipramine to rat brain: a presynaptic marker for noradrenergic uptake site. J. Neurochem. 38: 889-895 (1982).

Rider, J.A., Ellinwood, L.E. and Coon, J.M. Production of tolerance in rats to Octamethyl Pyrophosphoramide. Proc. Soc. Exp. Biol. Med. 81: 455-459 (1952).

Riker, W.F.,Excitatory and anti-curare properties of acetylcholine and related quaternary ammonium compounds at the neuromuscular junction. Pharmocol Rev. 5:1-86 (1953).

Ringdahl, B. and Jenden, D.J. Pharmacological properties of oxotremorine and its analogs. Life Sci. 32: 2401-2413 (1983).

Rosengarten, H. and Friedhoff, A.J. Enduring changes in dopamine receptor cells of pups from drug administration to pregnant and nursing rats. Science 203: 1133-1135 (1979).

Rosenthal, H. A graphic method for the determination and presentation of binding parameters in a complex system. Anal. Chem. 20: 525-532 (1967).

Russell, R.W., Overstreet, D.H., Cotman, C.W., Carson, V.G., Churchill, L., Dalglish, F.W. and Vasquez, B.J. Experimental tests of hypotheses about neurochemical mechanisms underlying behavioral tolerance to the anticholinesterase diisopropylfluorophosphate. J. Pharmacol. Exp. Ther. 192: 73-85 (1975).

Russell. R.W., Overstreet,D.H. and Netherton, R.A., Sex-linked and other genetic factors in the development of tolerance to the anticholinesterase, DFP. Neuropharmacol. 22: 75-81 (1983).

Scatchard, G. The attractions of proteins for small molecules and ions. Ann. N.Y. Acad. Sci. 51: 660-672 (1949).

Schwab, B.W., Studies of disulfoton tolerance in rats. Ph.D. thesis, University of Texas Health Science Center at Houston, 1981.

Schwab, B.W., Hand, H., Costa, L.G., Murphy, S.D. Reduced muscarinic receptor binding in tissues of rats tolerant to the insecticide disulfoton. Neurotoxicol. 2: 635-647 (1981).

Schwab, B.W., Costa, L.G. and Murphy, S.D. Muscarinic receptor alterations as a mechanism of anticholinesterase tolerance. Toxicol. Appl. Pharmacol. 71: 14-23 (1983).

Schwartz, R.D. and Kellar, K.J. Nicotinic cholinergic receptor binding sites in the brain: regulation in vivo. Science 220: 214-216 (1983).

Schwartz, J.C., Llorens Cortes,C., Rose, C., Quach, T.T. and Pollard, H. Adaptive changes of neurotransmitter receptor mechanisms in the central nervous system. In: "Molecular and cellular interactions underlying higher brain functions", Progress in Brain Research, vol. 58 (J.P. Changeaux, J. Glowinski, M. Imbert and F.E. Bloom,Eds.) Elsevier, 1983, pp. 117-129.

Seeman, P. Brain dopamine receptors. Pharmacol. Rev. 32: 229-313 (1980).

Seeman, P., Chau-Wong, M., Tedesco, J. and Wong, K. Brain receptors for antipsychotic-drugs and dopamine: Direct binding assays. Proc. Natl. Acad. Sci. USA 72: 4376-4380 (1975).

Sershen, H., Reith, M.E.A., Banay-Schwartz, M., and Lajtha, A. Effects of prenatal administration of nicotine on amino acid pools, protein metabolism, and nicotine binding in the brain. Neurochem. Res. 7: 1515-1522 (1982).

Seth, P.K., Agrawal, A.K. and Bondy, S.C. Biochemical changes in the brain consequent to dietary exposure of developing and mature rats to chlordecone (Kepone). Toxicol. Appl. Pharmacol. 59: 262-267 (1981a).

Seth, P., Hong, J.S., Kilts, C.D., and Bondy, S. Alteration of Cerebral neurotransmitter receptor function by exposure of rats to manganese. Toxicol. Lett. 9: 247-254 (1981b).

Seth, P.K., Alleva, F.R., Balazs, T. Alteration of high-affinity binding sites of neurotransmitter receptors in rats after neonatal exposure to streptomycin. Neurotoxicol. 3: 13-20 (1982).

Shain, W. and Carpenter, D.O., Mechanisms of synaptic modulation. Int. Rev. Neurobiol. 22: 205-250 (1981).

Shamoo, A.D., MacLennan, D. and Eldefrawi, M.E. Differential effects of mercurial compounds on excitable tissue. Chem. Biol. Interact. 12: 41-52 (1976).
Siiteri, P.K. Receptor binding studies. Science 223: 191-193 (1984).
Silbergeld, E.K. Neurochemical and ionic mechanisms of Lead neurotoxicity. In: "Mechanism of actions of neurotoxic substances (Prasad, K.N. and Vernadakis, A., Eds.) Raven Press, New York 1982, pp. 1-23.
Silbergeld, E.K. Erythrosin B is a specific inhibitor of high affinity [^{3}H]-ouabain binding and ion transport in rat brain. Neuropharmacol. 20: 87-90 (1981).
Silbergeld, E.K., Hruska, R.E., Miller, L.P. and Eng, N. Effects of Lead in vivo and in vitro on GABAergic Neurochemistry. J. Neurochem. 34: 1712-1718 (1980).
Siman, R.G. and Klein, W.L. Cholinergic activity regulates muscarinic receptors in central nervous system cultures. Proc. Natl. Acad. Sci. USA 76: 4141-4145 (1979).
Simon,E.J., Hiller, J.M. and Edelman, I. Stereospecific binding of the potent narcotic analgesic [^{3}H]-etorphine to rat brain homogenate. Proc. Natl. Sci. USA 70: 1947-1949 (1973).
Sivam, S.P., Norris, T. C., Lim, D.K., Hoskins, B. and Ho, I.K. Effect of acute and chronic cholinestrase inhibition with diisopropylfluorophosphate on muscarinic, dopamine, and GABA receptors of the rat striatum. J. Neurochem. 40: 1414-1422 (1983).
Smit, M.H., Ehlert, F.J., Yamamura, S., Roeske, W.R. and Yamamura, H.I. Differential regulation of muscarinic agonist binding sites following chronic cholinesterase inhibition. Eur. J. Pharmacol. 66: 379-380 (1980a).
Smit, M.H., Ehlert, F.J., Roeske, W.R. and Yamamura, H.I. Decreased agonist and antagonist binding to the muscarinic cholinergic receptor following chronic cholinesterase inhibition. Fed. Proc. 39: 388 (1980b).
Snyder, S.H. Brain peptides as neurotransmitters. Science 209: 976-983 (1980).
Snyder, S.H. Drug and neurotransmitter receptors in the brain. Science 224: 22-31 (1984).
Staatz, C.H., Bloom, A.S. and Lech, J.J. Effects of pyrethroids on [^{3}H] Kainic acid binding to mouse forebrain membranes. Toxicol. Appl. Pharmacol. 64: 566-569 (1982).
Sumner, P.R. and Hirsch, J.D. Trimethyltin induced changes in [^{3}H]-QNB binding in various rodent brain areas. Soc. Neurosci. Abstr. 8: 310 (1982).
Terenius, L. Characteristics of the "receptor" for narcotic analgesics in synaptic plasma membrane fraction from rat brain. Acta Pharmacol. Toxicol. 32: 377-384 (1973).
Ticku, M.K. and Olsen, R.W. Cage convulsants inhibit picrotoxinin binding. Neuropharmacol. 18: 315-318 (1979).

Tilson, H.A. The neurotoxicity of acrylamide: an overview. Neurobehav. Toxicol. Teratol. 3: 445-461 (1981).

Titeler, M. Understanding receptor-binding assays. In: "Research Methods in Neurochemistry", vol. 5 (N. Marks and R. Rodnight, Eds.), Plenum Press, NY, 1981, pp. 29-73.

Uphouse, L., McLean, S. and Russell, M. Stability of CNS binding sites uner various conditions. Neurotoxicol. 2: 533-540 (1981).

Von Burg, R., Northington,F.K. and Shamoo,A. Methylmercury inhibition of rat brain muscarinic receptors. Toxicol. Appl. Pharmacol. 53: 285-292 (1980).

Waku, K. and Nakazawa, Y. Toxic effects of several mercury compounds on SH and non-SH enzymes. Toxicol. Lett. 4: 49-55 (1979).

Wenger, G.R., McMillan, D.E. and Chang, L.W. Behavioral toxicology of acute trimethyltin exposure in the mouse. Neurobehav. Toxicol. Teratol. 4:157-161 (1982).

Williams, L.T. and Lefkowitz, R.J. Alpha-adrenergic receptor identification by [^{3}H] dihydroergocryptine binding. Science 192: 791-793 (1976).

Williams, L.T. and Lefkowitz, R.J. Receptor binding studies in adrenergic pharmacology, Raven Press, NY, 1978.

Winder, C. and Kitchen, I. Lead Neurotoxicity: A review of the biochemical, neurochemical and drug induced behavioral evidence. Progr. Neurobiol. 22: 59-87 (1984).

Wu, P.H., Phillis, J.W., Balls, K. and Rinaldi, B. Specific binding of 2-[^{3}H] chloroadenosine to rat brain cortical membranes. Can. J. Physiol. Pharmacol. 58: 576-579 (1980)

Yamada, S., Isogai, M., Okudaira, H. and Hayaski, E. Regional adaption of muscarinic receptors and choline uptake in brain following repeated administration of diisopropylpfluorophosphate and atropine. Brain Res. 268: 315-320 (1983a).

Yamada, S., Isogai, M., Okudaira, H. and Hayuashi, E. Correlation between cholinesterase inhibition and reduction in muscarinic receptors and choline uptake by repeated diisopropylfluorophosphate administration: antagonism by physostigmine and atropine. J. Pharmacol. Exp. Ther. 226: 519-525 (1983b).

Yamamura, H.I. and Snyder, S.H. Muscarinic cholinergic receptor binding in rat brain. Proc. Natl. Acad. Sci. USA 71: 1725-1729 (1974).

Yamamura, H.I., Enna, S.J. and Kuhar, M.J. Neurotransmitter receptor binding. Raven Press, N.Y., 1978.

Yamawaki, S., Segawa, T. and Sarai, K. Effects of acute and chronic toluene inhalation on behavior and [^{3}H]-serotonin binding in rat. Life Sci. 30: 1997-2002 (1982).

Yim, G.K.W., Holsapple, M., Pfister, W.R. and Hollingworth, R.M. Prostaglandin Synthesis inhibited by formamidine pesticides. Life Sci. 23: 2509-2516 (1978).

Young, A.B. and Snyder, S.H. Strychnine binding associated with glycine receptors of the central nervous system. Proc. Natl. Acad. Sci. USA 70: 2832-2836 (1973).
Young, E., Olney, J. and Akil, H. Selective alterations of opiate receptors subtypes in monosodium glutamate-treated rats. J. Neurochem. 40: 1558-1564 (1983).
Zivin, J. A. and Waud, D. R. How to analyze binding, enzyme and uptake data: The simplest case, a single phase. Life Sci. 30: 1407-1422 (1982).

THE USE OF NEUROTRANSMITTER INDICES AND THE DEOXYGLUCOSE TECHNIQUE TO ASSESS NEUROTOXIC EFFECTS

Edith G. McGeer

Kinsmen Laboratory of Neurological Research

University of British Columbia, Vancouver, Canada

INTRODUCTION

In this chapter we will review briefly the types of indices which can be used to detect toxic effects on specific neurotransmitter systems and some of the difficulties associated with their use. We will also mention the use of deoxyglucose in animals and the possible application of some of the newer imaging methods to a study of the effects of neurotoxins on the human brain *in vivo*. Relatively few literature references are given since the material is such a general summary; pertinent literature on individual neurotransmitter systems may be found in various textbooks[1,2].

NEUROTRANSMITTER INDICES

There are two major classes of indices available: those for the presynaptic neuron and those aimed at measuring postsynaptic receptors.

A. Postsynaptic Receptors

Measurement of high affinity binding of labeled transmitters or selective agonists or antagonists has become a very popular tool in neuroscience, largely because of the ease of the measurements. In practice, a brain membrane fraction is prepared and portions incubated with low concentrations (10^{-7}-10^{-9}M) of a radioactive ligand of high specific activity in the presence (tube A) or absence (tube B) of a much higher concentration ($\sim 10^{-4}$M) of an unlabeled ligand. The specific, saturable, high affinity binding is taken as the difference between the total binding (tube B) and the non-specific non-saturable binding (tube A). Suitable high affinity ligands are now available for most neurotransmitter systems.

It should be noted, however, that such data are extremely difficult to interpret. One reason is that the treatment of the tissue and the assay conditions can have enormous effects upon the number of binding sites found. The presence of ions such as sodium, calcium or magnesium, or of other additives such as guanyl phosphates, can affect the results markedly. Repeated washing of the tissue with a detergent such as Triton X may, in some cases (e.g. a GABA binding site), markedly increase the measurable number of sites, possibly by removal of an endogenous inhibitor; alternatively such treatment may diminish the number of measurable sites. Freezing is generally thought not to affect binding and yet one of the glutamate binding sites is lost on freezing tissue[3]. Even postmortem delay causes changes in some binding[4], although most of the literature suggests that postmortem delay has little effect on binding activity.

Another factor that complicates interpretation of binding data is the existence of multiple types of receptors for a single neurotransmitter and multiple localizations of these various types[5]. We are all familiar with the concept of pharmacologically distinct nicotinic and muscarinic receptors for acetylcholine. Two to four pharmacologically distinct sites have been described for each known neurotransmitter with the exception, so far, of glycine and some of the peptides. Many of these binding sites are found not only on postsynaptic neurons but on presynaptic nerve endings, where they appear to regulate the release or synthesis of the same neurotransmitter (autoreceptor) or of a different one; they can also occur on glia and blood vessels. The best known example of the autoreceptor is probably that on dopamine neurons in the striatum but such autoreceptors have now been reported for many of the neurotransmitters. An example of the heterogeneous type of presynaptic receptor is the existence of the so-called GABA-B site on noradrenergic nerve endings where GABA apparently acts to inhibit the release of noradrenaline[6]. Noradrenergic receptors have been reported on both glia and blood vessels with their action on the latter contributing to the control of cerebral circulation. Similar locations have been reported for other transmitter binding sites such as those for histamine, acetylcholine, etc.

There may be endogenous or exogenous inhibitors or modulators of binding. The best demonstrated example is the interaction of benzodiazepines with GABA binding sites but many of the peptide neurotransmitters may modulate the binding of other substances.

It is important to remember in interpreting binding data that the binding sites are not necessarily equivalent to physiological receptors. The physiological receptors are very probably high affinity binding sites but the converse is not necessarily true.

It is also important to remember that data on the binding of a given neurotransmitter or its analogs cannot be easily interpreted in terms of the functioning of the presynaptic neuron. It has been argued that excessive functioning of the presynaptic neuron might be revealed by a subsensitivity (decreased number) in the binding sites with the opposite being true in the case of presynaptic hypofunction. Although supersensitivity and subsensitivity can be induced in many neuronal systems by chronic pharmacological denervation, it seems clear that major losses of many presynaptic systems can occur without significant changes in the "postsynaptic binding sites". Thus, for example, in Alzheimer's disease, some centers report losses in cholinergic indices in the frontal cortex of 85-90% with no significant change in binding of the muscarinic antagonist ^{3}H-QNB[7].

At the same time it is clear that some neurotoxins such as α-bungarotoxin, for example, might have profound effects on postsynaptic receptors with little or no effect on presynaptic indices. Hence, binding assays are certainly worthwhile but should be regarded with caution.

Some other factors which affect the interpretation of both pre- and postsynaptic indices are discussed in Section C.

B. Presynaptic Indices

The best indices for judging the functioning of a neuron are turnover or release of neurotransmitter. Measurement of these indices is, however, technically demanding and generally the levels of the neurotransmitter, a specific synthetic enzyme or the high affinity uptake of the neurotransmitter or a precursor into the presynaptic synaptosome are measured. Changes in the activity of a neuronal system can occur without changes in these indices but they do reflect the integrity of the neuronal system.

All three indices are not applicable to every neuronal system (Table 1). Thus, for example, the activity of a specific synthetic enzyme can only be used where a specific enzyme has been identified. This is the case for neuronal systems using GABA, acetylcholine, histamine, dopamine, noradrenaline and serotonin (Table 1) but not for systems using glutamate, aspartate, glycine or one of the numerous peptide neurotransmitters. Choline acetyltransferase (ChAT) and glutamate decarboxylase (GAD), the specific enzymes involved, respectively, in the synthesis of acetylcholine and GABA are very easy to assay and are frequently used as indices of the neuronal integrity of these systems. The specific synthetic enzymes for the catecholamines and serotonin are somewhat more difficult to assay but can be done in any reasonably established laboratory.

Table 1. Neurotransmitters and the Useful Presynaptic Indices

Neurotransmitter		Type of Index: Level	Enzyme[2]	Uptake	Histochemical[6] or Immunohistochemical
Amino acids	Glu/Asp[1]			✓	(I)
	Glycine			✓	
	GABA	✓	GAD	✓	✓, I
Amines	Acetylcholine	✓	ChAT	✓[3]	✓, I
	Histamine		HD	✓[3]	I
	Dopamine	✓[4]	TyH	✓	✓, I
	Noradrenaline	✓[4]	TyH, DβH	✓	✓, I
	Serotonin	✓[4]	TpH	✓	✓, I
Peptides[5]		✓			I

1. It is often difficult to distinguish neurons using glutamate from those using aspartate so the term Glu/Asp is convenient.
2. GAD = glutamate decarboxylase; ChAT = choline acetyltransferase; HD = histidine decarbxylase; TyH = tyrosine hydroxylase; DβH = dopamine-β-hydroxylase; TpH = tryptophan hydroxylase.
3. Uptake of precursor rather than neurotransmitter.
4. Levels of the metabolites are often measured and considered possible indicators of turnover.
5. Over two dozen peptide neurotransmitters have now been reported in mammalian brain.
6. Histochemical procedures of AChE and GABA transaminase are relatively easy and may be used to study, respectively, cholinergic and GABAergic systems; they are, however, not definitive for such systems. Immunohistochemical procedures, indicated by I, depend on availability of suitable antibodies; an immunohistochemical procedure has been reported for glutamate neurons[8] but may not be definitive.

Histidine decarboxylase (HD), the specific enzyme involved in the synthesis of neuronal histamine, is relatively difficult to assay because the activity so far detected in brain is small. Enzyme activities have the advantage over levels and uptake of being generally less sensitive to factors such as postmortem delay. GAD is, however, rather sensitive to premortem coma or anoxia[9] and this is a point to remember in connection with its measurement.

The levels of neurotransmitters are satisfactory only where the given substance is limited to the neurotransmitter pool. Thus (Table 1), the levels of glutamate, aspartate and glycine are not good indices to the neurotransmitter pools since these amino acids serve many other uses in brain and exist in almost every structure. For this reason the regional distribution of the amino acids is rather uniform and does not reflect the distribution of the amino acid neurons[10]. The level of histamine is also not a good guide because histamine exists in mast cells in brain as well as in histaminergic neurons. The level is, however, the only presynaptic index so far found to the many peptide systems.

High affinity uptake into synaptosomes is a useful index in all non-peptidergic systems. In the case of acetylcholine and histamine the high affinity uptake system is for the precursors, choline and histidine, respectively; in the cases of the other non-peptide transmitters (Table 1) the uptake is of the neurotransmitter itself. The uptake is characterized by being sodium dependent and generally has a K_d of the order of 10^{-6}M. It should be measured on synaptosomal fractions rather than crude homogenates since there is frequently a glial uptake which may contaminate the results. For the same reason, uptake into brain slices is not as definitive as into the synaptosomal fraction. The high affinity uptake systems are dependent upon synaptosomal integrity and hence are lost on long standing of the tissue or homogenates or on freezing unless special precautions are used.

C. General Considerations Relative to Neurotransmitter Indices

There are a number of points which should be considered when addressing pre- or postsynaptic indices. These include:

1. Dose response
2. Regional differences
3. Selectivity
4. Reference base
5. Secondary effects
6. Miscellaneous problems

1. Dose response. Biochemical assays can frequently be used very easily to obtain a dose response curve when studying any neurotoxic material. The curves in some cases are extremely steep, as illustrated in Figure 1 for kainic acid injections into the neostriatum of rats. The reproducibility of the biochemical indices is usually sufficiently good that rather small differences between groups can be detected. In general the radioactive assays of enzyme activities and neurotransmitter uptake are designed so that the test results are at least 10 times the blank. In some binding assays, however, the specific binding may be a relatively small fraction of the total binding and, in such cases, good discrimination between experimental groups may be difficult to achieve. A limiting factor in studying the brain in many instances is the reproducibility of the dissection technique but, as discussed below, measurements on whole brain are generally not desirable.

2. Regional differences. Many neurotoxins, even on systemic administration, may have markedly different effects in different brain regions. If the whole brain is analyzed, significant abnor-

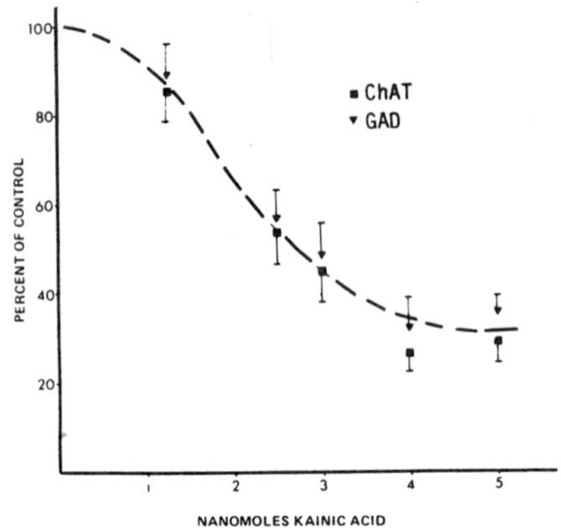

Fig. 1. Typical dose-response curves for GAD and ChAT activities in kainic acid-injected neostriata.

malities may be missed. Thus, for example, when dimethylmercury is administered systemically to neonatal rats, there is a significant effect on GABAergic neurons in the cortex but none in the thalamus (Table 2). When sampling regions for biochemical assay, it is important to remember that the distribution of transmitter systems is not uniform throughout most brain nuclei. Thus, for example, ChAT activities are markedly different in different layers of the cortex[11]. Nuclei such as the caudate-putamen or thalamus show heterogeneous distributions of neurotransmitter indices. The reproducibility of the dissection technique used must therefore be emphasized.

The existence of these marked regional differences in the brain emphasizes the importance of using various histological techniques, both to reveal structural changes which may be correlated with changes in the biochemical indices examined and, even more importantly, to allow a rapid survey to identify regions of interest. Various histochemical or immunohistochemical techniques are applicable to histological examination of specific neurotransmitter systems (Table 1) and autoradiographic methods allow a histological examination of binding sites. These can be quantitated to some degree but, once regions of interest are identified by such techniques, biochemical methods are generally more sensitive for quantitative work.

3. Selectivity. A question of importance which is often neglected in studies of neurotoxins is that of selectivity. Histological examination is again useful as a means of searching for signs of non-specific tissue destruction.

For biochemical analysis, it is better to measure indices of several different neurotransmitter systems rather than several

Table 2. ChAT and GAD Activities as a Measure of Regional Difference and Selectivity in Rat Experiments with Various Neurotoxins (As Percent of Control)

	After Systemic Me_2Hg In Neonates		After Local Injection of AF64A Into Basal Forebrain	
	Cortex	Thalamus	Basal Forebrain	Cortex
ChAT	96%	96%	29%	38%
GAD	49%	71% (N.S.)	56%	110%

indices of a single neurotransmitter system. In a study of a perspective cholinergic neurotoxin, for example, one might measure acetylcholine levels, choline uptake and ChAT activity but these would all be indicators of the integrity of the presynaptic cholinergic neuron. It would be better to measure only one of these indices and use the available tissue for measurements on other neurotransmitter systems. GAD is often a useful index since GABAergic systems are ubiquitous in brain and seem fairly sensitive to various insults. Measurements of ChAT and GAD were used, for example, to demonstrate the relative selectivity of dimethylmercury on the GABAergic system in the cortex (Table 2) and the relative non-selectivity of local injections of the mustard derivative AF64A into the medial basal forebrain (Table 2). It should be emphasized that, given results such as those in Table 2 on the methylmercury treated animals, it still cannot be said that methylmercury is a selective neurotoxin for the GABAergic system; many other neurotransmitter systems may also be affected.

4. Reference base. Neurotransmitter indices are usually expressed per gram of tissue or per mg of protein. The former is less satisfactory than the latter because it is influenced by edema or drying of tissues. Both may be unsatisfactory, especially in animals with chronic lesions. Such chronic lesions can induce shrinkage of the tissue which may conceal a significant loss of a neurotransmitter system in a given nucleus. Thus, for example, kainic acid injections into rat neostriatum cause a destruction of local cholinergic and GABAergic neurons which can be detected in the short term by pronounced losses in ChAT and GAD (Table 3). After several months, however, the neostriatum shrinks and ChAT and GAD activities expressed on a per gram of tissue or per mg of protein base return to near normal; total activity per striatum is still markedly reduced (Table 3). The question of a completely suitable reference base has not been resolved.

5. Secondary effects. It is generally important to measure the neurochemical effects of a neurotoxin at various times after

Table 3. Effect of Reference Base and Degeneration en Cascade on Some Neurotransmitter Indices in Rat Neostriata Following Local Injections of 2.5 nmoles of Kainic Acid (Percent of Control)

	At 10 Days	At 8 Months
ChAT:		
per mg protein	53%	86%
per neostriatum	48%	55%
Glutamate uptake:		
per mg protein	128%	95%
per striatum	115%	61%

administration in order to differentiate primary from secondary and other confusing effects. Some of these possibly confusing effects can be illustrated by data on the neurochemical changes following intrastriatal injections of kainic acid where the primary effect is destruction of the neurons which are postsynaptic to the glutamatergic corticostriatal tract (see Chapter). Injections of kainic acid may also, however, cause release of neurotransmitters such as noradrenaline from nerve endings so that there may be a decrease in the levels in the acute phase; such decreases are sometimes misinterpreted as indicating destruction of the neurons using that transmitter[12]. On the other hand, when the postsynaptic neuron is destroyed, the postsynaptic membranes may remain attached to presynaptic nerve endings for considerable periods of time[13] so that binding studies conducted shortly after the injections may indicate the persistence of these binding sites. In some cases such data have been used to argue against the existence of such binding sites on the postsynaptic neuron. However, binding assays carried out in chronic animals show the disappearance of these sites.

On the other hand, secondary changes can occur in the chronic animal which are not part of the primary neurotoxic effect. The phenomenon of degeneration en cascade is well established in the central nervous system. This means simply that when neurons in a functional circuit are destroyed, degeneration of other neurons in the chain may occur subsequently, due probably to the loss of trophic factors normally produced by the primarily destroyed neurons. In the kainic acid lesioned neostriatum, for example, the glutamatergic corticostriatal tract is not initially affected but, after some months, it begins to die back (Table 3). Degeneration of thalamostriatal neurons and of axons of passage in the lesioned striatum can also be seen in the chronic animal[14]. Binding sites generally show even greater plasticity than indices of presynaptic neuronal activity. In assessing the meaning of neurochemical data in neurotoxicology, therefore, it must be remembered that the brain is a plastic and highly interactive system.

6. Miscellaneous problems. The effects of postmortem delay, method of sacrifice, freezing or other handling of tissue on the neurotransmitter index or indices chosen must be established. In addition, it should be remembered that many neurotransmitter indices show circadian rhythms so that it is well to keep animals under a carefully controlled light schedule and sacrifice them at a standardized hour of the day. There may be seasonal rhythms as well in the catecholamines[15] and in many of the peptide neurotransmitters[16]. Hemispheric asymmetry and sex and strain differences have also been reported for a number of transmitter systems so these sources of experimental variability should be kept in mind.

DEOXYGLUCOSE TECHNIQUES

The deoxyglucose (DG) technique developed by Sokoloff[17] is a method for measuring the regional glucose metabolism in brain. It depends upon the generally accepted premise that deoxyglucose is taken up and phosphorylated in a manner comparable to glucose but the deoxyglucose phosphate is not metabolized further. If labeled deoxyglucose is used, the accumulation of the label in a particular brain region gives a measure of the glucose metabolic activity in that region and autoradiograms prepared from brain sections allow a rapid survey of regional metabolism. This is useful in identifying regions of interest in work with neurotoxins as well as in many other fields of neuroscience. ^{14}C-Deoxyglucose gives much better resolution than the ^{3}H-derivative although the latter has been used[18-20]. The brain can also be dissected and the amount of radioactivity in extracts of various regions determined by liquid scintillation counting[21]; this, however, does not permit the fine degree of regional localization possible in radioautograms.

This procedure may reveal regions which are functionally affected by a neurotoxin even if no permanent damage occurs, but the timing of the studies is again important because of the compensatory mechanisms of the brain. Thus, for example, a DG study in rats conducted at the time of an intrastriatal injection of kainic acid will show increased metabolism in the striatum with decreases in the habenula and substantia nigra, the latter being probably due to overactivation of inhibitory striatal projections to these nuclei. A DG study carried out 3-4 days after such a kainic acid injection will show decreased metabolism in the lesioned striatum but increased metabolism in the substantia nigra and habenula, due probably to removal of the inhibitory influences[22]. If the DG study is performed three months after the kainic acid injection, the lesioned striatum will still show decreased metabolism but metabolism in the substantia nigra and habenula will be near normal due to compensatory changes in brain functioning.

In another example of the use of the DG technique in neurotoxicology, Ben-Ari and his coworkers[23] have shown that systemic injections of kainic acid cause, in the acute phase, a much increased metabolism in those brain areas which later show neuronal loss and decreased metabolism.

An interesting aspect of the deoxyglucose technique is that analogous in vivo studies can now be done in man using one of the new imaging techniques; these techniques have not yet been applied in neurotoxicology but should be considered as valuable weapons in the neuroscientific armamentarium.

IMAGING TECHNIQUES[24]

A. Positron Emission Tomography (PET)

Positron emitting isotopes such as ^{11}C, ^{15}O or ^{18}F are typically of short half-life. When they decay, the positron emitted will travel only a short distance in tissue (a few mm) before annihilation by collision with an electron. Two gamma rays are given off at almost exactly 180^0 and these can be detected by, for example, NaI crystals. If a battery of detectors is suitably arranged in a tomograph, the point of origin of the gamma rays can be determined by computer techniques. The radioactive exposure is very low because of the short half-lives; it has been estimated that the typical scan exposes the patient to about as much extra radiation as encountered in an over-the-pole flight between Europe and America.

This method can, in theory, be used to pinpoint the regional distribution of any drug or to measure regional brain or body chemistry for which a suitable positron-labeled indicator can be synthesized. In practice, PET work has so far been largely limited to studies in the brain or heart of blood flow and metabolic rates (using $^{15}O_2$ or ^{18}F-fluorodeoxyglucose). Some success is now being achieved in studying dopamine metabolism using ^{18}F-6-fluorodopa[25] and initial reports are appearing on studies of the dopamine receptor using ^{11}C-spiperone. Interesting results have been reported in a number of neurological disorders including Parkinsonism, dystonia, epilepsy and Alzheimer's disease but the full potential of PET will only slowly be realized.

B. Nuclear Magnetic Imaging (NMI)

PET is useful for studying brain chemistry but gives poor anatomical resolution. NMI is a computer assisted tomographic method which gives far better tissue and pathological detail than does a computed tomography (CT) X-ray scan and involves no ionizing radiation at all[26]. Small cracks in myelin can, for example, be seen in multiple sclerosis cases and the absence of hazard means that repeated scans can be done to follow the progress of the disease. NMI can be used to obtain images throughout the brain and spinal cord. Presently NMI depends upon the differences in relaxation times of hydrogen atoms in different molecular forms (e.g. water or lipids). It is possible, however, that NMI techniques will be developed to image phosphorus atoms or other, including exogenous, atoms and these may give information on various aspects of brain chemistry as well as tissue pathology.

SUMMARY

There are many new techniques in the neurotransmitter and allied fields which should be useful in neurotoxicology. Many are suitable only for animal studies but some of the developing imaging techniques should provide new insights into neurotoxic effects in humans.

REFERENCES

1. "Basic Neurochemistry", G.J. Siegel, A.W. Albers, B.W. Agranoff and R. Katzman, eds., Little Brown & Co., Boston, (1981).
2. P.L. McGeer, J.C. Eccles and E.G. McGeer, "Molecular Neurobiology of the Mammalian Brain", Plenum Press, New York, 1978.
3. A.C. Foster and G.E. Fagg, Acidic amino acid binding sites in mammalian neuronal membranes: their characteristics and relationship to synaptic receptors, Brain Res. Rev. 7:103 (1984).
4. P.J. Whitehouse, D. Lynch and M.J. Kuhar, Effects of postmortem delay and temperature on neurotransmitter receptor binding in a rat model of the human autopsy process, J. Neurochem. 43:553 (1984).
5. S.H. Snyder and R.R. Goodman, Multiple neurotransmitter receptors, J. Neurochem. 35:5 (1980).
6. N.G. Bowery, A. Doble, D.R. Hill, A.L. Hudson, M.J. Turnbull and R. Warrington, Bicuculline-insensitive GABA receptors on peripheral autonomic nerve terminals, Eur. J. Pharmacol. 71:53 (1981).
7. E.,G. McGeer, Neurotransmitter systems in aging and senile dementia, Prog. Neuro-Psychopharmacol. 5:435 (1981).
8. J. Storm-Mathisen, A.K. Leknes, A.T. Bore, J.L. Vaaland, P. Edminson, F-M.S. Haug and O.P. Ottersen, First visualization of glutamate and GABA in neurones by immunocytochemistry, Nature 301:517 (1983).

9. P.L. McGeer and E.G. McGeer, Enzymes associated with the metabolism of catecholamines, acetylcholine and GABA in human controls and patients with Parkinson's disease and Huntington's chorea, J. Neurochem. 26:65 (1976).
10. P.L. McGeer and E.G. McGeer, Amino acid neurotransmitters. In: "Basic Neurochemistry", G.J. Siegel, A.W. Albers, B.W. Agranoff and R. Katzman, eds., Little Brown & Co., Boston, pp. 233-254 (1981).
11. H. Kimura, E.G. McGeer, F. Peng and P.L. McGeer, Cholinergic systems in the cat cortex studied by choline acetyltransferase immunohistochemistry, in: "Structure and Function of Peptidergic and Aminergic Neurons", Y.Sano, Y. Ibata and E.A. Zimmerman, eds., Japan Science Societies Press, Tokyo, pp. 263-274 (1983).
12. S.T. Mason and H.C. Fibiger, On the specificity of kainic acid. Science 204:1339 (1979).
13. J.W. Olney, Neurotoxicity of excitatory amino acids, in: "Kainic Acid as Tool in Neurobiology", E.G. McGeer, J.W. Olney and P.L. McGeer, eds., Raven Press, New York, pp. 95-122 (1978).
14. E.G. McGeer, P.L. McGeer, T. Hattori and S.R. Vincent, Kainic acid neurotoxicity and Huntington's disease, Adv. Neurology 23:577 (1979).
15. A. Carlsson, L. Svennerholm and B. Winblad, Seasonal and circadian monoamine variations in human brains examined post mortem, Acta Psychiatrica Scand. 61 (suppl. 280):75 (1980).
16. B. Krisch, Two types of luliberin-immunoreactive perikarya in the preoptic area of the rat, Cell Tissue Res. 212: 443 (1980).
17. L. Sokoloff, M. Reivich, C. Kennedy, M.H. Des Rosiers, C.S. Patlak, K.D. Pettigrew, O. Sukurada and H. Shinohara, The [^{14}C]deoxyglucose method for the measurement of local cerebral glucose utilization: theory procedure and normal values in the conscious and unconscious albino rat, J. Neurochem. Res. 28:897 (1977).
18. G.M. Alexander, J. Schwartzman, R.D. Bell, J. Yu and A. Renthal, Quantitative measurement of local cerebral metabolic rate for glucose utilizing tritiated 2-deoxyglucose, Brain Res. 223:59 (1981).
19. A.F. Ryan and F.R. Sharp, Localization of [^{3}H]2-deoxyglucose at the cellular level using freeze-dried tissue and dry-looped emulsion, Brain Res. 252:177 (1982).
20. C.R. Gallistel and S. Nichols, Resolution-limiting factors in 2-deoxyglucose autoradiography. I. Factors other than diffusion, Brain Res. 267:323 (1983).
21. R.C. Meibach, S.D. Glick, D.A. Ross, R.D. Cox and S. Mayani, Intraperitoneal administration and other modifications of the 2-deoxy-D-glucose technique, Brain Res. 195:167 (1981).
22. H. Kimura, E.G. McGeer and P.L. McGeer, Metabolic alteration in an animal model of Huntington's disease using the

^{14}C-deoxy-glucose method, J. Neural Transm., Suppl. 16:103 (1980).
23. Y. Ben-Ari, E. Tremblay, D. Riche, G. Ghilini and R. Naquet, Electrographic, clinical and pathological alterations following systemic administration of kainic acid, bicuculline or pentetrazole: metabolic mapping using the deoxyglucose method with special reference to the pathology of epilepsy, Neuroscience 7:1361 (1981).
24. G.L. Brownell, T.F. Budinger, P.C. Lauterbur and P.L. McGeer, Positron tomography and nuclear magnetic resonance imaging, Science 215:619 (1982).
25. E.S. Garnett, G. Firnau and C. Nahmias, Dopamine visualized in the basal ganglia of living man, Nature 305:137 (1983).
26. S.W. Young, "Nuclear Magnetic Resonance Imaging: Basic Principles", Raven Press, New York (1984).

RECENT ELECTROPHYSIOLOGICAL TECHNIQUES IN EXPERIMENTAL NEUROTOXICOLOGY

Philip L. Chambers

Department of Pharmacology and Therapeutics
University of Dublin
Trinity College
Dublin 2 Ireland

INTRODUCTION

Neurotoxicology has always been eclectic in its search for techniques for use in the detection of toxic changes in the nervous system. The newer electrophysiological techniques as discussed here, should be seen in the sense of new in application or a novel approach using techniques which are probably already established in neurophysiology. Neurophysiology has been the main source of ideas for the development of toxicological studies based upon the central and peripheral nervous systems.

Much of that which should be presented in this short review as new and novel approaches in fundamental research developments has been mentioned in earlier papers which appear in this volume and it would be redundant to report on these developments again. Moreover this chapter does not set out to be exhaustive in its overview of the topic but indicates some of the new uses of old and established techniques and suggests newly arrived techniques which, although not yet applied in neurotoxicology, may have advantages and provide advances in the future.

THE PROBLEM

There are really two aspects to neurotoxicology. The first has been dealt with in detail in the earlier part of this book. These are the in depth studies of the means by which known neurotoxicants exert their effects. It is an exciting and satisfying area of research which often throws further light on the fundamental processes of neurochemistry and neurophysiology. In the main, such studies are carried out on established chemicals and agents with economic implications which results in financial support at a high level. The cost of such studies would be financially prohibitive in many countries.

There is however another aspect of neurotoxicology, one which exercises many toxicologists. It is the simple question set by industry and by governmental agencies. Is this new candidate chemical, for whatever purpose it may have been synthesized, neurotoxic? The in depth studies have to be set aside initially and the proximate question of neurotoxicity has to be answered quickly and decisively if decisions are to be made on the future for such a chemical or drug.

SUGGESTIONS FOR AN ANSWER

A schematic approach to answer this question is set out in Fig 1. This schema is not intended to be exhaustive but it should provide indications of adverse reactions and functional changes either by the acute application of the chemical or, by longer application *in vivo*, the possible chronic effects which may be produced.

The application of electrophysiological techniques is particularly aimed at the detection of functional changes in the nervous system. Changes in transmission would be detected either as a diminution in the response or as an augmentation of the response, increased firing or decreased firing of neurones, depolarization or hyperpolarization. The use of the findings from the *in vivo* and *in vitro* test should indicate the position and extent of the functional damage. This information can be interpreted as direct tissue damage or some form of transmission fault as shown in the scheme in Fig 2.

A crude indication of the probable site of action of the candidate chemical can be provided by adequate polygraphic recordings of the onset of toxic effects even in the fully anaesthetised small mammal where the electroencephalogram, electromyogram, electrocardiogram, respiration, blood pressure, both arterial and venous, are simultaneously displayed.

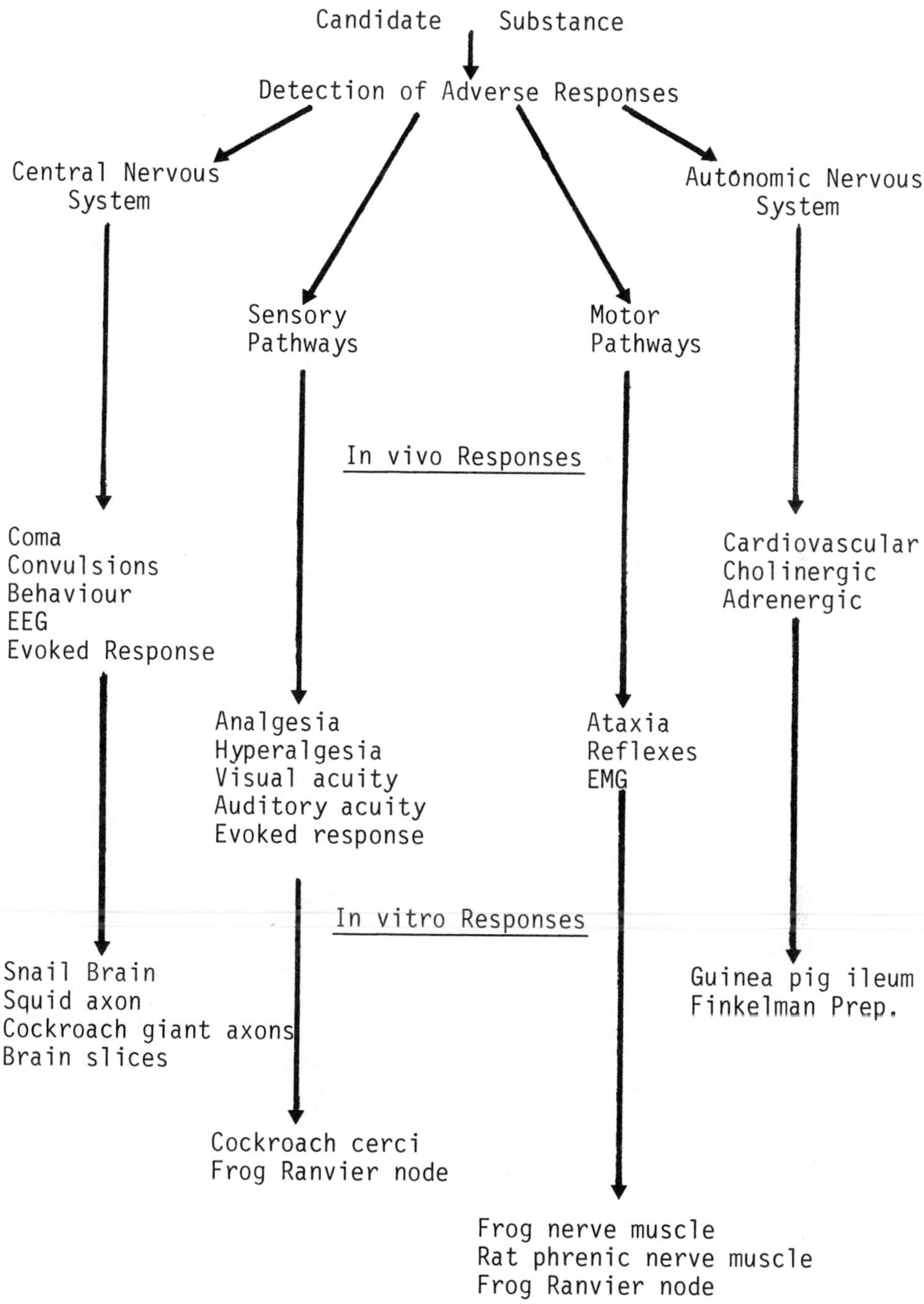

Figure 1 IS THIS SUBSTANCE NEUROTOXIC?

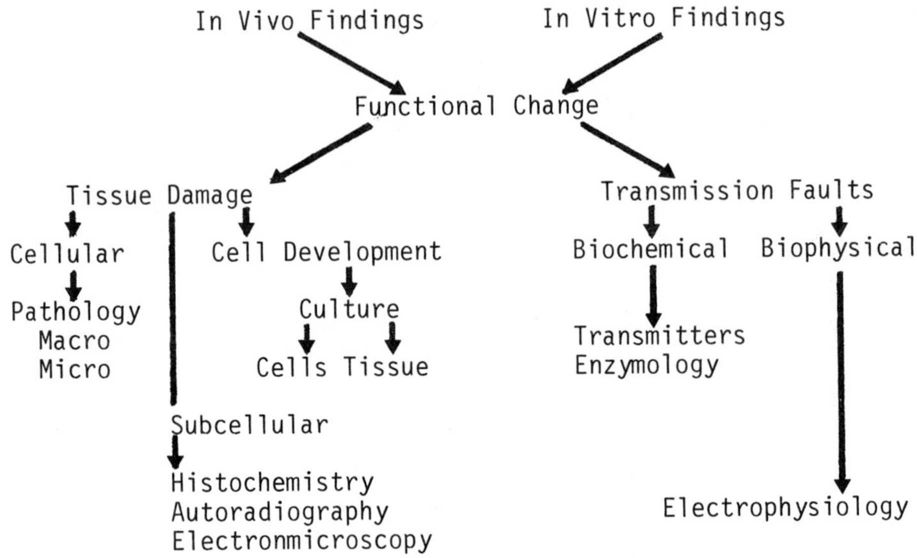

Figure 2 DEVELOPMENT OF TEST PROCEDURES

NOVEL TECHNIQUES

Since this article sets out to look at the problem of screening for neurotoxic action it deals with techniques used primarily for this purpose which also provide some indication of the mode of action of the toxicant. Fox et al (1982) have presented a review of electrophysiological techniques of use in neurotoxicology. Their article deals with electroencephalography, evoked potentials, spinal cord reflexes, perikaryal function, dorsal root ganglion and motor neurones and their use in the study of the toxic changes in the central nervous system. In considering toxic effects on the peripheral nervous system, nerve conduction velocities and peripheral nerve terminal function are discussed.

A simple and relatively inexpensive technique for the evaluation of drug activity at central and peripheral synapses, which can be applied either to acute or chronic studies in toxicology, has been devised by Buckle and Spence (1981). By recording the electromyogram from the muscles of both hind limbs on stimulation of the sciatic nerve in mice, the effects on monosynaptic and crossed polysynaptic reflexes can be assessed. It is also possible to distinguish between the effect on neuromuscular transmission and on nerve conduction by examining the different effects on re-excitation of the motor neurones.

Those interested in toxic effects at the auditory level should refer to the recent paper of Henderson et al (1983) which deals with auditory evoked potentials and behaviour thresholds in the noise-exposed chinchilla. Auditory brainstem evoked responses have been shown to be useful particularly in chronic studies.

The evoked potential response has received much attention in recent years. One criticism of the non-invasive recording of potentials from the scalp is that the evoked volume currents are markedly attentuated as they pass through the intracerebral space and intervening tissues to the scalp. The development of super-conducting devices has made it possible to detect extremely weak magnetic fields near the scalp which can be evoked by auditory, visual or somatic stimuli. These transient changes of the brain magnetic field in its temporal wave form are similar to the electrical potential changes seen at the pial surface of the brain, according to Okada et al (1981). A recent paper by Kaufman et al (1981) deals in detail with the relationship between the evoked changes in magnetic fields and evoked changes in potential. A superconducting quantum interference device (SQUID) connected to a gradiometer is used to detect the extremely weak magnetic fields. Magnetic fields fluctuating at frequencies less than 1 kHz are not attenuated by the media that intervene between their source in the active neural tissue and the scalp. The intervening tissues are thus transparent to the signals which are of biological interest. At present this is a costly venture but it can be expected that this approach will be used in studies on the effects of toxicants on the evoked magnetic fields as has been the case with evoked potentials.

The use of isolated systems for the study of neurotoxic responses has grown in recent years. Acute effects are easily studied in the in vitro preparations classically used in physiology and pharmacology. Reference to some of these has been made earlier in Fig 1. The Squid axon has received attention earlier in this volume (c.f J. Van Den Bercken). Since the time of Hodgkin and Huxley (1939) this preparation has been used in fundamental neurophysiology research as well as providing evidence of the mode of action of toxicants (cf. Narahashi and Lund (1979)).

Walker (1968) has made use of the snail brain. Intracellular recordings after ionophoretic applications to these large cells is relatively easy to accomplish. Multibarrelled micropipettes, as used by Curtis (1964), can be of use in this and other preparations when the toxicant is capable of being ionized.

Application of the mannitol gap technique has been applied to the isolated nerve cord of the cockroach (Periplaneta americana L.). This technique provides a means of recording the electrical responses at the 6th abdominal ganglion without the use of microelectrodes. Both synaptic and axonal transmission activity may be recorded. The technique was first introduced by Callec and Sattelle in 1973. Sattelle (1977) and Chambers and Rowan (1982) have reported on the use of this preparation in neurotoxicological studies. Rowan and Chambers (1982) have recently published an assessment of the use of this technique. The 6th abdominal ganglia is capable of being driven by sensory nerves of the cerci; both GABA and cholinergic receptors are believed to be present at the synaptic sites of the ganglion.

The single isolated node of Ranvier has received attention recently from Mitolo-Chieppa and Carratu (1984) as a means to study the toxic effects of some aminoglycoside antibiotics on this unprotected portion of the otherwise medullated nerve fibre. The technique of isolating a single node of Ranvier in an air gap was introduced by Stampfli (1959). Mitolo-Chieppa and Carratu were able to show increases in the duration of the stimulated action potential in the presence of neomycin, streptomycin, gentamycin, kanamycin, sisomycin and amikacin as well as a slight increase in the threshold to stimulation. This air gap _in vitro_ technique can be applied to both motor and sensory medullated nerves (Stampfli, 1979).

One method of _in vitro_ electrophysiological study that is rapidly gaining the interest of toxicologists and pharmacologists utilizes isolated hippocampal slices. These slices may be used for acute studies where the agent is applied _in vitro_ to the tissue. They may also be used in chronic studies after long term treatment with the candidate toxicant. Changes in response to stimulation or other acutely applied agents with known effects on the cells of the hippocampus can then be examined. Extracellular or intracellular recordings can be made in this preparation. Dingledine et al (1980), Olpe and Schellenberg (1980), Mueller et al (1981), Ferrendelli et al (1983) and Anwyl and Rowan (1984) have all described this technique and it is presently of particular interest to workers in the field of antidepressant activity. The slices are superfused and evoked responses can be recorded from the pyramidal cell layer (CA1 region) by stimulation of the stratum radiatum.

A more interesting, albeit more expensive, method of recording from the hippocampal slice has been described by Grinvald et al (1982). By use of voltage-sensitive membrane-bound dyes and photodetectors, the spread of the evoked electrical activity in the hippocampal slice was detected. The limitation of the restricted number of electrodes which can be used in the tissue to be analysed and the fact that intracellular recording is not possible from the finer elements of the tissue, such as the axons, make this method of optical monitoring very attractive. Particularly this is so where the spread of the wave of activation is to be followed. Attention is drawn to the work of Ross et al (1977) and Waggoner (1979) in the development of this technique for the optical measurement of membrane potentials. The development of this technique is still at an early state and it is to be expected that some direct action of the dyes may occur at the neuronal membrane. The advantages and disadvantages are dealt with in the paper of Grinvald et al (1982). It is to be expected that with more sensitive dyes the attraction to this technique will increase.

CONCLUSION

The broad range of techniques now in vogue and the development of new approaches to this area in which scientific interest is so active has set major problems in a review as short as this. It is hoped that the short bibliography presented along with the references will help to lead the interested toxicologist to an awareness of the growth areas in neurotoxicology.

REFERENCES

Anderson, P.A.V. and Schwab, W.E., 1983, Action potential in neurons of motor nerve net of cyanea coelenterata, J. Neurophysiol (Bethesda), 50 (3) : 671.

Anwyl, R. and Rowan, M.J., 1984, Neurophysiological evidence for tricyclic antidepressant-induced decreased beta-adrenergic responsiveness in the rat hippocampus, Brain Res., 300:192.

Baker, P.F., Hodgkin, A.L. and Shaw, T.I., 1961, Replacement of the protoplasm of a giant nerve fibre with artificial solutions, Nature, 190:885.

Baker, P.F., Hodgkin, A.L. and Shaw, T.I., 1962, Replacement of the axoplasm of giant nerve fibres with artificial solutions, J. Physiol., 164:330.

Bierkamper, G.G. and Goldberg, A.M., 1978, Vascular perfused rat phrenic nerve-hemidiaphragm: A model system for studying the physiological and neurochemical aspects of neuromuscular transmission, J. Electrophysiol Tech., 6:40.

Blagova, O.E., Budantsev, A.Y., Sytinsky, I.A. and Lajtha, A., 1982, Changes of neurochemical and electrophysiological indices of rat brain under ethanol intoxication, Neurochem Res., 7 (11):1335.

Bobbin, R.P., May, J.G. and Lemoine, R.L., 1979, Effects of pentobarbital and ketamine on brain stem auditory potentials latency and amplitude intensity functions after intraperitoneal administration in rats, Arch Otolaryngol., 105 (8) : 467.

Britt, R.H. and Rossi, G.T., 1982, Quantitative analysis of methods for reducing physiological brain pulsations, J. Neurosci Methods, 6 (3) : 219.

Buckle, P.J. and Spence, I., 1981, A simple in vivo method for evaluating drug action at central and peripheral synapses, Nauyn-Schmiedeberg's Arch Pharmacol, 315:211.

Callec, J.J. and Satelle, D.B., 1973, A simple technique for monitoring the synaptic actions of pharmacological agents, J. exp Biol., 59:725.

Chambers, P.L. and Rowan, M.J., 1982, The toxicity of p Benzoquinone on the central nervous system of the cockroach, Arch Toxicol Suppl., 5:107.

Curtis, D.R., 1964, Electrophysiological methods in "Physical techniques in biological research", W.L.Nastuk, ed., Academic Press, London.

Dingledine, R., Dodd, J. and Kelly, J.S., 1980, The 'in vitro' brain slice as a useful neurophysiological preparation for intracellular recording, J. Neurosci Meth., 1:323.

Ferrendelli, J.A., McKeon, A.C. and Klunk, W.E., 1983, The evoked and spontaneous activity of hippocampal slices in-vitro, Exp Neurol, 82 (3):663.

Finkleman, B., 1930, On the nature of the inhibition in the intestine, J. Physiol., 70:145.

Fox, D.A., Lowndes, H.E. and Bierkamper, G.G., 1982, Electrophysiological techniques in neurotoxicology, in "Nervous System Toxicology", C.L. Mitchell, ed., Raven Press, New York.

Fox, J.M., Neumcke, B., Nonner, W. and Stampfli, R., 1976, Blocking of gating currents in myelinated nerve by UV radiation. Pfluegers Arch Eur J. Physiol., 362 (Suppl), R29.

Fournier, E.P., Roux, F., 1980, Limits of the use in neurotoxicology of cellular models developed in neurobiology, in "Advances in Neurotoxicology", L. Manzo, ed., Pergamon Press, Oxford.

Fukuda, J. and Kameyama, M., 1980, A tissue culture of nerve cells from adult mammalian ganglia and some electro physiological properties of the nerve cells in-vitro, Brain Res., 202 (1):249.

Gioanni, Y., Everett, J. and Lamarche, M., 1983, The trans cortical reflex triggered by cutaneous or muscle stimulation in the cat with a penicillin epileptic focus relative importance of regions 3A and 4, Exp Brain Res., 51 (1):57.

Grinvald, A., Manker, A. and Segal, M., 1982, Visualization of the spread of electrical activity in rat hippocampal slices by voltage sensitive optical probes. J. Physiol., 333;269.

Hagiwara, S. and Tasaki, I., 1958, A study on the mechanism of impulse transmission across the giant synapse of the squid, J. Physiol., 143-114.

Henderson, D., Hamernik, R.P., Salvi, R.J., Ahroon, W.A., 1983, Comparison of auditory-evoked potentials and behavioral thresholds in the normal and noise-exposed chinchilla. Audiology 22 : 172-180.

Hodgkin, A.L. and Huxley, A.F., 1939, Action potentials recorded from inside a nerve fibre, Nature, 144:740.

Hooisma, J., 1982, Tissue culture and neurotoxicology, Neurobehav Tox and Terat., 4, 617.

Jordan, J.E., Haining, J.L. and Mishra, S.K., 1982, Evoked potential spectral and cerebral blood flow changes induced by ethanol. Electroencephalogr Clin Neurophysiol., 53(6). 90P.

Jule, Y. and Szurszewski, J.H., 1983, Electrophysiology of neurons of the inferior mesenteric ganglion of the cat, J. Physiol., 344:277

Kaila, K., 1982, Cellular neurophysiological effects of phenol derivatives, Comp Biochem Physiol., 73:2231.

Kato, E., Anwyl, R., Quandt, F.N. and Narahashi, T., 1983, Acetyl choline induced electrical responses in neuroblastoma cells, Neuroscience, 8 (3):643.

Kaufman, L., Okada, Y. and Brenner, D., 1981, On the relation between somatic evoked potentials and fields, Intern J. Neurosci., 15:223.

Kostopoulos, G., Avoli, M., Pellegrini, A. and Gloor, P., 1982, Laminar analysis of spindles and of spikes of the spike and wave discharge of feline generalized penicillin epilepsy, Electroencephalogr Clin Neurophysiol., 53 (1):1.

Lothman, E.W. and Collins, R.C., 1981, Kainic acid induced limbic seizures metabolic behavioral electroencephalographic and neuropathological correlates, Brain Res., 218-299.

Manalis, R.S., Cooper, G.P. and Pomeroy, S.L., 1984, Effects of lead on neuromuscular transmission in the frog Rana pipiens, Brain Res., 294:95.

Mitolo-Chieppa, D. and Carratu, M.R., 1984, Aminoglycoside Antibiotics: A study of their Neurotoxic Effects at peripheral Nerve Fibres. Arch. Toxicol. Suppl. 7: 464-466.

Mueller, A.L., Hoffer, B.J. and Dunwiddie, T.V., 1981, Noradrenergic responses in rat hippocampus: evidence for mediation by alpha and beta receptors in the 'in vitro slice'. Brain Res 214 : 113-126.

Narahashi, T. and Anderson, N.C., 1967, Mechanism of excitation block by the insecticide allethrin applied externally and internally to squid giant axon. Toxic appl. Pharm., 10:529.

Narahashi, T., 1974, Chemicals as tools in the study of excitable membranes, Phys Rev., 54:813.

Narahashi, T. and Lund, A.E., 1979, Giant axons as models for the study of the mechanism of action of insecticides, in "Insect Neurobiology and Pesticide Action (Neurotox 79)". Society of Chemical Industry, London.

Okada, Y., Kaufman, L., Brennar, D. and Williamson, S.J., 1981, Analysis of field potentials in the central nervous system, in "Handbook of Electroencephalography and Clinical Neurophysiology", Vol 2B, A. Remond ed., Elsevier, Amsterdam.

Olpe, H.R. and Schellenberg, A., 1980, Reduced sensitivity of neurons to noradrenaline after chronic treatment with antidepressant drugs. Europ. J. Pharmacol., 63 : 7-13.

Posthuma, J., Visser, S.L. and De Rijke, W., 1983, Peripheral nerve conduction visual evoked potentials and Vitamin B-1 serum levels in chronic alcoholics, Clin Neurol Neurosurg., 85 (4) : 267.

Ross, W.N., Salzberg, B.M., Cohen, L.B., Grinvald, A., Davila, H.V., Waggoner, A.S. and Wang, C.H., 1977, Changes in absorption, fluorescence, dichroism and birefringence in stained giant axons: Optical measurement of membrane potential, J. Membrane Biol., 33:141.

Rowan, M.J. and Chambers, P.L., 1982, The assessment of Neurotoxicity using the Cockroach Nerve Cord, Neurobehav Tox and Terat., 4:605.

Sattelle, D.B., 1977, A simple assay for the actions of toxic agents on synaptic transmission in the insect CNS. in "Crop Protection Agents: Their biological evaluation", N.R. McFarlane, ed., Academic Press, London.

Schaeffler, L., Imbach, P., Ruedeberg, A., Vassella, F. and Karbowski, K., 1982, Conventional and spectral electroencephalographic analysis in children treated with cytotoxic agents. Eur J Cancer Clin Oncol., 18 (9):827.

Schaeppi, U., Teste, M. and Siegenthaler, U., 1982, Sensory and motor maximum nerve conduction velocity in the peripheral and central nervous system of the beagle dog, Agents Actions., 12 (4):566.

Schafer, D.F., Brody, L.E. and Jones, E.A., 1979, Visual evoked potentials an objective measurement of hepatic encephalopathy in the rabbit, Gastroenterology., 77 (5) : A38.

Schrier, B.K., 1982, Nervous system cultures as toxicologic test systems. in "Nervous System Toxicology", C.L. Mitchell, ed., Raven Press, New York.

Schrivastav, B.B., Narahashi, T., Kitz, R.J. and Roberts, J.D., 1976, Mode of action of Trichloroethylene on squid axon membranes, J Pharmacol Exp Ther., 199:179.

Sokoll, M.O. and Dieke, F.P.J., 1969, Some effects of streptomycin on frog nerve, Arch Int Pharmacodyn., 177:332.

Stampfli, R., 1959, Is the resting potential of Ranvier nodes a potassium potential? Ann N.Y. Acad Sci., 81:265.

Stampfli, R., 1979, Electrophysiological signs which make it possible to distinguish between motor and sensorial nerve fibers, J. Physiol., (Paris) 75:41A.

Taghavy, A., Reinhardt, G. and Hermes, K., 1976, Effects of ethanol on scalp visual evoked potentials, Electroencephalogr Clin Neurophysiol., 41 (6) : 656.

Waggoner, A.S., 1979, Dye indicators of membrane potential, Ann Rev Biophys Bioeng., 8:47.

Walker, R.J., 1968, Intracellular microelectrode recording from brain of helix, in: "Experiments in Physiology and Biochemistry", G.A. Kerkut, ed., Academic Press, London and New York.

Young, S.H. and Poo, M., 1983, Spontaneous release of transmitter from growth cones of embryonic neurones, Nature, 305:636.

Zaczek, R., Nelson, M. and Coyle, J.T., 1981, Kainic acid neurotoxicity and seizures, Neuropharmacology, 20 (2) : 183.

INDEX

Acetylcholinesterase, 207-209,247
aging, 209
as a peptidase, 222,223

Aconitine, 88

Acrylamide, 5,163-173
acute intoxication, 166
autonomic nervous system effects, 166, 169
behavioral toxicity, 57
damage to Pacinian corpuscles, 169,170
effect on axonal transport, 6, 171,172
effect on receptor system in brain, 57,58,59,326
encephalopathy, 166
enzyme inducers and, 77
experimental animal studies with, 168-170
interaction with glutathione, 34
metabolic activation of,57,75, 77
neurofilamentous accumulation induced by, 6,171
peripheral neuropathy,171,172
and plasma testosterone levels, 48
and prolactin, 52

Acute intermittent porphyria, 25, 31,32

Adenosine receptors, 309, 332

Adenosine triphosphatase (Na,K-dependent) and lead toxicity, 194

Adrenergic system see also Cathecolamine system
effect of azidinium derivatives on, 115

Adrenoreceptors, 309
effect of trimethyl tin on, 328
organophosphate interaction with, 220

AF64A, 115,116,357

Age
and chloroquine retinopathy, 140
and exposure to lead, 194, 259-262
neurobehavioral toxicity, variables related to,292, 297-305
and organophosphate intoxication, 6,214

Alcohol see Ethanol

Aldicarb, 323

Allethrin, 91,95,96,97
electrophysiological effect in frog nerve, 94
and sodium tail current,99, 100
structure, 92

Aluminium, 179

Amblyopia in toxic disease
digitalis, 143
ethambutol, 143
quinine, 141

Aminoacids
as excitotoxins, 107-121
regional distribution in brain, 355

γ-Aminobutyric acid (GABA)
brain levels, paraoxon-induced changes in, 219
and lead toxicity, 261

neuronal indices and kainic acid toxicity, 111,112,113
and organophosphates, 219-220, 230,247,323
and prenatal exposure to antidepressant drugs, 300

γ-Aminobutyric acid receptors, 305
manganese-induced changes in,56
and prenatal exposure to diazepam, 302
and pyrethroids, 103
in rat striatum, decrease caused by DFP, 219

Aminocarb, 323

Aminoglycoside antibiotics, 370

Aminooxyacetic acid, 219

3,4-Aminopyridine, 88

4-Aminoquinoline retinotoxicity, 141

Amitraz, 324

Amitriptyline, 300

Amphetamine
and kainic acid, 113
paradoxical effect in lead exposed animals, 261,265

Amygdala, 118
and kainic acid induced seizures, 118

Analgesia, organophosphate-induced, 226

Angiotensin II, 223,310

Angiotensin converting enzyme, 111,112

Anoxia, neuropathy related to, 7

Antianxiety drugs, 302

Antidepressant drugs, 300-301

Antimitotic agents, 46

Antioxidants, 69

Apomorphine, 299
behavioral effect in methyl mercury-treated animals, 298
and kainic acid toxicity,113

Arcuate nucleus and excitotoxins, 120

Arsenic, 25,29,164,177-182
cerebrovascular damage induced by, 10,13,14
concentration in root ganglion cells, 180
metabolism, 180
neuropathy, 5,7-8,9,10,178-180
pentavalent, 178
trivalent, 178

Arsenolysis, 178

Arsphenamine, 178

Aspartate, 354

Astrocytes, 11,13,14

Autoreceptors, 352

Avoidance behavior, 287,290

Axon, 4,24,28

Axonal transport, 6,26
toxin-induced disturbances of, 6,46,171

Axonopathy in toxic disease, 25
acrylamide, 171
thallium, 186-187
organophosphates, 228, 247-253

Azidinium derivatives, 115

Baclofen, 114,306

Basal ganglia
  degeneration in manganese poisoning, 179
  as a target of kainic acid toxicity, 111

Batrachotoxin, 88

ß,ß'-iminodipropionitrile, 25

Behavioral teratology, 297-302

Behavioral toxicity
  assessment of, 51,279-293
  conditioning procedures, 291
  kainic acid, 51
  lead, 259-261,270
  neurochemical correlates, 297-302

Benzodiazepine drugs
  metabolites of, 74
  in organophosphate-induced seizures, 219

Benzodiazepine receptors, 308
  and methyl mercury, 328
  and prenatal diazepam administration, 301
  and prenatal toxicity of diphenylhydantoin, 332

Beir-beri, 25,29

Benserazide, 70

Bicycli phosphorus esters see Organophosphates

Bioresmethrin, 96

Blood-brain barrier, 11,12,46
  in developing brain, 15
  and organotin toxicity, 46

Blood-retina barrier, 133

Bombesin, 223

Brain
  activation of organophosphates in, 206,207
  adaptation to toxic injury, 44
  biochemistry and toxic disease, 12-15
  capillaries, 12,16
  development and neurotoxic agents, 15-16,196
  energy requirement, 45,75
  morphological targets of toxic damage, 10,11
  proteolipid content, 46

α-Bungarotoxin, 308,323

Butyryl-cholinesterase see Cholinesterase

Cadmium, 179,329

Caffeine, 331,332

Calcitonin, 310

Calcium
  lead interaction with, 194, 197,261
  metabolism, 267-269

Calcium channels, 88
  and lead toxicity, 268-269

Calcium protein binding, 194

Calmodulin, 269

Calomel, 190

Carbachol, 319,320

Carbamates, 323

Carbaryl, 323

Carbidopa, 70
Carbon disulphide, 25,36
  depression of corneal reflex by, 164
  intoxication, Parkinsonism in, 14
  metabolic activation of, 75,82
  neuropathy, 5,6,82
  non-neural effects, 10

Carbon monoxide, 5,7
  cerebrovascular damage by, 16
  encephalopathy, 13
  long-term behavioral effects, 45

Cassava, 7

Catecholamine system
  enzyme assay, 353
  role in lead toxicity, 261
  and organophosphates, 220
  and perinatal exposure to methyl mercury, 298

Cerebellum, 10
  and acrylamide intoxication, 166,167
  and methyl mercury toxicity, 189,190
  neurological examination, 166

Chemical warfare agents, 204

Circadian cycle in behavioral toxicity testing, 288

Chlordecone, 325
  endocrine effects, 48
  and serotonin metabolism in brain, 54
  and striatal spiroperidol binding, 58

Chlordiazepoxide, 302,332

Chlordimeform, 324

Chloroform, 47

Chloroquine retinopathy, 134, 135-141
  experimental animal models, 135,139
  predisposing factors in, 140

Chlorpyriphos, 204

Cholecystokinin, 223,310
  and kainic acid toxicity, 112,113

Choline acetyltransferase, 221
  assay of, 353

Cholinergic system
  action of azidinium choline derivatives on, 115,116
  action of kainic acid on, 111,112,113,116
  and kindling, 118
  and metal toxicity, 261,326-330
  tolerance to organophosphates and, 217-218,322

Cholinesterase
  as a peptidase, 223
  reactivation of, 209

Cismethrin, 92,95,96
  and sodium tail current, 98,99

Cis-platinum, 142

Clioquinol, 164

Clonidine, 220

Cockroach nerve cord technique, 370

Cognitive behavior, toxin-affecting, 289-291

Colchicine, 5
behavioral effects, 46
inhibition of tubulin polymerization by, 5

Color vision disturbances
in chloroquine intoxication, 135,139
digitalis-induced, 143

Convulsions in toxic disease
acrylamide, 168
bicyclic phosphorus esters, 229-230,247
folic acid, 110
kainic acid, 117
organophosphates, 219
pyrethroids, 92

Corticosteroids, retinal damage by, 143

Cyanide, 5
effect on brain metabolism, 45

Cyanogenetic agents, 72

Cyanopyrethroids, 92
action on GABA receptors, 103
poisoning, 92

Cypermethrin, 91,95,96
and sodium tail current, 99

Cyphenothrin, 93

Cystathioninase, 32,33

Cystathionina synthetase, 32,33

Cystathioninuria, 32,33

Cytosine arabinoside, 46

Cytotoxic drugs, retinal toxicity of, 135,142

DDT, 102,103

Decamethrin, 321

Deltamethrin, 91,94,96,97
and sodium tail current,
structure, 92

2-Deoxyglucose technique, 12, 359-360

Desipramine, 301

DFP, 225,322

Diazepam
behavioral teratogenic effects, 301
and excitotoxins, 110

Dichlorvos, 322

Dicrotophos, 322

Dieldrin, 325,326

Diethyldithiocarbamate, 82

Digitalis, 135,143

Digitoxin, 143

Dimercaptopropanol, 180

Dimethylsulphoxide, 53

Diphenylhydantoin
behavioral teratogenic effects, 289
receptor binding disturbance induced by, 332
and serum folates, 119

Disulfiram
metabolic activation, 82-83
neuropathy, 82

Disulfoton, 216,319
tolerance to, 320,321

Dithiocarbamates, 83

DMSO see Dimethylsulphoxide

l-DOPA, 70
psychotic reactions to, 74

Dopamine, 354
indices and kainic acid toxicity, 112,113
release, effect of organophosphates on, 220

Dopamine receptors, 309
action of acrylamide on, 58,59,330
action of ethanol on, 332
and methyl mercury, 328
and neuroleptic drugs, 319

Dopaminergic system, 14
and lead toxicity, 261-267
and neuroleptic drugs, 57
and prenatal exposure to haloperidol, 299-300
role in tolerance to organophosphates, 218

Dorsal root ganglia, 8,14

DSP4, 115

Dying-back process in toxic neuropathies
acrylamide, 169
metals, 179
organophosphates, 228

Electroencephalogram
in lead exposed children, 259
in organophosphate poisoning, 211,215,218

Electromyography, 165

Electroretinography and toxic disease, 164
4-aminoquinoline, 14
chloroquine, 135,139
organophosphates, 215
quinine, 141

Encephalopathy, 13,14
neurological examination, 164

Endocrine status and behavioral testing, 51

Energy metabolism disorders and neurotoxicity
acrylmide, 172
arsenic, 180
excitatory aminoacids, 108,109
peripheral neuropathy, 5, 28-30
phenothiazine-induced retinotoxicity, 147

Enkephalins, 223
and kainic acid toxicity, 111,112
and lead toxicity, 261

Erethism in mercury intoxication, 189

Erythrosin B, 333

Ethambutol, 135,143

Ethanol, 331,332
neuropathy, 5,7

Ethyl-eptbo, 229

Evoked potentials, 164,165,369

Excitotoxins, 107-121
and animal models of human disease, 107-121
hypothalamic-pituitary effects, 120-121
mode of action, 108-110
as neurobiological tools, 108
structure, 108

Fenfluramide, 261

Fenfluthrin, 96

Fenithrothion, 207

Fenpropathrin, 93,95,96

Fenthion, 215

Fenvalerate, 92,93,96
and sodium tail current, 98,99

Flurazepam, 74

Folic acid, 108,110
brain levels and seizure, 119

Fredreich's disease, 25

Fucogangliosides, 140

Funduscopy, 134

GABA _see_ γ-Aminobutyric acid

Ganglioside metabolism, 139,140

Glutamate, 48,108,120,332
effect on testosterone levels, 48
and Huntington's disease, 114
release and kainic acid toxicity, 109

Glutamate decarboxylase, 61
assay of, 353

Glutamate-obese mouse, 121

Glutamate receptors, 109,352
action of ibotenic acid on, 110

Glutamatergic pathways, 354
and kainic acid toxicity, 109

Glutamine synthetase, 13

γ-Glutamyl-cysteine synthetase, 31,33

Glutathione, 27
and acrylamide, 31
interaction with dihaloalkanes, 73
metabolism and peripheral neuropathy, 31
protective effect against reactive metabolites, 69,76
synthesis, 33

Glutathione epoxide transferase, 77

Glutathione synthetase deficiency, 32,33

Glyceraldehyde-3-phosphate dehydrogenase, 77

Glycine, 230,354
receptors and acrylamide toxicity, 58,59

Granule cells, 189,190

Grayanotoxin, 88

Halogenated hydrocarbons, 16

Haloperidol, 113,299,332

Hemiballismus, 114

2,5-Heptadione, 80

Hexacarbons, 35
neurofilamentous neuropathy induced by, 81

2,5-Hexandiol, 80

2,5-Hexandione, 5,36,80
effect on axonal transport, 6
nerve regeneration, impairment by, 38

n-Hexane, 79-81

Hippocampal slices, 370

Hippocampus, 10
damage by organotins, 47,291
ibotenic aid induced lesion in, 110
and kainic acid toxicity, 117
lead accumulation in, 262

Histamine, 354, 355

Homocysteine, 33

Homocysteinuria, 32,33

Huntington's disease, 110-113
  biochemical changes in, 112
  excitotoxins and, 113

Hydrogen disulphide, 82

Hydroxychloroquine, 141

6-Hydroxydopamine, 115

Hydroxyquinolines, 141

5-Hydroxytryptamine see Serotonin

Hyperactivity, 289
  in lead exposed animals, 260
  and prenatal exposure to ionizing radiation, 283

Hypotaurine, 114

Hypothalamus, 10
  and chlordecone, 48
  and kainic aid, 16

Ibotenic acid, 107,110
  cholinergic effects, 116
  structure, 108

ß,ß'-Iminodipropionitrile (IDPN), 6

Imipramine, 300

Indomethacin, 135,143

Insecticides
  pyrethroids, 91-103
  organophosphates, 203-246,247-253
  receptor binding abnormalities caused by, 320-326

Interstitial myocardial necrosis, 119-120

Intracerebral grafts, 113,114

Ion channels, 87-88
  and lead toxicity, 268-269
  and pyrethroids, 96-102

Isocitric dehydrogenase, 147

Isoniazid, 25
  interaction with pyridoxal phosphate, 33
  metabolic activation, 72,73
  neuropathy, 31

Isopropyl-iptbo, 229

Isoproterenol, 319

Kainic Acid, 107, 108
  and animal models of Parkinson's disease, 115
  behavioral toxicity, 113
  biochemical effects, 112
  2-deoxyglucose technique study of, 359,360
  effect on blood pressure in dogs, 120
  epileptogenic activity, 117
  interstitial myocardial necrosis induced by, 119-120
  mechanism of action, 109

Kepone see Chlordecone

Kindling, 119

Lathyrism see Neurolathyrism

Lead, 179,194-197,259-270
  accumulation in nerves, 197
  blood levels, 193,194,195,260
  and calcium metabolism, 261,267-269
  cerebrovascular damage induced by, 13,14,196
  and drug responsivity in animals, 261

effect on testosterone
levels, 48
electroencephalographic effects, 259
encephalopathy, 179,195-196,260
goitrogenic effects, 16
metabolism, 194
and muscarinic receptors,
326,327
neuropathy, 5,179,196-197
neurotransmitter changes induced by, 261
neuropsychological dysfunction
in children, 259
and nitrendipine binding sites
in striatum, 267-268
and plasma prolactin, 265,266
prenatal effects, 270
testicular effects, 259
tooth levels, 259
toxicity, animal models of,
260,262

Leptophos, 5,6

Lindane, 325

Lipofuscinosis, 135

Lipoic acid and arsenic toxicity,
25,180

Lung, activation of organophosphates in, 206

Lupanine, 88

Lysosomes, 13,14

Maculopathy, 134
in chloroquine intoxication,
135,140

Manganese, 179
effect on testosterone
levels, 48
neurochemical changes in
neonatal brain, 59
Parkinsonism induced by, 14
receptor-neurotransmitter
changes induced by, 53,54,
56,329
testicular effects, 48

Mannitol gap technique, 370

Melanin, 133,135,139

Meperidine, 72

Mercury, 179,187-193
clinical effects, 188-189
effect on receptor system,
327-328
metabolic activation, 72
metabolism, 188
organic, see methyl mercury
peripheral neuropathy, 5

Methanol, 72

n-Methyl-d-aspartic acid, 110

Methyl bromide, 13

Methylchlorpyrifos, 207

Methyl-n-butyl ketone (MnBK),
79-81

Methyl mercury, 187
behavioral teratogenic
effects, 298-299
clinical effects, 188-190
damage to granule cells, 14
distribution of neural
lesions, 189-190
effects on receptor-neurotransmitter systems, 323,
327,328,356
effect on tubulin, 5
metabolism, 188
neuropathy, 190

selective cell injury, 192
visual toxicity, 8,164

Methyl nitrosourea derivatives, 142

Methylphenidate, 261

n-Methyl-4-phenyl-1,2,3,6-tetrahydropyridine see MPTP

Metronidazole, 29

Mianserin, 301

Microtubules, 26,35,36,46
and vincristine neuropathy, 37-38

Minamata disease, 187

Mipafox, 6

Misonidazole, 29

Mitochondria
damage in thallium intoxication, 8,186
and lead toxicity, 269

Mitotic inhibitors, 15,16

MnBK see Methyl-n-butyl ketone

Monocrotophos, 322

Morphine glucoronide, 73

Motor function tests, 285,288

Movement disorders and excitotoxins, 110-115

MPTP, 14,115

Myelin, 11,14

Myopathy, organophosphate-induced, 215-216,247

Naloxonazine, 310

Naloxone, 114
reversal of organophosphate-induced analgesia, 225,226

Neostigmine, 319

Nerve conduction velocity in neurotoxic disease, 165
acrylamide, 168
arsenic, 179
lead, 196

Nerve gases, 204

Neuroendocrine system, 47-51
as a toxicity target during development, 16,292

Neurofilaments, 4,6
and toxic peripheral neuropathy, 5,6,35-37,81,171

Neurolathyrism, 108,165

Neuroleptic drugs, 57,319
behavioral teratogenic effects, 299-300

Neuromuscular junction, 4,93

Neuropathy (central), 10-15
anatomical targets, 10-12
and anoxia, 7
classification, 13

Neuropathy (peripheral), toxin-induced
acrylamide, 167
arsenic, 9,10
biochemical aspects of, 4-5
classification, 5
disulfiram, 82
hexarbaons, 35,81
isoniazid, 31
methyl mercury, 8
molecular pathology, 23-29
morphology, 4

organophosphates, 228-229, 247-253
thallium, 5,7-8,186-187
vincristine, 36

Neuropeptides, 310
and excitotoxins, 112
and organophosphate toxicity, 221-227

Neurotensin, 310

Neurotoxic agents, 5,13 (see also individual agents)
adaptive responses to, 60
aminoacids as, 107-121
definition, 45
membrane effects of, 87-88
metabolic activation, 67-83

Neurotoxicity assessment, 163-173
animal models of human disease, 107-121,167-170
biochemical contributions to, 43-60
2-deoxyglucose technique in, 12,359-360
electrophysiological studies, 165,365-371
in human disease, 164-167
morphological techniques, 168-170
neurobehavioral procedures, 279-293,297-302
neurotransmitter indices, 351-359
problems in experimental design, 51
radioligand binding assays, 307-334

Neurotoxicity target esterase (NTE), 5,6,228,249-250
aging, 249
distribution on body tissues, 229,250
in limphocytes, 252
and monitoring of exposure to organophosphates, 229,252

Neurotransmitters, 12 (see also the individual systems)
adaptive changes in neurotoxic states, 55-59
and kainic acid toxicity, 112
and lead toxicity, 261-267
and methyl mercury, 298-299
and peripheral neuropathy, 4
presynaptic indices, 353-355
and pyrethroids, 325

Nicotine, 331,332

Nipecotic acid, 333

Nitrendipine, 268,334

Nitrofurantoin, 29

5-Nitroimidazole, 25,29

Norpethidine, 77

NTE see Neurotoxicity target esterase

Nuclear magnetic imaging, 361

Nucleus accumbens, 263

Obesity syndrome, 120

3,6-Octanedione, 80

Octopamine, 324

ODAP see ß-n-Oxalyl-l- α,ß-diaminopropionic acid

Oligodendrocytes, 11,14

Open-field, behavior, 289

Opiate receptors, 308-310,318

and prenatal exposure to glutamate, 332

Opiates, endogenous
and lead toxicity, 261
organophosphate interaction with, 225

Optic nerve, toxic damage to,
clioquinol, 164
hydroxyquinolines, 141
organophosphates, 215

Oral contraceptives, 142-143

Organic solvents, 88

Organochlorine pesticides, 48

Organolead compounds, 47
effect on muscarinic receptors, 323
effect on testosterone levels, 48
metabolic activation, 47

Organophosphate compounds, 203-246
activation of, 78-79,206,251
antinociceptive effect, 226
bicyclic compounds, 323
biochemical monitoring, 252-253
chemistry, 204-205
detoxication reactions, 207
effect on axonal transport, 6
historical development, 203-204
interaction with neurotransmitters, 54,219-221,230
metabolism, 205-207
and neuropeptides, 221-227
non-neural effect, 211,230
physico-chemical reactivity, 204-205
site of action, 207-209
structure-activity relationship, 251
symptoms of poisoning, 210-216
tolerance to, 216-218,322
visual toxicity, 215

Organophosphate-induced delayed neuropathy, 228-229,247-253
clinical aspects, 248
electrophysiological changes, 248
experimental animal model, 248-249
initiation mechanism, 249-250
outbreaks of human disease, 248
pyramidal involvement, 248
screening tets, 250-251

Organotins, 179,333 (see also individual agents)
behavioral teratogenic effects, 289
neural targets of, 46

Organotypic cultures in neurotoxicology, 69

Ornithine decarboxylase, 48

ß-n-Oxaly-1- α,ß-diaminopropionic acid (ODAP), 108

Oxotremorine, 321,322

Oximes, 209,330

Pacinian corpuscles, 169,170

Paraoxon, 204
effect on GABA levels in brain, 219
effect on skeletal muscle, 215-216

Paraoxonase, 207

Parathion, 203

Parkinscn's disease
animal models of, 115
chemicals inducing, 13,14,57

d-Penicillamine, 180

Permethrin, 96,97
and sodium tail current, 98,99

Pethidine, 77

Phenothiazines
lipofuscinosis induced by, 135,148
retinotoxic effects, 135, 144-148

Phenylmethylsulphonyl fluoride, 225

Phenytoin see Diphenylhydantoin

Physostigmine, 113

Phosphofructokinase, 77

Phosphonates, 249,252

Phosphotionates, 78

Pilocarpine, 113

Pink disease, 190

Positron emission tomography (PET), 360

Potassium
channels, 87,88
and thallium toxicity, 183

Pralidoxime, 219

Preweaning behavior, chemicals affecting, 292

Prolactin, 302
and acrylamide toxicity, 52

Pronase, 88

Protein
metabolism in melanocytes, chloroquine affecting, 139
synthesis, disorders in mercury intoxication, 192

Prussian blue, 7

Psychiatric disturbances in toxic disease
carbon disulphide, 82
disulfiram, 82
l-DOPA, 74
organophosphates, 211,212
thallium, 187

Psychotropic drugs, behavioral teratogenic effects, 299-302

Purkinje cells, 11
loss in acrylamide intoxication, 169

Pyrethroids, 88,91-103
effect on sodium channel gating, 97-102
effect on receptor-neurotrasmiter systems, 325
mode of action, 93-103
occupational exposure, 92
repetitive activity, 93-96
structure-activity relationship, 91-92
symptoms of poisoning, 91-92

Pyridoxal phosphate, 25,31,32

Pyridoxine, 25,172

Pyroglutamate, 114

Pyruvate and toxic neuropathies, 29,30,172

Quinine, 135
retinotoxicity, 141-142

Quinolinic acid, 108,110
and Huntington's disease, 114

Receptor assay in neurotoxicology, 307-334,351-353

Reproductive behavior, chemicals affecting, 291

Retina as a target for toxic agents, 133-149,164,215

Riboflavin, 25,29,30,187

Ribosomes, 179,192

Ruthenium red, 269

Sarin, 204
analgesic action, 226
electroencephalographic changes induced by, 218

Saxitoxin, 88,333

Scopolamine, 113

Scorpion toxins, 88

Sea anemone toxins, 88

Selenium, 76

Senile dementia, excitotoxins and, 116,117

Serotonin
and lead toxicity, 261
presynaptic indices, 354
receptors and neurotoxic agents, 58,59,309
striatal levels in manganese intoxication, 53
turnover in organophosphate intoxication, 221

Serotoninergic system effect of toluene on, 331
and organophosphate toxicity, 220,221
and prenatal exposure to antidepressant drugs, 300

Snake venoms, 44

Sodium channel, 87,88
DDT and, 102,103
gating, pyrethroids affecting, 97-102

Soman, 219,226

Somatostatin, 223
and kainic acid toxicity, 113
and senile dementia, 116,117

Sparsomycin, 142

Sparteine, 88

Streptomycin, 332

Substance P, 223,310
and kainic acid toxicity, 11, 112,113

Substantia nigra, 112,113

Sulfur mustards, 73

Sulpiride, 264

Tabun, 204

Tamoxifen, 142

Taurine, 14,114

Temporal lobe epilepsy, 117

Tetraethylammonium, 88

Tetraethyl lead see Organolead compounds

Tetraethyl pyrophosphate, 203

Tetram, 322

Tetrodotoxin, 88,333

Thallium, 25,29,164,179,182-187

acute poisoning, 184-185,186
biological effects, 185
distribution in tissues, 184
interaction with riboflavin, 30
mechanism of toxicity, 187
metabolism, 182-184
peripheral neuropathy, 5,7-8, 186-187
potassium-like effects, 8,183

Thiamine, 5,26,27
and carbon disulphide neuropathy, 7

Thiapride, 264

Thioridazine, 147-148

Thyroid gland, 116

Thyrotropin releasing hormone, 112,113

Tilorone, 142

α-Tocopherol, 31,34-35

TOPC see triorthocresylphosphate

Toluene, 165,331

Toxaphene, 325

Triethyl lead see Organolead compounds

Triethylphosphate, 227

Triethyl tin, 46,179
behavioral teratogenic effects, 291
encephalophathy, 13,14
myelinotoxicity, 46

Trichloroethylene, 164

Trimethyl tin, 179,291
receptor system changes induced by, 328-329

Triorthocresylphosphate, 5,6,56

Triorthotolylphosphate, 207

Tubulin, 5,8,46

Vanadium, 329

Vasoactive intestinal polypeptide, 223,310

Veratridine, 88

Viloxazine, 301

Vinblastine, 46

Vincristine, 5,164

VIP see Vasoactive intestinal polypeptide

Visual evoked potentials see Evoked potentials

Visual motor integration, lead induced impairment in, 259

Visual system damage
assessment, 164,287
methyl mercury induced, 8,14
organophosphate-induced, 215
retinotoxicity, 133-149

Voltage clamp technique, 87, 93,97

Werding-Hoffman disease, 25

Wernicke's encephalopathy, 29

Xenopus laevis lateral-line sense organ, 93,95,96